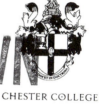

ADVANCES IN PERSONALITY SCIENCE

ADVANCES IN PERSONALITY SCIENCE

Edited by
Daniel Cervone
Walter Mischel

THE GUILFORD PRESS
New York   London

© 2002 The Guilford Press
A Division of Guilford Publications, Inc.
72 Spring Street, New York, NY 10012
www.guilford.com

Printed in the United States of America

This book is printed on acid-free paper.

Last digit is print number: 9 8 7 6 5 4 3 2 1

Library of Congress Cataloging-in-Publication Data

Advances in personality science / edited by Daniel Cervone, Walter Mischel.
    p. cm.
    "Originated at the inaugural conference of the Association for Research in
Personality, held in San Antonio, Texas, in 2001"—Pref.
    Includes bibliographical references and index.
    ISBN 1-57230-737-4
    1. Personality—Congresses. I. Cervone, Daniel. II. Mischel, Walter.
BF698 .A3294 2002
155.2—dc21
                                             2001056918

About the Editors

Daniel Cervone, PhD, is Associate Professor of Psychology at the University of Illinois at Chicago. He has been a visiting faculty member at the University of Washington and the University of Rome "La Sapienza," and a fellow at the Center for Advanced Study in the Behavioral Sciences. He is coauthor of *Personality: Determinants, Dynamics, and Potentials*, with Gian Vittorio Caprara, and coeditor of *The Coherence of Personality*, with Yuichi Shoda.

Walter Mischel, PhD, is the Robert Johnston Niven Professor of Humane Letters in Psychology at Columbia University, to which he came after 20 years as a professor at Stanford University. Currently he holds an NIMH MERIT award and is the editor of the *Psychological Review*. He is the author of the classic monograph, *Personality and Assessment*, as well as *Introduction to Personality*, and has published over 150 articles and book chapters. Dr. Mischel, a past president of the Division of Social and Personality Psychologists, is the recipient of the Distinguished Scientific Contribution Award of the American Psychological Association, has won the Distinguished Scientist Award 2000 of the Society of Experimental Social Psychologists, and was elected a Fellow of the American Academy of Arts and Sciences.

Contributors

Daniel Cervone, PhD, Department of Psychology, University of Illinois at Chicago, Chicago, Illinois

Paul T. Costa, Jr., PhD, National Institute on Aging, National Institutes of Health, Baltimore, Maryland

Nathan A. Fox, PhD, Institute for Child Study, University of Maryland, College Park, Maryland

Elena L. Grigorenko, PhD, PACE Center and Child Study Center, Yale University, New Haven, Connecticut; Department of Psychology, Moscow State University, Moscow, Russia

Patricia H. Hawley, PhD, Department of Psychology, Southern Connecticut State University, New Haven, Connecticut

Wendy Heller, PhD, Department of Psychology, University of Illinois at Urbana–Champaign, Champaign, Illinois

Nancy S. Koven, MA, Department of Psychology, University of Illinois at Urbana–Champaign, Champaign, Illinois

Michael Lewis, PhD, Institute for the Study of Child Development, University of Medicine and Dentistry of New Jersey, Robert Wood Johnson Medical School, New Brunswick, New Jersey

Scott LeeTiernan, BS, Department of Psychology, University of Washington, Seattle, Washington

Todd D. Little, PhD, Department of Psychology, Yale University, New Haven, Connecticut

Robert R. McCrae, PhD, National Institute on Aging, National Institutes of Health, Baltimore, Maryland

Gregory A. Miller, PhD, Department of Psychology, University of Illinois at Urbana–Champaign, Champaign, Illinois

Walter Mischel, PhD, Department of Psychology, Columbia University, New York, New York

Jack B. Nitschke, PhD, Department of Psychology, University of Wisconsin–Madison, Madison, Wisconsin

Andrzej Nowak, PhD, Center for Complex Systems, University of Warsaw, Warsaw, Poland; Department of Psychology, Florida Atlantic University, Boca Raton, Florida

Louis A. Schmidt, PhD, Department of Psychology, McMaster University, Hamilton, Ontario, Canada

Jennifer I. Schmidtke, PhD, Department of Psychology, University of Illinois at Urbana–Champaign, Champaign, Illinois

Yuichi Shoda, PhD, Department of Psychology, University of Washington, Seattle, Washington

Carolin J. Showers, PhD, Department of Psychology, University of Oklahoma, Norman, Oklahoma

Steven K. Sutton, PhD, Department of Psychology, University of Miami, Coral Gables, Florida

Jean M. Twenge, PhD, Department of Psychology, San Diego State University, San Diego, California

Robin R. Vallacher, PhD, Department of Psychology, Florida Atlantic University, Boca Raton, Florida

Michal Zochowski, PhD, Department of Physics, University of Michigan, Ann Arbor, Michigan

Preface

This volume originated at the inaugural conference of the Association for Research in Personality, held in San Antonio, Texas, in 2001. The conference featured a particularly telling moment. In remarks to attendees, the president of the Association, David Watson of the University of Iowa, requested a show of hands: "How many of you consider yourself to be traditional personality psychologists?" Very few hands went up (though scattered catcalls directing one or another member to stick their hands in the air could be heard). More remarkable than the response—"traditional" having such a negative connotation in this context—was Watson's prescience in asking the question. The audience was committed to advancing a psychology of personality. But the traditional subfield of personality psychology, he discerned, seemed insufficient to the task.

A second conference happening also speaks to the rationale for this volume. A number of presenters began by noting that they had "never been to a personality conference before." Yet their presentations inevitably addressed the most central questions in the study of personality. It was only arbitrary disciplinary boundaries that had separated their work from discourse in the traditional field. The presenters attacked questions of individuality and individual differences by drawing on bodies of knowledge in diverse disciplines: molecular genetics, child and lifespan developmental psychology, historical analyses of social change, mathematical analyses of nonlinear dynamical systems, neuroscience, evolutionary psychology, social cognition—as well as methods originating in the psychology of personality. Even more striking than the diversity and range of methods were the underlying unities—the common concerns—that seemed to motivate so much of the research: an attempt to understand, in detail, how interactions among biological and psychological systems and between persons and the environments in which they develop give rise to the enduring behavioral and affective expressions that define the individual and distinguish individuals from one another. Latent within the superficially diverse presentations was a coherent interdisciplinary science of personality. Maintaining traditional disciplinary boundaries would obscure this fact, causing interconnected advances in the study of persons to be shunted off to separate professional conferences and publication outlets. By allowing these boundaries to be fuzzy, the interconnections become apparent. One comes to appreciate that fundamental advances in the study of personality are today found in diverse branches of the psychological, biological, and social sciences and that, despite their diversity, these advances are beginning to yield a surprisingly coherent portrait of everyone's fundamental target of investigation: the individual, whole person.

It is the strength of these conference presentations and the great excitement they generated that motivated this volume. The presentations made clear to us that the time had arrived to call for a personality science: an integrative interdisciplinary study of personhood, individual differences, and human diversity. This volume is a first step in this enterprise.

*   *   *

The preparation of this volume greatly benefited from the efforts of colleagues both at the University of Illinois at Chicago and at other institutions who volunteered to provide feedback on initial drafts of chapters. For these efforts, we wish to thank Daniele Artistico, Tracy Caldwell, Karen Crane, Simon Jencius, David Kenny, Sunyoung Oh, Heather Orom, Brent Roberts, Bill Shadel, and Melissa Steineck. We thank our contributors for their professionalism in meeting the project's tight production deadlines. We also express our appreciation to Seymour Weingarten of The Guilford Press for his support. Finally, Daniel Cervone wishes to thank his students and colleagues at the University of Illinois at Chicago for their assistance at various stages in the production of the work and the Steering Committee of the Association for Research in Personality for the honor of chairing its inaugural conference.

DANIEL CERVONE
WALTER MISCHEL

Contents

ADVANCES IN PERSONALITY SCIENCE

CHAPTER 1

Personality Science

DANIEL CERVONE
WALTER MISCHEL

Academic disciplines rarely cut nature at its joints. Instead, advances in knowledge force modifications of traditional disciplinary boundaries. These modifications come in three varieties. Sometimes subareas within traditional disciplines become so specialized that they function as unique fields with their own professional associations, journals, and academic departments. The multiple branches of contemporary physics or chemistry illustrate this. Sometimes the intersection of two traditional disciplines becomes a focus of such intense investigation that the point of intersection becomes a stand-alone field. Biochemistry is an example.

The third variety of disciplinary development is of greatest interest here. Investigators from multiple fields occasionally recognize that they are interested in the same phenomena and that scientific understanding can best be advanced through a concerted interdisciplinary effort. Cognitive science is the classic example. As of the 1960s, the psychological subfield of cognitive psychology was a vibrant enterprise that had made significant progress on many of its core problems (Neisser, 1967). The pace of future progress accelerated, however, only when psychologists fully joined forces with anthropologists, computer scientists, linguists, neuroscientists, and philosophers who shared their interest in the acquisition and representation of knowledge (Gardner, 1985). By participating in an interdisciplinary effort, cognitive psychologists were able to capitalize on theoretical and methodological tools available in neighboring fields. Conversely, scholars in these fields could draw on the wisdom of the cognitive psychologist. If traditional disciplinary boundaries had been maintained, scientific progress in the study of cognition would have been retarded. The revolution that did occur illustrates the remarkable synergy that can be generated when there is an opportune convergence among diverse disciplines that view the same basic phenomena from different vantage points and at different levels of abstraction and analysis—and when the moment is right.

The basic premise of this book is that personality psychology stands today at such a moment, reminiscent of where cognitive psychology stood a third of a century ago. Personality psychology currently is a vibrant field of study, as the growth of professional organizations, journals, and handbooks attests (e.g., Pervin & John, 1999). Its investigators can justly claim to have made progress on some of their discipline's core questions, as reviews of the field make clear (Caprara & Cervone, 2000; Mischel & Shoda, 1998). However, maintaining sharp disciplinary boundaries between personality psychology and neighboring fields is not a path to more rapid progress. The phenomena that interest the personality psychologist also attract the attention of the social, clinical, developmental, cultural, and cognitive psychologist (cf. Brewer, Kenny, & Norem, 2000). Of equal importance, they attract the efforts of psychiatrists, anthropologists, neuroscientists, sociologists, molecular biologists, and philosophers who investigate human nature and the multiplicity of differences among individuals. An insular view of personality psychology today would bear the same costs as an insular view of cognitive psychology would have a generation ago. Insularity breeds ignorance of scientific developments that might advance one's scientific agenda, while also making one vulnerable to positing theoretical positions that are untenable if viewed in the light of findings from other disciplines.

The nature of the gains that were made by cognitive psychology is particularly instructive to the student of personality. The study of cognition did not merely develop into one of many successful subspecialties within psychology. Instead, it moved to the center stage of the entire psychological enterprise. Investigators throughout the psychological sciences gained greater understanding of their domains of interest by drawing on theoretical languages and methodological tools developed in the cognitive laboratory. Questions of the architecture of the mind and the nature of its workings became organizing themes for the discipline. Cognitive psychologists thus found themselves at the hub of a vast disciplinary and interdisciplinary effort. Their influence only grew as they proved able to meet the fundamental challenge of providing rigorous methods for studying mental systems.

Today one can identify an even greater challenge. It is to understand the psychological architecture of whole, intact persons: those thinking and feeling, motivated yet conflicted, self-obsessed yet social beings in whom cognitive systems reside. The task is complicated by the need to understand not only cognitive systems but also their noisy neighbors: affective systems that variously inform, inhibit, and impel the organism. A particularly exciting development is that work in multiple fields seems increasingly to converge on this complex challenge. A brief survey of the psychological sciences reveals fundamental advances in the understanding of individuals and the differences among them; these advances include work on human motivation (Higgins & Kruglanski, 2000), emotions and individual differences in affective experience (Ekman & Davidson, 1994; Lazarus, 1999; Lewis & Haviland-Jones, 2000), temperament and self-regulation (Posner & Rothbart, 2000; Rothbart, Ahadi, & Evans, 2000), the dynamics of cognitive and affective intrapersonal processes (Tesser & Schwarz, 2001), coherence in cognitive and behavioral systems (Thagard, 2000), autobiographical memory, self-concept, and personal identity (Bruner, 1990; Leary & Tangney, in press), health psychology (Davison & Pennebaker, 1996; Miller, Shoda, & Hurley, 1996), and the development of persons across the span of life (Baltes, Lindenberger, & Staudinger, 1998; Brandtstädter & Lerner, 1999). A look outside the discipline reveals similar strides; these include work on the molecular-genetic roots of temperament (Cloninger, Adolffson, & Svrakic, 1996; cf. Herbst, Zonderman, McCrae, & Costa, 2000), the biological bases of consciousness (Damasio, 1999; Edelman & Tononi, 2000), nonconscious influences on behavior (Bechara, Damasio, Tranel, & Damasio, 1997; Damasio, 1994), the nature of self-concept and personal identity (Harré, 1998; Taylor, 1989), and the reciprocal interplay of biological and sociocultural factors in the development of persons (Durham, 1991; Ehrlich, 2000; Lewontin, 2000).

Whether each of the investigators responsible for these advances happens to be familiar with Allport (1937) or not, their contributions address the very questions that drove him to write his classic personality text: How can we best conceptualize the enduring patterns of thought, feeling, and social behavior that characterize individuals over time and across situations? How can we relate knowledge of psychological subprocesses (motivation, emotion, theories of mind, self-theories, interpersonal relations, life narratives) to the more molar levels of analysis that are required to capture the whole person, contextualized within his or her social world? What is the interplay among biological and social factors in the growth and maturity of the individual? How do distinct cognitive, emotional, and motivational processes come to function as coherent psychological systems that contribute to coherence in experience and action? At this point in our history, the classic problems of personality are no longer the sole province of the personality psychologist. Investigators from multiple disciplines work toward their solution. A coherent organization of these interdisciplinary efforts may advance a science of personality in much the same manner as the science of cognition was advanced a generation ago.

This volume, then, is a call for a personality science, that is, for an interdisciplinary study of the determinants and development of individuality, individual differences, and intraindividual coherence in personal functioning. This enterprise's ingredients are already visible, it is developing with remarkable speed, and it now seems virtually waiting to be recognized, articulated, and nurtured. The contributions to the book consist of advances in the study of personality that derive both from within and outside the traditional discipline of personality psychology. The volume thus illustrates the gains to be made by combining insights from multiple theoretical perspectives and empirical methods into a cumulative science of persons.

Four aspects of our appeal for a personality science are of particular note. First, we are not calling here for novel forms of personality research that currently do not exist. Instead, we wish to call attention to and to stimulate interactions among developments that already are well under way. Our basic premise is that extant work in multiple subdisciplines of psychology, as well as in disciplines beyond psychology, informs the classic concerns of the personality psychologist. The construct of personality, despite its resistance to simple definition, is a valuable one for identifying the fundamental target of these research developments: the coherent, enduring, distinguishing features of whole persons and the processes that underlie them.

Second, endorsing a personality science does not inherently imply the endorsement of one versus another theoretical perspective in the current field of personality psychology. Any theoretical perspective should benefit from the consideration of interdisciplinary sources of evidence, and any well-developed theory should be able to withstand the scrutiny of a diverse set of scholars. A personality science may unify the study of persons and individual differences, but not by forcing diverse perspectives under one omnibus theoretical umbrella. Personality psychology currently harbors theories that differ from one another in fundamental ways. It likely will continue to do so. The advantage of an interdisciplinary personality science is not that it will serve as a theoretical melting pot but that it will foster advances in all theoretical perspectives as investigators become obliged to refine their positions in the face of a more diverse range of empirical findings and theoretical challenges. As Geertz (2000) put it, the "deployment of distinct inquiries . . . [that] force deep-going reconsiderations upon one another" is what "drive[s] the enterprise erratically onward" (p. 199).

Third, our use of the term personality *science* should be understood by way of the analogy to cognitive science, in which *science* is meant to signify a multidisciplinary research-based effort. It is not meant to restrict the study of personhood to any particular set of methodologies or to reduce persons to a stereotypically "scientific" collection of variables and formulae. On the contrary, we urge sensitivity to the potential limitations of some traditional scientific methods. The most distinguishing feature of persons is that they construct meaning by reflecting on themselves, the past, and the future. Many writers have questioned the assumptions that meaning construction can be adequately captured by the traditional methods of natural science or that persons can be construed as a collection of quantifiable personality variables that index essential qualities of the individual (Geertz, 1973, 2000; Polkinghorne, 1988; Shweder, 2000; Shweder & Sullivan, 1990; Taylor, 1989). They discourage the positing of abstract global tendencies, urging instead that personal qualities be studied within the specific physical, social, and cultural contexts that comprise the individual's life (Kagan, 1998)—a theme that has been sounded by a variety of scholars throughout the history of the field (Shweder, 1999). These concerns are as much a part of personality science as are investigations that happily make these assumptions.

Fourth and finally, one might ask about a potential cost of embracing a broadly focused personality science. Might this not blur the distinction between the study of personality and the study of psychology as a whole, with the result that a science of personality loses its unique raison d'être? In answering this question, one must recognize where the true costs lie. It is far more important to advance a science of personhood than to defend the boundaries of an academic discipline, and the discipline must be evaluated according to whether it promotes a scientific understanding of persons. In this regard, the notion of personality, at least as it was construed by virtually all of the major personality theorists of the 20th century, does have one unique advantage. It calls attention to the consistency, coherence, intrapersonal organization, and uniqueness of the individual's psychological life in a way that no other branch of the psychological sciences does (Cervone & Shoda, 1999; McAdams, 1997). A major trend in the recent history of the study of mind is to identify mental mechanisms that function independently from one another and that are common to all people (Pinker, 1997). Whatever gains are derived from this development, it remains that the psychological features that define the individual appear not to be functionally independent but coherently interconnected. We generally experience our lives, and those of others, not as independent bursts of output from encapsulated mental organs but as coherent streams of interrelated psychological events, as William James (1890) so clearly recognized at the founding of the field of psychology. Furthermore, we experience ourselves and others not as redundant exemplars of human universality but as incontrovertibly unique beings.

Whether one calls the study of these beings personality, personalistics (Stern, 1930/1961), personology (Murray, 1938), or the study of personhood (Harré, 1998), a scientific field that targets coherent individuals and the differences among them can serve a critical integrative function within the psychological and social sciences.

That said, we note that the specific terminology of "personality" also bears a potential cost. In the recent era, much effort in personality psychology has been directed toward identifying interindividual-difference dimensions that capture variations in the population in global dispositional tendencies. Results robustly indicate that interindividual differences can be usefully characterized according to a small set of dimensions along which one may rank individuals according to their overall, average tendency to display each of a variety of categories of experience and action (John & Srivastava, 1999). Work in this area has progressed to such a degree that some tend to equate the notion of personality with the study of these global tendencies and thus to judge that developments outside of the study of such broad interindividual differences fall outside of the field of personality. In principle, investigators can define their terms and organize their disciplines however they wish. But the problem with this narrow definition of personality psychology is that it would require yet another discipline to address the within-person dynamics, psychological coherence, and life-course development of individual persons or selves— precisely the phenomena that attracted the attention of the founders of personality psychology (Hall & Lindzey, 1970). Even investigators who have contributed to the study of global interindividual-difference dimensions now urge that "personality researchers should take deviations from the traditional linear model seriously and exploit their inherent information about within-personality organization" (Asendorpf, Borkenau, Ostendorf, & Van Aken, 2001, p. 196)—a theme that we also have sounded (Cervone, Shadel, & Jencius, 2001; Cervone & Shoda, 1999; Mischel & Morf, in press; Mischel & Shoda, 1995, 1998). We envision a personality science that addresses within-person dynamics and coherence while simultaneously drawing on and contributing to the study of individual differences in personal tendencies.

PERSONALITY SCIENCE: WHY BOTHER?

Many personality psychologists may rightly feel that they already are flooded with an excess of scientific information within their own discipline. Why, they may ask, should they confront the greater deluge entailed by an interdisciplinary perspective? Gestures toward interdisciplinarity may sound nice. They have a pleasantly warmhearted ring to them. But the hardheaded investigator needs concrete reasons for investing the effort required by an expansion of traditional disciplinary boundaries.

An interdisciplinary perspective does not conflict with specialization and, on the contrary, can be especially timely and opportune as specialization increases in the growth of a field. Its unique advantage is the special synergy that can arise from the heuristic interplay among disciplines and subdisciplines that address overlapping phenomena and problems at different levels of analysis and with different methods and vantage points. The potential gains to be realized from a broad perspective are inherently appealing to the psychologist committed to understanding the coherent functioning of the whole person with increasing depth.

Interdisciplinarity is not merely an appealing option but an obligation when investigations in other disciplines address issues that are core concerns of one's own. As we have noted, such is already the case for the personality psychologist. A broad consideration of work in other disciplines yields a variety of discoveries. Often one finds empirical results that converge with, and thus complement, standard findings in personality psychology. At other times, one may encounter findings that illuminate phenomena that have received insufficient empirical attention within the traditional field. On yet other occasions, work in other fields may conflict with findings or theoretical conceptions held by many personality psychologists. Such instances present a particular challenge when the conflicting ideas are those of scholars in other disciplines who bring unique, specialized expertise to the particular issues under study.

To illustrate these points, we note here five issues of central importance to personality science that are informed by research in other disciplines. We focus in this section primarily on work conducted outside of the field of psychology. We return to the relevance of multiple subdisciplines within psychology to the study of individuals and individual differences when we overview the contributions to this volume later in the chapter.

Conscious and Unconscious Processes

A question at the heart of the earliest comprehensive psychological conception of personality, psychoanalytic theory, was the interplay of conscious and unconscious mental processes (Freud, 1900/1953). Today, these questions are addressed by an extraordinarily wide range of scholars in psychology (e.g., Bargh, 1997; Kihlstrom, 1999), philosophy (e.g., Dennett, 1991, Searle, 1998), and neuroscience (e.g., Edelman & Tononi, 2000; Damasio, 1999). Neuroscience research yields particularly compelling evidence of an aspect of personality dynamics envisioned by the psychoanalyst, namely, unconscious affective input into what otherwise might appear to be conscious, rational decision processes (Bechara et al., 1997). Such work is an obvious case of research conducted outside of the academic discipline of psychology that directly informs historic concerns in the psychological study of personality processes.

Mental Architectures for a Psychology of Persons: Modularity? Innateness?

One of the most noted developments in the recent history of personality psychology is the growth of evolutionary personality psychology. The basic contention in a major branch of this work (Buss, 1999; Tooby & Cosmides, 1990) is that the mind consists of a collection of evolved, domain-specific modular mechanisms, each of which is constrained to process only select forms of environmental input and to generate a limited number of equally domain-linked behavioral outputs. Evolutionary psychology is itself a major example of interdisciplinarity in personality science, as the field, of course, combines traditional psychological analyses with the insights of evolutionary biology. Yet those who wish to base an analysis of personality on the modular "Swiss army knife" mental architecture implied by this approach would seem compelled to consider evidence from another field that also is directly concerned with evidence of the evolutionary heritage of mind and personal capacities—namely, archaeology. Mithen's (1996) review of archaeological evidence leads him to conclude that notions of modularity are necessary but distinctly insufficient to account for the mental abilities of Homo sapiens sapiens. A modular mental architecture may have characterized the mind of some of our evolutionary ancestors. The archaeological record, however, indicates that our species developed not only modular capabilities but also critically, domain-general processing mechanisms that enable us to combine information from multiple domains when reasoning about ourselves, our creations, and the natural world. Neuropsychological research provides evidence that is consistent with this conclusion. Analyses of the frontal lobes, the last of the brain regions to evolve, reveals little sign of modularity of neural architecture, although modularity is evident in older brain regions such as the thalamus (Goldberg, 2001). More generally, the personality psychologist who is interested in the evolutionary origin of personal capacities and behavioral tendencies or who wishes to posit innate modular mechanisms as basic units of analysis in conceptualizing persons is compelled to consider a particularly wide range of evidence, some of which may raise conceptual issues that commonly are skirted in evolutionary accounts of personal functioning (Cervone, 2000; Cervone & Rafaeli-Mor, 1999). Hawley and Little (Chapter 7, this volume) provide an instructive example of how agentic action can be explained by reference to both evolved tendencies and self-referent cognitive processes that develop through social experience.

Interactionism

Personality psychologists have long debated the merits of interactionism, that is, the notion that individual experience and action should be understood not as the product of separate personal and situational factors but as the result of dynamic interactions between aspects of personality and situations (Magnusson, 1999; Magnusson & Endler, 1977). Work in biology bears on this issue by providing such strong evidence of organism–environment interactions as to quell debate. Lewontin (2000) explains that genetic and environmental influences are intertwined, with the results of ontogenetic development being "contingent on the sequence of environments in which it occurs" (p. 20). Research on plant growth proves illustrative. As Lewontin summarizes, when cloned samples of seven different individuals of a given plant species were grown at different elevations, there was little cross-environment consistency in the rank ordering of the size of mature plants. An individual plant that flourished at one altitude may have exhibited below-average growth in another. Plant growth thus must be represented not in terms of the average growth tendencies of an individual organism but via "norm of reaction" graphs that plot phenotypic properties of a given genotype as a function of the environment in which the organism develops; plant growth, then, is understood through . . . if . . . then contingencies, with the plant achieving a certain size in relation to other plants only if particular environmental conditions are present (cf. Mischel & Shoda, 1995).

Numerous other forms of research compellingly document the interactions among environmental circumstances and the development of biological systems; these include work on the plasticity of neural systems (Edelman, 1992; Kolb & Whishaw, 1998), the experiential activation of genetic mechanisms (Gottlieb, 1998), and the reciprocal interplay of cultural and biological factors in human evolution (Durham, 1991). Such considerations led Ehrlich (2000) to conclude that the interaction of genetic endowment and environmental experience is so profound that the psychologist's typical strategy of partitioning phenotypic variance in behavioral characteristics into separate genetic versus environmental causes makes no more sense than "trying to separate the contributions of length and width to the area of a rectangle" (p. 6) or asking which areas of the rectangle are primarily due to length and which primarily due to width. In this instance, then, work outside of the discipline would appear to suggest a redirection of activities in the psychology of personality away

from questioning the general merits of interactionism and toward understanding the multiple cognitive, behavioral, and physiological mechanisms
through which interactions come about. Such activity is, of course, well
under way and is illustrated by a number of contributions to this volume.

Work in additional fields of study contributes to making principles
of interactionism a common ground for a great many students of individuality and individual differences (Caprara & Cervone, 2000). In cultural anthropology, people primarily are understood in terms of the processes of meaning construction through which they understand and
organize their lives; these processes are grounded in and maintained by
the social practices of a culture (Geertz, 1973). Work in cultural psychology (Kitayama & Markus, 1999; Shweder & Sullivan, 1993) similarly
reveals how cultural contexts and practices contribute to people's sense
of personal coherence and to the basic issue of what it means to be a
person; recent findings are of particular cross-disciplinary relevance in
that they suggest that cultural variations do not entail merely quantitative shifts in psychological content but qualitative variations in the psychological processes that are invoked by tasks of social inference (Nisbett,
Peng, Choi, & Norenzayan, 2001). Finally, although it involves a form
of evidence that rarely is considered in psychological science, work in lit-
erary criticism provides a compelling argument for interactionism. Readers
are seen to create meaning in texts through their interpretive activities,
which in turn reflect the beliefs and interpretive styles of the communities of which they are a part (Fish, 1980). Reader and text thus are no
longer separate entities; there is no textual meaning that exists independently of the reader. Because any social situation can be construed as a
text that is interpreted by a reader (see Shweder & Sullivan, 1990), this
argument dissolves the traditional distinction between situations (construed as entities with properties that existence independently of persons)
and persons (construed as a collection of essential qualities that exist independently of situations), forcing one to a wholly interactionist position.

Biological Bases of Personality and Individual Differences

A question of enduring interest to the personality psychologist is that of
the biological bases of personality and individual differences. What biological mechanisms are most central to primary aspects of personality?
Traditionally, speculation and research in personality psychology has
plumbed lower level brain regions such as the brain stem and limbic system when searching for fundamental sources of personality variation (e.g.,
Eysenck, 1990) and has employed animal models to study variations in
affective experience that may cut across species (see Pickering & Gray,
1999). Enormous progress in understanding the architecture and emotion-

related functioning of limbic regions such as the amygdala has been made (LeDoux, 1996). Nonetheless, it has become increasingly clear that higher level brain regions also are central to the emotional experiences and expressions of humans (Davidson, 1992; Metcalfe & Mischel, 1999; Posner & DiGirolamo, 2000; see also Chapters 3–5, this volume), who reflect on their experiences, evaluate them in relation to personal goals, and attempt to inhibit affective impulses when it is socially appropriate to do so. Advances in the neurosciences highlight the need to focus on cortical regions in the search for biological bases of individual differences. Work on the frontal lobes, which are centrally involved in the unique human capacities for proactive, goal-directed action, suggest that they "have more to do with our 'personalities' than any other part of the brain" (Goldberg, 2001, p. 122). If so, this would appear to constrain the claim that the basic "structures of personality" are preserved across human and non-human species (Gosling & John, 1999).

Causal Status of Dispositional Constructs

A basic goal in personality psychology is the understanding of personality dispositions, that is, people's individuating, enduring tendencies to display particular classes of experience and action. Although investigators agree on the importance of explaining dispositional tendencies, they differ in the forms of explanation that they pursue (Cervone, 1997, 1999). A major point of debate is the causal status of dispositional constructs. Some see dispositional constructs as serving merely a descriptive function (Buss & Craik, 1983; Wright & Mischel, 1987). Others suggest that the dispositional variables that compose taxonomies of individual differences can be granted causal status; in this view, dispositions are causally responsible for observed consistencies in social behavior. This question, too, has been taken up in another discipline, namely, the philosophy of science. Harré (1998) rejects the notion that dispositional constructs provide causal explanations, noting that dispositions (in the study of personality or any other science) refer to observable properties that must be explained, not in terms of other dispositions but by reference to causal powers that are possessed by an entity, and that dispositional constructs that may prove useful in constructing a classificatory taxonomy cannot also serve an explanatory function, because classificatory and explanatory constructs differ fundamentally. (A fern may be classified as a plant and may be disposed to display plant-like activities such as photosynthesizing, but one would not explain the dispositional tendency by claiming that the fern possesses "plantness" that causes photosynthesis. One would refer, instead, to chemical structures possessed by the fern that enable the chemical reactions we call photosynthesis.) Whatever one's slant on this issue, personality psychologists who are interested in the causal status of dispositional constructs are obliged to consider analyses of the issue by scholars with expertise in scientific explanation (see also Shaffer, 1996). An interdisciplinary personality science calls attention to such obligations.

Note that this critique applies only to cases in which dispositional constructs refer simultaneously to two things: a phenotypic tendency and the purported cause of that tendency. Conceptual problems are eliminated once one specifies a stable system of biological or psychological processes that gives rise to the overt behavioral tendency that requires explanation. Dispositional tendencies, such as rejection sensitivity (Ayduk et al., 2000) or narcissism (Morf & Rhodewalt, 2001), for example, have been successfully analyzed in terms of underlying cognitive-affective systems that give rise to the distinctive behavioral signatures of personality that define the dispositional category (Mischel & Shoda, 1998). Problems of circularity are avoided in that none of the individual cognitive or affective processes directly corresponds to the overt tendency that is to be explained; no individual process is "rejection-sensitivityness" (see Cervone, 1997, 1999). This volume is replete with examples in which well-specified physiological or cognitive-affective systems are shown to explain overt tendencies in experience and action.

THE HISTORY OF PERSONALITY PSYCHOLOGY: ISOLATION AND (OCCASIONAL) INTERDISCIPLINARITY

As the broadest of the subfields of academic psychology, one might expect that personality psychology historically would have been the most fully attuned to and enmeshed with developments throughout the field. This, however, has not been the case. Indeed, the opposite has sometimes been true. The field has been often been marked by a unique degree of isolationism from the rest of the psychological discipline; as Hall & Lindzey (1970, p. 4) observed, "personality theory has never been deeply embedded" in the rest of the field. Even within the discipline, theories have developed in isolation from one another. Cattell (1990), for example, proclaimed his research career, which proved so instrumental to later developments (John & Srivastava, 1999), to be "an extraordinary tale of isolation from," as he perceived it, "the random mainstream of personality speculation" (1990, p. 101).

The risks inherent in such isolationism are particularly well illustrated by the history of psychoanalytic theory. The psychoanalytic community expressed explicit disinterest in having their work evaluated according to the methodological standards of the broader science of psychology or in integrating their ideas with knowledge rising in that discipline. The costs of this choice are now painfully apparent. Despite the brilliance of some initial speculations, psychoanalytic theory yielded a "view of unconscious mental life . . . that, to date, has found little or no support in empirical science" (Kihlstrom, 1999, p. 436) and spawned a personality assessment technology whose level of support can be characterized similarly (Lilienfeld, Wood, & Garb, 2000). The latter failure in particular entailed significant costs, not only to our science but also to society.

One stellar counterexample to this trend was the work of Henry Murray and his associates at the Harvard Psychological Clinic and the university's interdisciplinary Department of Social Relations (Kluckhohn & Murray, 1949; Murray, 1938). Murray, whose own training was in medicine and biochemistry, organized a remarkable interdisciplinary group of investigators. They explored the internal dynamics of personality, the social and cultural contexts in which persons developed, and clinical techniques for learning about individuals in depth and for improving their psychological conditions. This effort did not ultimately succeed because it was premature. Investigators at the time were operating primarily at molar levels of analysis that proved difficult to integrate in a productive manner. The contemporaneous cognitive science center at Harvard succeeded because the timing was right; cognitive psychologists, linguists, and information scientists had developed detailed models of their phenomena that could be integrated fruitfully. Contemporary developments in understanding the physiological, cognitive, and affective systems possessed by the individual and the interpersonal, social, and cultural contexts in which they develop and function suggest that the time may finally be right to advance the science of persons envisioned by Murray.

THE CONTRIBUTIONS TO THIS VOLUME

This volume is organized into three parts. Before reviewing each of them, we note that contributions throughout the text speak to questions of personality development, the study of which has a curious history within personality psychology. In the early days of the field, psychoanalytic theorists centered much of their investigation on the question of how, during the early years of life, personality develops in dynamic interaction with the social and interpersonal environment (Adler, 1927; Freud, 1900/ 1953). Subsequent work extended these efforts to consider development across the life course (Erikson, 1963). In retrospect, it is obvious that these efforts were hampered by inadequate empirical methods and a tendency to overestimate the influence of early life experiences on later development (Kagan, 1998; Mischel, 1968; see also Chapter 6, this volume). Nonetheless, this work was valuable in calling attention to interactions between the developing person and the social world—a critical question that subsequently was taken up in alternative theoretical languages (e.g., Bandura & Walters, 1963). A great strength of the contemporary field is that it provides rich data and sophisticated analyses of how physiological systems (Gunnar, 2000), cognitions (Bugental & Johnston, 2000), and behavioral strategies (Sulloway, 1996, 2001) develop in interaction with the social and family environment and how psychological dynamics shift systematically across the life span (Heckhausen & Dweck, 1998). Yet a singular oddity of the contemporary field is that this valuable knowledge base insufficiently penetrates the academic discipline of personality psychology. In part, this fact reflects institutional factors; different professional conferences and publication outlets exist for investigators who self-identify as developmental as opposed to personality psychologists. Scientific efforts that have direct bearing on one another thus become isolated. But this division also reflects trends within personality psychology, which in recent years has seen theoretical conceptions that so strongly discount the impact of environmental experience on the developing person that the very "concept of personality development is an oxymoron" (Zelli & Dodge, 1999, p. 97). A great challenge for the contemporary field is to marry the compelling evidence of temporal stability in dispositional tendencies with the equally compelling evidence that persons develop through dynamic interactions with the social world.

Biological Bases of Individual Differences: Cortical Activity, Affect, and Motivation

The contributions to Part I of this volume address individual differences in psychobiological systems that contribute to personality characteristics, as well as the genetic and environmental bases of these systems. Grigorenko's (Chapter 2) enlightening review of research on genes and personality documents advances in both behavior-genetic analyses of molar personality traits and molecular-genetic analyses of the relations between genetic variability in neurotransmitter systems and overt personality characteristics. Her findings challenge commonly accepted assumptions in the field. For example, do genetic factors contribute robustly to the similarity of monozygotic twins, whereas as family and environment contribute little? Grigorenko's findings force the sophisticated conclusion: It depends. In a recent behavior-genetic analysis conducted with more than 700 Russian families, shared family–environment factors contributed significantly to variation in the majority of the traits studied. In contrast, in a large subsample of the population (218 families in which at least one parent had a criminal record), genetic factors did *not* contribute significantly to variation in 13 of 15 traits. Grigorenko's analysis of genes and neurotransmitter systems highlights the enormous complexities involved in relating these systems to phenotypic qualities that distinguish personalities from one another: Personality characteristics will not reflect the action of a single neurotransmitter system, if only because neurotransmitter systems interact with one another; gene expression and surface-level behavioral characteristics are not stable but fluctuate across development in interaction with environmental conditions; and even the dependent measure to select for study is not obvious, because measures of global personality characteristics may obscure contextualized behavior patterns that have a partly genetic basis. No stronger case could be made for fully incorporating the knowledge base of contemporary genetics into the science of personality.

Schmidt and Fox (Chapter 3) provide a comprehensive and synthetic account of the biological bases of temperamental shyness. Their "frontal activation–neuroendocrine–experiential hypothesis" explains temperamental shyness in terms of interactions among (1) the frontal cortex and the forebrain limbic area, (2) serotonergic systems that regulate activity in these regions (and whose molecular genetic bases are beginning to be understood), and (3) socialization processes that have the potential to alter a child's brain systems and affective tendencies. The psychobiological systems, then, prove to be highly plastic. Social factors such as parenting style and experience in day care are found to alter children's temperament classifications.

Heller, Isom, Nitschke, Koven, and Miller (Chapter 4) present a neuropsychological model of individual differences in two primary components of emotional states: valence and arousal. A compelling convergence of findings involving both electroencephalograph (EEG) and blood flow measures of cortical activity indicates that differential activation in the left versus right hemispheres, as well as in frontal versus posterior regions of the brain, is robustly correlated with these two emotional components. Their findings lead to a distinction between two aspects of anxiety: (1) worry, or anxious apprehension, and (2) anxious arousal, or panic. Individuals who are prone to one versus the other class of emotional experience are found to display enhanced activation in different brain regions.

Sutton's findings (Chapter 5) similarly reveal that differential hemispheric activity is associated with different affective and motivational characteristics. Individuals are found to exhibit stable individual differences in EEG measures of asymmetry in anterior brain regions. These measures of brain activity are strongly correlated with self-report measures of behavioral inhibition versus activation–approach. Findings also indicate that EEG asymmetry relates to self-motivated performance, supporting the contention that different frontal brain regions function as elements of incentive versus threat motivation systems. An intriguing feature of this work is that advances in the understanding of brain functioning lead naturally to a theoretical position that has classically interactionist qualities. Incentive and threat systems are responsive to environmental signals of reward and threat, respectively, and different environments naturally will feature different configurations of signals. Both the brain and the external world thus contribute to overt motivational qualities.

These latter three analyses of individual differences in neurobiological systems have an interesting relation to individual-difference analyses that involve self-report or observer-report questionnaire data. Factor analyses of such data robustly yield a factor of Neuroticism, defined by characteristics that include the tendency to be anxious, worrying, high-strung, touchy, nervous, and emotional (John & Srivastava, 1999). Neuroticism, in this work, appears to be a psychologically unitary entity that all individuals possess to a greater or lesser degree. The contributions in this volume, though, raise alternative possibilities. For example, Schmidt and Fox do not conceive of temperamental shyness as a continuous dimension; instead, they posit that a distinct class of children, constituting 10–15% of the population, are consistently inhibited in social situations (see also Kagan, 1994). Recent work employing statistical techniques designed to identify distinct classes in nature (Meehl, 1992) provides initial evidence in support of this claim (Woodward, Lenzenweger, Kagan, Snidman, & Arcus, 2000). It is also noteworthy that Schmidt and Fox do not conceive of inhibitedness as a global tendency but as a quality that specifically manifests itself in social situations, particularly those involving novelty. The work of Heller and colleagues also varies from the standard conceptualization of neuroticism. They suggest that worry and anxious emotional arousal are best considered not as aspects of neuroticism but as separate constructs, because these two tendencies relate to separate neural networks. They note that traditional self-report indices of neuroticism thus mix together indices of two constructs that are physiologically distinct. Sutton's work similarly raises fundamental questions about the conceptualization and assessment of differences among individuals. His findings indicate that a key issue in affective functioning is not the sensitivity of a single, isolated affective system but the *relative* sensitivity of one system versus another; their relation is important because the systems are mutually inhibitory. This finding implies that individuals who possess the same threat-system sensitivity, for example, may differ in their tendency to display threat-related behaviors because of the functioning of a second personality system. There is, then, no simple, isomorphic mapping of the genotypic threat system to phenotypic behavioral tendencies. (Lewis, Chapter 6, and Nowak and colleagues, Chapter 12, raise a similar conceptual point about the relations between phenotype and genotype.) Note that the functional relations between positive/incentive and negative/threat affect systems explored by Sutton commonly are not addressed in traditional lexical analyses of individual differences; in these analyses, investigators generally search for factors that are orthogonal to one another at the level of the population and rarely address the possibility that these factors are dynamically related at the level of the individual.

Personality Development in Its Social Context

Lewis begins Part II of the volume in Chapter 6 by addressing three conceptual models that guide theory and research on personality development: trait, environmental, and interactional models. While noting that no model alone is sufficient to explain fully the development of the individual, Lewis's analyses of how individuals adapt to current environmental conditions and how developmental outcomes reflect the "goodness-of-fit" between characteristics of the child and environmental demands (cf. Wright & Mischel, 1987) underscore the utility of environmental and interactional conceptions. He challenges investigators to include measures of environmental context in studies of the longitudinal stability of personality characteristics and to control for the effects of contextual stability prior to concluding that unchanging properties of persons are singly responsible for observed stability in behavioral tendencies.

Hawley and Little (Chapter 7) analyze personality agency and person-by-context interactions at two conceptual levels. Hawley's resource control theory provides an evolutionary perspective that highlights two domains of life that individuals must manage simultaneously: meeting personal needs and establishing social relationships. Children who develop both coercive and prosocial strategies for meeting these needs are found to be socially successful and well liked by their peers. Little (in press) action control theory provides a developmental account of how personal actions give rise to perceptions of personal agency and how agency and control judgments change, in a domain-linked manner, across the life course.

Twenge (Chapter 8) explores the possibility that social changes in the United States across the 20th century influenced the personalities of its inhabitants. Specifically, different birth cohorts, who experienced different sociocultural environments, are found to exhibit different mean levels of dysphoric affect (anxiety, depression), as well as different views of self and related personality dispositions (including individualism, self-esteem, and extraversion). As Twenge notes, these results—which often include remarkably large effect sizes—directly contradict the hypothesis that self-reported personality characteristics may be unaffected by socio-historical conditions. Instead, they motivate future research on how social conditions, which can vary so dramatically across both time and cultures, influence the developing person. Interestingly, Twenge also notes that her findings suggest that traditional twin studies underestimate the potential impact of environmental conditions and thus overestimate the overall percentage of variability in phenotypic characteristics that may be due to genetic factors by virtue of the fact that such studies generally include only one birth cohort.

Costa and McCrae (Chapter 9) provide a valuable reminder that, whatever the evidence for dynamic development in individual functioning, some measures of personality characteristics yield remarkably high degrees of stability. In their contribution, they ask whether, at the level of the population, mean levels of self-reported global personality dispositions vary across the life course. Although some changes are observed, particularly across the transition from adolescence to adulthood, findings generally yield striking evidence of stability in mean trait levels. Data collected in the United States, in Europe, and in East Asian nations yield highly similar developmental curves.

Personality as a Complex System: Social-Cognitive and Affective Dynamics

The contributors to Part III of the volume treat personality as a complex system of cognitive and affective elements that develops and functions in interaction with the social environment. In so doing, they take part in a major trend in the recent history of research in the physical and social sciences, namely, the widespread application of principles of nonlinear dynamical systems (see especially Chapter 12). In this regard, the chapters are a paradigm case of interdisciplinarity in personality science.

Shoda and LeeTiernan (Chapter 10) solve a problem that is of critical importance, although it sometimes goes unrecognized. A variety of theoretical systems in the psychological sciences posit mechanisms through which people adapt to specific features of the environment. Because any complex social environment contains multiple features, if the theoretical system is to make testable predictions, it must grapple with the problem of identifying which of the various situational features a person is attending to and encoding. The failure to solve this problem raises difficulties in scientific explanation for theories ranging from behaviorism (Chomsky, 1959) to evolutionary psychology (Cervone, 2000). Drawing on their cognitive-affective processing system (Mischel & Shoda, 1995) and on the personal construct theory of Kelly (1955), Shoda and

LeeTiernan devise a novel "virtual situations paradigm" to address this problem. Through it, they are able to identify which features of social situations are uniquely salient to a given individual. This featural analysis enables the prediction of coherent patterns of cross-situational variability in behavior, or coherent behavioral signatures (Mischel & Shoda, 1995; Shoda, 1999), that are observed when the individual encounters a novel set of circumstances.

Showers (Chapter 11) presents a dynamic model of self-structure that highlights a key feature of self-concept, namely, the evaluative organization of the multifaceted aspects of self. Some individuals are found to possess a compartmentalized self-concept in which positively and negatively valenced attributes are organized into conceptually distinct self-aspect categories. Others exhibit an evaluatively integrated self-concept; they tend to experience a mix of positive and negative personal attributes in any given context. Findings indicate that type of self-concept organization is related to mood and self-esteem in interaction with the personal importance of positive and negative self-beliefs. Importantly, the organization among multiple aspects of self is open to change—the self-concept is dynamic—and the capacity to change in a flexible, adaptive manner is found to contribute to psychological health. Results from a prospective study of depression suggest that people who are most capable of flexibly changing their type of self-organization when facing stressful circumstances experience lower levels of negative mood.

In Chapter 12, Nowak, Vallacher, and Zochowski apply the principles and the mathematics of nonlinear dynamical systems to the question of how people develop stable personal qualities. They posit that stable dispositions emerge, in part, as a result of social interactions in which individuals strive to synchronize their actions with one another. If, in this process, a given level or type of action is sustained over a prolonged period, it becomes a stable parameter in the complex cognitive-affective system that is the individual's personality. The stable parameter can be understood as a structure of personality that fosters enduring, distinct patterns of behavior. The authors present results from computer simulations of synchronized interactions that vividly illustrate the emergence of personal stability.

As Nowak et al. explain, nonlinear dynamical systems principles force a profound rethinking of traditional conceptions of personality structure and dispositions. In this regard, two features of dynamical systems particularly stand out. First, a dynamical system may have multiple stable equilibria that foster conflicting types of behavior in different contexts; as Nowak et al. note, personality consistency thus may be manifested in stable patterns of variability in action; aggregated mean levels of behavior may, for many individuals, be relatively meaningless as a characterization of their personality tendencies or structure (cf. Mischel & Shoda, 1995, 1998). Second, dynamical systems can organize into patterns that are idiosyncratic; furthermore, individuals may idiosyncratically identify their own characteristic action tendencies. As a result, personality consistency may be organized, at the level of the individual, around a mix of both normatively common and highly idiosyncratic personal attributes (cf. Cervone, 1997; Cervone et al., 2001).

PREPARING FOR THE FUTURE

Our call for an interdisciplinary personality science entails one obstacle that we have yet to raise. It involves the training of our students, the next generation of personality scientists. If personality science is to serve an integrative function in the study of human individuality and diversity, then the personality scientist's training must be atypically broad, spanning multiple areas of psychology, as well as neighboring fields. It is difficult not only to provide such training but also to motivate the student to engage in it during an era that often seems to value productivity above scholarly breadth. The students' need to acquire increasingly specialized technical and quantitative skills only makes the challenge more difficult. Yet if our field is to advance, our students must be at least as well versed in the human sciences as in the statistical sciences. An enhanced valuing of interdisciplinarity in graduate training is required to protect that endangered yet essential species of psychologist: the generalist.

Those who long for such developments but doubt their feasibility may again take solace from a look back to the history of cognitive psychology. The growth of cognitive science made course work in computer science, linguistics, and neuroscience a routine part of graduate training for students in cognitive psychology.

A look further back in history also is encouraging. The greatest figure in the founding of psychology, William James, also was its greatest generalist. And broad, Jamesian training seemed to promote exactly the scientific mission we call for now. The first volume of the series *A History of Psychology in Autobiography* featured a contribution by Mary Whiton Calkins (1930/1961), whose educational introduction to psychology was an individualized tutorial with James in the year of the publication of his *Principles of Psychology* (1890). In the career that followed, Calkins promoted a "science . . . of conscious, experiencing, functioning beings, that is, of persons or selves" (1930/1961, p. 44) that was integrated with, rather than isolated from, more atomistic branches of the discipline. Because psychological functions—perceiving, remembering, learning, acting, interacting—are performed not by isolated mechanisms but by whole, intact persons, the study of the "person, as related to its environment, physical and social" (Calkins, 1930/1961, p. 42) is the natural center point of psychological science (cf. Stern, 1930/1961). Such a science of persons, she concluded decades ago, "is imperatively needed today for the grounding and the upbuilding of the . . . eclectic disciplines roughly grouped as the social sciences" (p. 62). We concur in this conclusion, and the contributions to this volume are one step in meeting this need. It is easy to hear James and Calkins saying "it's about time."

REFERENCES

Adler, A. (1927). *Understanding human nature.* New York: Greenberg.

Allport, G. W. (1937). *Personality: A psychological interpretation.* New York: Holt.

Asendorpf, J. B., Borkenau, P., Ostendorf, F., & Van Aken, M. A. G. (2001). Carving personality description at its joints: Confirmation of three replicable personality prototypes for both children and adults. *European Journal of Personality, 15,* 169–198.

Ayduk, O., Mendoza-Denton, R., Mischel, W., Downey, G., Peake, P. K., & Rodriguez, M. (2000). Regulating the interpersonal self: Strategic self-regulation for coping with rejection sensitivity. *Journal of Personality and Social Psychology, 79,* 776–792.

Baltes, P. B., Lindenberger, U., & Staudinger, U. (1998). Life-span theory in developmental psychology. In W. Damon (Series Ed.) & R. Lerner (Vol. Ed.), *Handbook of child psychology: Vol.1. Theoretical models of human development* (5th ed., pp. 1029–1144). New York: Wiley.

Bandura, A., & Walters, R. (1963). *Social learning and personality development.* New York: Holt, Rinehart & Winston.

Bargh, J. A. (1997). The automaticity of everyday life. In R. S. Wyer, Jr. (Ed.), *Advances in social cognition* (Vol. 10, pp. 1–61). Mahwah, NJ: Erlbaum.

Bechara, A., Damasio, H., Tranel, D., & Damasio, A. (1997). Deciding advantageously before knowing the advantageous strategy. *Science, 275,* 1293–1295.

Brandtstädter, J., & Lerner, R. M. (Eds.). (1999). *Action and self-development: Theory and research through the life span.* Thousand Oaks, CA: Sage.

Brewer, M. B., Kenny, D. A., & Norem, J. K. (Eds.) (2000). Personality and social psychology at the interface: New directions for interdisciplinary research [Special issue]. *Personality and Social Psychology Review, 4*(1).

Bruner, J. (1990). *Acts of meaning.* Cambridge, MA: Harvard University Press.

Bugental, D. B., & Johnston, C. (2000). Parental child cognitions in the context of the family. *Annual Review of Psychology, 51,* 315–344.

Buss, D. M. (1999). Human nature and individual differences: The evolution of human personality. In L. A. Pervin & O. P. John (Eds.), *Handbook of personality: Theory and research* (2nd ed., pp. 31–56). New York: Guilford Press.

Buss, D. M., & Craik, K. H. (1983). The act frequency approach to personality. *Psychological Review, 90,* 105–126.

Calkins, M. W. (1961). Mary Whiton Calkins. In C. Murchison (Ed.), *A history of psychology in autobiography* (Vol. 1, pp. 31–62). New York: Russell and Russell. (Original work published 1930)

Caprara, G. V., & Cervone, D. (2000). *Personality: Determinants, dynamics, and potentials.* New York: Cambridge University Press.

Cattell, R. B. (1990). Advances in Cattellian personality theory. In L. A. Pervin (Ed.), *Handbook of personality: Theory and research* (pp. 101–110). New York: Guilford Press.

Cervone, D. (1997). Social-cognitive mechanisms and personality coherence: Self-knowledge, situational beliefs, and cross-situational coherence in perceived self-efficacy. *Psychological Science, 8,* 43–50.

Cervone, D. (1999). Bottom-up explanation in personality psychology: The case of cross-situational coherence. In D. Cervone & Y. Shoda (Eds.), *The coherence of personality: Social-cognitive bases of personality consistency, variability, and organization* (pp. 303–341). New York: Guilford Press.

Cervone, D. (2000). Evolutionary psychology and explanation in personality psychology: How do we know which module to invoke? *American Behavioral Scientist, 6,* 1001–1014.

Cervone, D., & Rafaeli-Mor, N. (1999). Living in the future in the past: On the origin and expression of self-regulatory abilities. *Psychological Inquiry, 10,* 209–213.

Cervone, D., Shadel, W. G., & Jencius, S. (2001). Social-cognitive theory of personality assessment. *Personality and Social Psychology Review, 5,* 33–51.

Cervone, D., & Shoda, Y. (1999). Beyond traits in the study of personality coherence. *Current Directions in Psychological Science, 8*(1), 27–32.

Chomsky, N. (1959). Review of *Verbal Behavior* by B. F. Skinner. *Language, 35,* 26–58.

Cloninger, C.R., Adolffson, R., & Svrakic, N. M. (1996). Mapping genes for human personality. *Nature Genetics, 12,* 3–4.

Damasio, A. R. (1994). *Descartes' error: Emotion, reason, and the human brain.* New York: Grosset/Putnam.

Damasio, A. R. (1999). *The feeling of what happens: Body and emotion in the making of consciousness.* New York: Harcourt Brace.

Davidson, R. J. (1992). Emotion and affective style: Hemispheric substrates. *Psychological Science, 3,* 39–43.

Davison, K. P., & Pennebaker, J. W. (1996). Social psychosomatics. In E. T. Higgins & A. W. Kruglanski (Eds.), *Social psychology: Handbook of basic principles* (pp. 102–130). New York: Guilford Press.

Dennett, D. C. (1991). *Consciousness explained.* Boston: Little Brown.

Durham, W. H. (1991). *Coevolution.* Stanford, CA: Stanford University Press.

Edelman, G. M. (1992). *Bright air, brilliant fire: On the matter of the mind.* New York: Basic Books.

Edelman, G. M., & Tononi, G. (2000). *A universe of consciousness: how matter becomes imagination.* New York: Basic Books.

Ehrlich, P. R. (2000). *Human natures: Genes, cultures, and the human prospect.* Washington, DC: Island Press.

Ekman, P., & Davidson, R. J. (Eds.). (1994). *The nature of emotion: Fundamental questions.* New York: Oxford University Press.

Erikson, E. (1963). *Childhood and society* (2nd ed.). New York: Norton.

Eysenck, H. J. (1990). Biological dimensions of personality. In L. A. Pervin (Ed.), *Handbook of personality: Theory and research* (pp. 244–276). New York: Guilford Press.

Fish, S. (1980). *Is there a text in this class?* Cambridge, MA: Harvard University Press.

Freud, S. (1953). The interpretation of dreams. In J. Strachey (Ed. and Trans.), *The standard edition of the complete psychological works of Sigmund Freud* (Vol. 4, pp. 1–338; vol. 5, pp. 339–621). London: Hogarth Press. (Original work published 1900)

Gardner, H. (1985). *The mind's new science: A history of the cognitive revolution.* New York: Basic Books.

Geertz, C. (1973). *The interpretation of cultures.* New York: Basic Books.

Geertz, C. (2000). *Available light: Anthropological reflections on philosophical topics.* Princeton, NJ: Princeton University Press.

Goldberg, E. (2001). *The executive brain: Frontal lobes and the civilized mind.* New York: Oxford University Press.

Gosling, S. D., & John, O. P. (1999). Personality dimensions in nonhuman animals: A cross-species review. *Current Directions in Psychological Science, 8*(3), 69–75.

Gottlieb, G. (1998). Normally occurring environmental and behavioral influences on gene activity: From central dogma to probabilistic epigenesis. *Psychological Review, 105,* 792–802.

Gunnar, M. R. (2000). Early adversity and the development of stress reactivity and regulation. In C. A. Nelson (Ed.), *The Minnesota symposia on child psychology: Vol. 31. The effects of early adversity on neurobehavioral development* (pp. 163–200). Mahwah, NJ: Erlbaum.

Hall, C. S., & Lindzey, G. (1970). *Theories of personality* (2nd ed.). New York: Wiley.

Harré, R. (1998). *The singular self: An introduction to the psychology of personhood.* London: Sage.

Heckhausen, J., & Dweck, C. S. (Eds.). (1998). *Motivation and self-regulation across the life span.* New York: Cambridge University Press.

Herbst, J. H., Zonderman, A.B., McCrae, R. R., & Costa, P. T. Jr. (2000). Do the dimensions of the Temperament and Character Inventory map a simple genetic architecture? Evidence from molecular genetics and factor analysis. *American Journal of Psychiatry, 157,* 1285–1290.

Higgins, E. T., & Kruglanski, A. W. (Eds.). (2000). *Motivational science: Social and personality perspectives* (pp. 202–214). Philadelphia: Taylor & Francis.

James, W. (1890). *Principles of psychology.* New York: Holt.

John, O. P., & Srivastava, S. (1999). The Big-Five Factor taxonomy: History, measurement, and theoretical perspectives. In L. A. Pervin & O. P. John (Eds.), *Handbook of personality: Theory and research* (2nd ed., pp. 102–138). New York: Guilford Press.

Kagan, J. (1994). *Galen's prophecy: Temperament in human nature.* New York: Basic Books.

Kagan, J. (1998). *Three seductive ideas.* Cambridge, MA: Harvard University Press.

Kelly, G. (1955). *The psychology of personal constructs.* New York: Norton.

Kihlstrom, J. F. (1999). The psychological unconscious. In L. A. Pervin & O. P. John (Eds.), *Handbook of personality: Theory and research* (2nd ed., pp. 424–442). New York: Guilford Press.

Kitayama, S., & Markus, H. R. (1999). Yin and Yang of the Japanese self: The cultural psychology of personality coherence. In D. Cervone & Y. Shoda (Eds.), *The coherence of personality: Social-cognitive bases of consistency, variability, and organization* (pp. 242–302). New York: Guilford Press.

Kluckhohn, C., & Murray, H. A. (1949). *Personality in nature, society, and culture.* New York: Knopf.

Kolb, B., & Whishaw, I. Q. (1998). Brain plasticity and behavior. *Annual Review of Psychology, 49,* 43–64.

Lazarus, R. S. (1999). *Stress and emotion: A new synthesis.* New York: Springer.

Leary, M. R., & Tangney, J. P. (Eds). (in press). *Handbook of self and identity.* New York: Guilford Press.

LeDoux, J. (1996). *The emotional brain: The mysterious underpinnings of emotional life.* New York: Simon & Schuster.

Lewis, M., & Haviland-Jones, J. M. (Eds.) (2000). *Handbook of emotions* (2nd ed.). New York: Guilford Press.

Lewontin, R. (2000). *The triple helix: Gene, organism, and environment.* Cambridge, MA: Harvard University Press.

Lilienfeld, S. O., Wood, J. M., & Garb, H. N. (2000). The scientific status of projective techniques. *Psychological Science in the Public Interest, 1*(2).

Little, T. D. (in press). Agency in development. In R. Silbereisen & W. H. Hartup (Eds.), *Expert views on human development.* East Sussex, England: Psychology Press.

Magnusson, D. (1999). Holistic interactionism: A perspective for research on personality development. In L. A. Pervin & O. P. John (Eds.), *Handbook of personality: Theory and research* (2nd ed., pp. 219–247). New York: Guilford Press.

Magnusson, D., & Endler, N. S. (Eds.) (1977). *Personality at the crossroads: Current issues in interactional psychology.* Hillsdale, NJ: Erlbaum.

McAdams, D. P. (1997). A conceptual history of personality psychology. In R. Hogan, J. Johnson, & S. Briggs (Eds.), *Handbook of personality psychology* (pp. 3–39). San Diego, CA: Academic Press.

Meehl, P. (1992). Factors and taxa, traits and types, differences of degree and differences in kind. *Journal of Personality, 60,* 117–174.

Metcalfe, J., & Mischel, W. (1999). A hot/cool-system analysis of delay of gratification: Dynamics of willpower. *Psychological Review, 106,* 3–19.

Miller, S. M., Shoda, Y., & Hurley, K. (1996). Applying cognitive-social theory to health-protective behavior: Breast self-examination in cancer screening. *Psychological Bulletin, 119,* 70–94.

Mischel, W. (1968). *Personality and assessment.* New York: Wiley.

Mischel, W., & Morf, C. (in press). The self as a psycho-social dynamic processing system: A meta-perspective on a century of the self in psychology. In M. Leary & J. Tangney (Eds.), *Handbook of self and identity*. New York: Guilford Press.

Mischel, W., & Shoda, Y. (1995). A cognitive-affective system theory of personality: Reconceptualizing situations, dispositions, dynamics, and invariance in personality structure. *Psychological Review, 102*, 246–286.

Mischel, W., & Shoda, Y. (1998). Reconciling processing dynamics and personality dispositions. *Annual Review of Psychology, 49*, 229–258.

Mithen, S. (1996). *The prehistory of the mind: The cognitive origins of art, religion and science*. London: Thames & Hudson.

Morf, C. C., & Rhodewalt, F. (2001). Unraveling the paradoxes of narcissism: A dynamic self-regulatory processing model. *Psychological Inquiry, 12*, 177–196.

Murray, H.A. (1938). *Explorations in personality*. New York: Oxford University Press.

Neisser, U. (1967). *Cognitive psychology*. Englewood Cliffs, NJ: Prentice-Hall.

Nisbett, R. E., Peng, K., Choi, I., & Norenzayan, A. (2001). Culture and systems of thought: Holistic versus analytic cognition. *Psychological Review, 108*, 291–310.

Pervin, L., & John, O. P. (Eds.). (1999). *Handbook of personality: Theory and research* (2nd ed.). New York: Guilford Press.

Pickering, A. D., & Gray, J. A. (1999). The neuroscience of personality. In L. A. Pervin & O. P. John (Eds.), *Handbook of personality* (2nd ed., pp. 277–299). New York: Guilford Press.

Pinker, S. (1997). *How the mind works*. New York: Norton.

Polkinghorne, D. (1988). *Narrative knowing and the human sciences*. Albany: State University of New York Press.

Posner, M. I., & DiGirolamo, G. J. (2000). Cognitive neuroscience: Origins and promise. *Psychological Bulletin, 126*, 873–889.

Posner, M. I., & Rothbart, M. K. (2000). Developing mechanisms of self-regulation. *Development and Psychopathology, 12*, 427–441.

Rothbart, M. K., Ahadi, S. A., & Evans, D. E. (2000). Temperament and personality: Origins and outcomes. *Journal of Personality and Social Psychology, 78*, 122–135.

Searle, J. R. (1998). *Mind, language, and society*. New York: Basic Books.

Shaffer, D. (1996). Understanding bias in scientific practice. *Philosophy of Science, 63* [Suppl.], 89–97.

Shoda, Y. (1999). Behavioral expressions of a personality system: Generation and perception of behavioral signatures. In D. Cervone & Y. Shoda (Eds.), *The coherence of personality: Social-cognitive bases of consistency, variability, and organization* (pp. 155–181). New York: Guilford Press.

Shweder, R. A. (1999). Humans really are different. [Review of J. Kagan, *Three seductive ideas*]. *Science, 283*, 798–799.

Shweder, R. A. (2000). The essential anti-essentialist [Review of the book *Available light: Anthropological reflections on philosophical topics*]. *Science, 290*, 1511–1512.

Shweder, R. A., & Sullivan, M. (1990). The semiotic subject of cultural psychology. In L. Pervin (Ed.), *Handbook of personality* (pp. 399–416). New York: Guilford Press.

Shweder, R. A., & Sullivan, M. A. (1993). Cultural psychology: Who needs it? *Annual Review of Psychology, 44,* 497–523.

Stern, W. (1961). William Stern. In C. Murchison (Ed.), *A history of psychology in autobiography* (Vol. 1, pp. 335–388). New York: Russell and Russell. (Original work published 1930)

Sulloway, F. J. (1996). *Born to rebel: Birth order, family dynamics, and creative lives.* New York: Pantheon Books.

Sulloway, F. J. (2001). Birth order, sibling competition, and human behavior. In H. R. Holcomb III (Ed.), *Conceptual challenges in evolutionary psychology: Innovative research strategies* (pp. 39–83). Dordrecht and Boston: Kluwer Academic.

Taylor, C. (1989). *Sources of the self: The making of modern identity.* Cambridge, MA: Harvard University Press.

Tesser, A., & Schwarz, N. (Eds.). (2001). *Blackwell handbook of social psychology: Intraindividual processes.* Malden, MA: Blackwell.

Thagard, P. (2000). *Coherence in thought and action.* Cambridge, MA: MIT Press.

Tooby, J., & Cosmides, L. (1990). On the universality of human nature and the uniqueness of the individual: The role of genetics and adaptation. *Journal of Personality, 58,* 17–67.

Woodward, S. A., Lenzenweger, M. F., Kagan, J., Snidman, N., & Arcus, D. (2000). Taxonic structure of infact reactivity: Evidence from a taxometric perspective. *Psychological Science, 11,* 296–301.

Wright, J. C., & Mischel, W. (1987). A conditional approach to dispositional constructs: The local predictability of social behavior. *Journal of Personality and Social Psychology, 53,* 1159–1177.

Zelli, A., & Dodge, K. A. (1999). Personality development from the bottom up. In D. Cervone & Y. Shoda (Eds.), *The coherence of personality: Social-cognitive bases of consistency, variability, and organization* (pp. 94–126). New York: Guilford Press.

PART I

BIOLOGICAL BASES OF INDIVIDUAL DIFFERENCES
Cortical Activity, Affect, and Motivation

CHAPTER 2

In Search of the Genetic Engram of Personality

ELENA L. GRIGORENKO

Is it not surprising that the worm *Caenorhabditis elegans* has 18,424 genes in its genome, the fruit fly *Drosophila melanogaster* 13,601, the plant *Arabidopsis* about 24,498, and humans only around 35,000 (Szathmáry, Jordán, & Pál, 2001)? Given the evolutionary distance between the worm *C. elegans* and humans, a reasonable assumption would be to expect a larger difference in the number of genes between two organisms. But, somehow, humans are what they are with a number of genes only two times as many as those of *C. elegans.*

Moreover, a number of genetic studies aimed at understanding genetic variation between humans and their primate cousins have unveiled yet another surprise of comparative genomics (a branch of modern science comparing the genomes of various species). It appears that human genomes differ only slightly—an estimated 1% to 2%—from those of great apes (Kaessmann, Wiebe, Weiss, & Pääbo, 2001). In short, the comparative genomics data suggest that there must be another, more sensible indicator of the complexity of genomes of different species than the mere number of genes.

The recent flurry of completed genome sequences for various species has indicated that there are significant differences in how genes are expressed and regulated between different species. Specifically, gene expression in liver and blood tissue appears to be very similar in chimps and humans, but the profiles of gene expression in the brain are markedly different; specifically, what is very special about the human brain are the accelerated patterns of gene activity (Kaessmann et al., 2001), the enhanced power of networks of genes (Szathmáry et al., 2001), and the sensitivity of these networks to proximal and distant environments (Anthony, 2001). In other words, the brain, which especially differentiates humans from their closest evolutionary relatives, is characterized by the enhanced power of genes expressed in the brain, the enhanced power of the networks organized by these genes, and the sensitivity of these networks to various environmental influences.

This idea that the complexity of the system is derived not only (or only partially) from the complexity of its elements but also from the complexity of interactions among these elements and between the system and its context is, of course, not new. In fact, the increasing impact of theories of complex dynamic systems is more and more obvious in the human sciences (Cilliers, 1998). And, certainly, for the field of personality, there is much benefit to be derived from complexity theories (Cervone & Shoda, 1999).

The purpose of this chapter is twofold. First, I provide a brief overview of the current state of affairs in the field, attempting to unveil the genetic etiology of personality. Summaries are presented for both behavior-genetic and molecular-genetic approaches. Second, I discuss a number of issues that should be considered for us to realize the enormous potential of research into the genetic basis of personality.

GENES AND PERSONALITY: A CAPSULE OVERVIEW

The question of the link between variability in genes and variability in personalities has been the focus of scientific interest for more than a century. As is typical for research on the etiology of psychological traits, the work has developed on two planes—the "normal" variability in personality traits and the "abnormal," exaggerated manifestation of certain traits (e.g., aggression, impulsivity, neuroticism) in psychiatric conditions—and by means of two methodologies—quantitative and molecular genetics. The field of behavior genetics has focused primarily on analyses of the overlap between the variability of genetic and personality traits in samples in which personality traits are more or less normally distributed, trying to establish a causal relationship between the two. The field of molecular genetics (or now, more specifically, molecular psychiatry) has primarily concentrated on finding gene variants that are possibly responsible for specific personality and personality-related disturbances in truncated samples, in which normal variability is suppressed and "psychiatry-spectrum" personality traits are embroidered. This division, although somewhat artificial and imprecise, structures the following review.

From the Viewpoint of Behavior Genetics

A growing body of data indicates an important contribution of genetic variability to variability of personality traits (Eaves, Eysenck, & Martin, 1989; Loehlin, 1992). These studies have used a variety of methodologies, the specifics of which depended on the nature of the recruited sample and on the type of instrument used. Sample-wise, the data were collected from twins reared apart (Bouchard, Lykken, McGue, Segal, & Tellegen, 1990; Pedersen, Plomin, McClearn, & Friberg, 1988; Tellegen et al., 1988) and twins reared together (Eaves et al., 1989; Heath, Cloninger, & Martin, 1994; Rose & Kaprio, 1988; Rose, Koskenvuo, Kaprio, Sarna, & Langinvainio, 1988), as well as from adoptive (Loehlin, Willerman, & Horn, 1982; Scarr, Webber, Weinberg, & Wittig, 1981) and biological families (Eaves, Martin, Heath, Hewitt, & Neal, 1990). Instrument-wise, most of the studies used self-reported data, but one study utilized ratings by informants (Heath, Neale, Kessler, Eaves, & Kendler, 1992). Theory-wise, the studies used instruments based on different personality theories: the Tridimensional Personality Questionnaire (Cloninger, Przybeck, & Svrakic, 1991, used in Heath et al., 1994; Cloninger, 1994); the revised Eysenck Personality Questionnaire (Eysenck, Eysenck, & Barrett, 1985, used in Eaves et al., 1989; Heath et al., 1994; Pedersen et al., 1988; Scarr et al., 1981); the Karolinska Scales of Personality (Gustavsson, 1997; used in Grigorenko, 2001); the NEO Personality Inventory (Costa & McCrae, 1985; used in Bergeman et al., 1993); and many others.

The body of behavioral-genetic research has produced a large amount of data. To illustrate, consider heritability estimates presented by Loehlin (1992) for the Big Five model. These heritability (h^2) and shared environment (c^2) estimates were calculated on a large twin sample that included both MZ (monozygotic) and DZ (dizygotic) twins under two different sets of modeling assumptions[1]—(1) the excess environmental similarity for MZ twins raised together (MZ twins share both genes and environments) and (2) the excess genetic similarity for MZ twins (MZ twins share not only main genetic effects but also interactive genetic effects). These estimates were as follows: (1) Extraversion, $h^2 = .36$ and $c^2 = .00$ (for model 1) and $h^2 = .49$ and $c^2 = .02$ (for model 2); (2) Agreeableness, $h^2 = .28$ and $c^2 = .09$ (for model 1) and $h^2 = .28$ and $c^2 = .11$ (for model 2); (3) Conscientiousness, $h^2 = .28$ and $c^2 = .04$ (for model 1) and $h^2 = .38$ and $c^2 = .07$ (for model 2); (4) Neuroticism, $h^2 = .31$ and $c^2 = .05$ (for model 1) and $h^2 = .41$ and $c^2 = .07$ (for model 2); and (5) Openness, $h^2 = .46$ and $c^2 = .05$ (for model 1) and $h^2 = .45$ and $c^2 = .06$ (for model 2). The mean values across the five traits were $h^2 = .34$ and $c^2 = .05$ (for model 1) and $h^2 = .42$ and $c^2 = .04$ (for model 2). Thus, although there were some differences in the obtained estimates depending on how MZ similarity was modeled, one major conclusion appeared to be unequivocal—whatever made MZ twins similar to each other involved the similarity in their genes, not the similarity in their environments.

A similar conclusion has been made in a summative analysis of a number of behavior-genetic studies of personality traits. Specifically, Bouchard (1994) has undertaken an exhaustive review of the current twin and adoptive studies and concluded that 30–60% of the variance in a number of personality traits is due to genetic factors. Similarly to many other traits investigated by means of behavior-genetic approaches, shared environment appears to be unimportant (7–10%), leaving nonshared environment accounting, on average, for the largest portion of the variance in personality.

This general picture, however, becomes much more complex when other factors important for understanding interindividual variability in personality traits are taken into account. Specifically, Viken, Rose, Kaprio, and Koskenvuo (1994) conducted developmental genetic analyses on Extraversion and Neuroticism scale scores from nearly 15,000 male and female Finnish twins, aged 18–53 years at baseline. The twins were tested on two occasions, 6 years apart. Not surprisingly, significant genetic effects on both traits were found, at all ages, in both men and women on each measurement occasion. However, the heritability estimates for the two traits showed developmental fluctuations and variable gender patterns. For Extraversion, heritability was invariant across gender but decreased from late adolescence to the late 20s, with a smaller additional decrease at about 50 years of age. For Neuroticism, heritability also decreased from late adolescence to late 20s and remained stable thereafter. For all ages after the early 20s, heritability of Neuroticism was significantly higher among women. Means for the two traits were gender dependent and, apparently, influenced by cohort and time of assessment, as well as by age. Moreover, there was little evidence of new genetic contributions to individual differences after age 30; in contrast, the researchers reported the emergence of significant new environmental effects at every age.

The overwhelming majority of behavior-genetic studies of personality traits have been conducted with self-reported measures. A significantly smaller but substantial body of behavior-genetic research has utilized behavioral ratings of relatives conducted by other relatives (e.g., parental ratings). There is, however, a rather small number of studies that have used observational indicators of behaviors and related personality traits. Miles and Carey (1997) conducted a meta-analysis on data from 24 genetically informative studies that utilized various (self-reported, parent-reported, and observation-based) personality measures of aggression. Overall, researchers have reported the presence of a strong overall genetic effect accounting for up to 50% of the variance in aggression. However, the estimates of h^2 and c^2 varied dramatically for different measures. Specifically, self-report and parental ratings showed genes and the family environment to be important in youth; the influence of genes increased but that of family environment decreased at later ages. However, observational ratings of laboratory behavior found no evidence for heritability and a very strong family environment effect. The importance of this observation is difficult to overestimate. Given that almost all substantive conclusions about heritability estimates of various personality traits have been drawn from self- or parental reports, the "nonfitting" pattern of the results obtained with observational ratings has to be reconciled with the existing body of the literature regarding the true correspondence (if any and ever) between self- and parent-reported personality traits and behaviors and the meaning of various heritability estimates for the understanding of the physiological links between the genes and behavior.

The study by Leve, Winebarger, Fagot, Reid, and Goldsmith (1998) makes a step toward such a reconciliation, although it adds even more complexity to the global picture of the correspondence between genes and behavior exhibited by various personalities. In their study, the genetic and environmental contributions to children's maladaptive behavior were assessed in a sample of young twin pairs (who ranged in age from 6 to 11 years). Interestingly, the researchers reported that genetic variation accounts for a majority of the variance in parent-reported child maladaptive behavior, whereas environmental variation accounts for the majority of the variance in the observational coding and global impressions of parent–twin interactive behavior. A new and exciting observation was made in this study—the researchers pointed out that the direct influence of one's interactive partner makes a significant impact on the expression of maladaptive behavior in an interactive setting; when controlling for the coparticipant's behavior, genetic variation increases and shared environmental variation decreases.

Yet another attempt to contextualize h^2 and c^2 estimates and to penetrate their somewhat abstract meaning has been made in the framework of a large family study (Grigorenko, 2001). In this study, heritability estimates for 15 personality traits (as assessed by the Karolinska Scales of Personality; Gustavsson, 1997) were obtained, initially, in a sample of 493 families representative of a general Russian population and then in a subsample of 218 families in which at least one of the parents had exhibited behaviors that resulted in criminal records. The estimates were obtained controlling for age, gender, and parent-reported indices of general family functioning. Although in the general sample, statistically significant heritability estimates were obtained for six traits (Somatic Anxiety, Muscular Tension, Socialization, Social Desirability, Detachment, and Monotony Avoidance), for only two of these traits (Detachment and Monotony Avoidance) were heritability estimates significant in the subsample. Moreover, this study pointed out the statistically significant effects of shared family environment for the majority of the traits (all but five in both the general sample and the subsample).

To conclude, it is difficult to come up with a one-sentence interpretation of the richness of the data accumulated in the framework of behavior-genetic research. Nevertheless, it might be worth trying. Thus, in brief, there appears to be evidence for associating the variance at the genetic level with the variance at the level of personality traits and behaviors exhibited by possessors of these traits. However, the very presence, as well as the strength, of this association varies depending on the gender and age of the possessor of a given personality trait, the trait itself, the way in which this trait has been assessed, the situation in which this trait is exhibited, and the broader genetic and environmental background in which this trait has developed and been socialized. Although the picture is complex, there is much enthusiasm in the field for trying to penetrate this complexity. We do know that there is a link between the variability in personality traits and genetic variability; the question is whether and to what degree we understand this link.

From the Viewpoint of Molecular Genetics

Having committed itself to looking for genetic mechanisms of personality, the field had to start somewhere. An obvious place was an attempt to find associations between genetic variability in neurotransmitter systems and personality traits and behavioral patterns. The first pioneering studies that investigated links between genetic profiles of the neurotransmitter systems and human behavior were carried out in the late 1970s. Recently, a number of publications have examined multiple interactions between common genetic polymorphisms in the genes involved in neurotransmitter systems and complex behavioral traits (e.g., Ebstein, Segman, Benjamin, Osher, & Belmaker, 1997; Netter, Henning, & Roed, 1996). In brief, the system of neurotransmitters is responsible for establishing neuronal communicational networks and carrying out the functions of signal detection and response. Thus neurotransmitters form chains of events, consisting mainly of recognition of binding sites and translating the recognition into second-order messages. These chains eventually affect behavior.

Although the functions "transmitting" and "behaving" are carried out by the same organism, the distance between a neurotransmitter molecule and a manifested behavior is huge. It is not measured in terms of traditional metrics but rather in terms of the number of interactions of various substrates (static interactions) and events (dynamic interactions) linking the two realities (the biochemical reality of neurotransmitter action and the social reality of human behavior). These interactions range from the interactions between molecules (any transmission requires at least two molecules) to the interactions between systems (e.g., modulation of events in the nervous system by actions of the endocrine system).

Prior to carrying out the review of molecular-genetic explorations of human personality, I review a number of postulates describing the reality of the neurotransmitter receptors' world (Russell, 1992).

First, the primary stimulus by which endogenous or exogenous chemicals affect subsequent physiological and behavioral functions consists of a physiochemical binding between a chemical and a specific receptor site on a biologically active macromolecule in the body.

Second, there exist a finite number of such receptor sites.

Third, the magnitudes of events that follow the co-occurrence of a chemical-receptor complex are related by some function to the number of sites occupied.

Fourth, the nervous system is capable of synthesizing receptors de novo. This synthesis is a part of the holistic pathway linking together various components of the neurotransmitter metabolic cycles.

Fifth, different transmitter systems are localized in different anatomical sites within the central nervous system.

These postulates (each of which is well supported by years of research and extensive literature) allow us to formulate a general assumption, namely the following: Each individual in a population has a definite threshold for responses to stimulation from both internal and external environments (Ashford, 1981; Rothman, Greenland, & Walker, 1980); thus receptors play primary roles in the physicochemical events that may eventually influence (or establish dynamic borders of reactivity) of behaviors.

Based on this general premise, we can delineate factors of interest that might be relevant to understanding the link between neurotransmitters and behaviors. These factors are (1) structure and density of neurotransmitter receptors and transporters, (2) efficiency of receptors in interacting with endogenous and exogenous reagents (so-called *ligands*— factors that bind to receptor molecules); and (3) interactions between receptors/transporters and neurotransmitter systems in general. Accepting the theoretical role for neurotransmitter systems specified previously, the question arises as to how we can empirically understand the role of these systems in personality. The most obvious (but not the only possible) step is to reformulate the general task of understanding the link of the variability at the genetic level with the variability at the level of personality into a number of more specific tasks. Particularly, we want (1) to describe various systems of neurotransmitters, understand their roles in carrying neural signaling (as it might be of relevance to personality), and describe the genetic variability occurring in these systems; and (2) to link this variability to variability in human behavior (potentially, at both individual and population levels).

What follows is a brief review of recent studies that establish associations or point out linkages between various genes involved in neurotransmitting and various personality traits and behaviors. The discussion focuses primarily on neurotransmitter receptors but also touches on genes involved in neurotransmittor transportation and metabolic pathways. There are nine systems of neurotransmitters (Cooper, Bloom, & Roth, 1996). Based on their biochemical functions, some of them appear to be more relevant to carrying out complex psychological functions than others—therefore, the body of the literature is uneven, concentrating on some neurotransmitting systems and barely touching others. For a number of historical and scientific reasons, the discussion of which lies outside of the spectrum of this chapter, there are three systems which, unarguably, have been in the center of researchers' attention for the past 10 years. They are the dopaminergic, serotonergic, and GABAergic systems. Thus the remaining part of this section will be devoted to a review of the documented and potential roles of these systems in human behavior.

However, it is important to issue a note of caution. Given what we know now about personality—a particularly complex psychological phenomenon—the hypothesis that personality depends on only one neurotransmitter system appears to be unlikely. Even such simple action as the stretch reflex (which involves only one afferent and an efferent neuron) interfaces with other systems by way of receptors on its cell surfaces. Thus I begin this review with the profound understanding that interactions among neurotransmitter systems are paramount to the very existence of living organisms.

The Dopaminergic System

Due to its connection with a wide number of neuropsychiatric and neurological conditions, the dopaminergic system has been extensively studied within the past decade. Its pervasiveness in the human brain is unarguable and has even been used as an explanatory factor in theories of the origins of human intelligence (Previc, 1999).

Dopaminergic pathways have been repeatedly implicated in the pathogenesis of a number of neuropsychiatric disorders (e.g., Tourette syndrome, attention-deficit/hyperactivity disorder [ADHD], conduct disorder). In addition, multiple sources of data indicate the involvement of the dopaminergic system in personality traits that have been shown to correlate with antisocial behaviors and various neuropsychiatric conditions (e.g., Comings et al., 1996).

Dopamine is predominantly localized in two systems that are characterized primarily by indirect projection to the cerebral cortex—the nigrostriatal system that emanates from cells in the substantia nigra and the mesolimbic system that emanates from cells in the ventral tegmentum area (Iversen, 1984). Table 2.1 summarizes the main genes involved in the dopaminergic system (symbols and identifications) and their locations in the genome. A number of genes whose polymorphisms have been featured in the literature recently are reviewed in more detail in the following subsections.[2]

DRD2 (Dopamine Receptor D2)

The presence of a polymorphism 40-bp repeat in the 3' untranslated region[3] (UTR) of the genes with repeat numbers ranging from 3 to 11 and Taq I restriction fragment length polymorphisms (RFLP) A and B allowed

TABLE 2.1. Dopaminergic System

Locus symbol	Gene description	Chromosomal location
	Dopaminergic synthesis enzymes	
TH	Tyrosine hydroxylase	11p15.5
DDC	Aromatic L-amino acid (DOPA) decarboxylase	7p11
	Dopaminergic degradative enzymes	
COMT	Catechol-O-methyl transferase	22p11.21-q11.23
MAO A	Monoamine oxidase A	Xp11.4-11.3
MAO B	Monoamine oxidase B	Xp11.4-11.3
	Dopamine transporters	
SLC6A3	Dopamine transporter (DAT) Solute carrier family 6, type 3	5p
SLC18A1	Vesicular monoamine transport (VMAT1)	8p21.3
SLC18A2	Vesicular monoamine transport (VMAT2)	10q26
	Dopamine receptors	
DRD1	Dopamine D1 receptor	5q35.1
DRD2	Dopamine D2 receptor	11q22-q23
DRD3	Dopamine D3 receptor	3q13.3
DRD4	Dopamine D4 receptor	11p15.5
DRD5	Dopamine D5 receptor	4p15–16

researchers to carry out a number of linkage and association studies for a number of neuropsychiatric conditions.

In the coding region, Cravchik, Sibley, and Gejman (1996) first reported that two of the variants altering amino acids (Pro310Ser and Ser311Cys) appeared to alter signal transduction properties of DRD2. In the regulatory region, Arinami, Gao, Hamaguchi, and Toru (1997) reported single nucleotide polymorphisms (SNPs). Moreover, there is a short tandem repeat polymorphism, in which the repeating component consists of four nucleotides; this tetranucleotide STRP was identified and reported by Kidd (K. Kidd, personal communication, April 1, 2001).

Blum et al. (1997) have studied the association between three dopaminergic genes (DRD2, DAT1, and DβH; see later in this section) and schizoid/avoidant behavior. The sample included "non-Hispanic, Northern, and Western European Caucasians with some exception" (p. 240); there was no clear distinction of ethnic background. The authors claimed that the study revealed an association between schizoid/avoidant behavior and the dopamine D2 receptor Taq A1 and a suggestive association between schizoid/avoidant behavior and 480-bp variable number tandem repeat (VNTR) 10/10 allele of the DAT1 genes.

Some molecular genetic studies have suggested a link between reward-dependent behaviors (e.g., heavy drinking, polysubstance abuse, carbohydrate bingeing, smoking, pathological gambling) and polymorphisms in DRD2, but these studies have generated mixed results, both suggesting (e.g., Blum, Cull, Braverman, & Comings, 1996; Blum, Sheridan, et al., 1996; Neiswanger, Hill, & Kaplan, 1993) and negating (e.g., Bolos et al., 1990; Gelertner et al., 1991; Suarez, Parsian, Hampe, Todd, Reich, & Cloninger, 1994) associations between genetic variation in DRD2 and these behaviors (for a review, see Noble, 1993).

DRD3 (Dopamine Receptor D3)

The Ball polymorphism in DRD3 has been examined for an association with bipolar affective disorder by Mitchell et al. (1993), Souery et al., (1996), and Gomez-Casero, Perez de Castro, Saiz-Ruiz, Llinares, and Fernandez-Piqueras (1996); with schizophrenia by Wiese et al. (1993), Sabate et al. (1994), Nanko et al. (1994), Inada et al. (1995), Tanaka et al. (1996), Asherson et al. (1996), Rietschel et al. (1996), Rothschild, Badner, Cravchik, Gershon, and Gejman (1996), and Griffon et al. (1996); with obsessive–compulsive disorder by Catalano et al. (1994); and with alcohol dependence by Sander et al. (1995). Among all these studies, a statistically significant association was found for schizophrenia in only two studies (Griffon et al., 1996; Basile et al., 1999); for alcohol dependence in one, but only where this was complicated by delirium (Lannfelt et al.,

1992); and for personality traits related to common mental disorders in one study (Henderson et al., 2000). All other association studies on DRD3 have produced negative results.

DRD4 (Dopamine Receptor D4)

DRD4 is characterized by substantial polymorphic variation in its coding region (Lichter et al., 1993; Chang, Ko, Lu, Pakstis, & Kidd, 1997; Chang & Kidd, 1997). It also appears that DRD4 has polymorphic regularity variation. Thus there are multiple polymorphisms known in this gene (Kamakura, Iwaki, Matsumoto, & Fukumaki, 1997; Seaman, Fisher, Chang, & Kidd, 1999).

The polymorphism in the exon 3 exists at two levels. First, there is an imperfect tandem repeat of 48 base pairs coding for 16 amino acids—alleles have been identified with 2 (32 amino acids) and 10 (160 amino acids) repeats. Second, the imperfect nature of the repeats is linked to more subtle variation—alleles with the same number of repeats can differ in the exact sequences or in the order of the variants of the 48-bp unit. Chang et al. (1997) undertook the survey of frequency of this allele in 36 different populations around the world. The authors identified 10 various repeats and reported significant frequency differences of various repeats between populations. The authors reported three most common alleles. Specifically, the 4-repeat allele was the most prevalent (with a global frequency of 64.3%) and was detected in every population studied; the range of frequencies was 0.16 to 0.96. The 7-repeat allele was the second most common (global mean = 20.6%), but the populations differed dramatically; this allele was found most frequently in the Americas (48.3%) but only occasionally in East and South Asia (1.9%). Similarly, the 2-repeat also exhibited substantial differences in population frequencies, with a global frequency of about 8.2% (third most common), being common in East and South Asia (18.1%) but rather uncommon in the Americas (2.9%) and Africa (1.9%). The occurrence of this repeat-number polymorphism within a coding region of the dopamine D4 receptor implies a possible functional relevance in signal transduction (Ren, Mayer, Cichetti, & Baltimore, 1993). The following three possible roles for variation in this protein domain have been proposed (Lichter et al., 1993): (1) different cytoplasmic loops change the conformation of transmembrane domains and alter the ligand bindings; (2) the repeat variation affects signal transduction by altering interactions with downstream intracellular proteins; or (3) the repeat variation has essentially no functional consequences. These potential properties of the exon 3 variants resulted in a number of linkage and association studies with different neuropsychiatric conditions. Investigations have been carried out with Parkinson's disease (Nanko,

Hattori, Ueki, & Ikeda, 1993), bipolar illness (Debruyn, Mendelbaum, et al., 1994), schizophrenia (Barr et al., 1993; Iversen, 1993; Macciardi et al., 1994; Nanko, Hattori, Ikeda, et al., 1993; Seeman, Guan, & Van Tol, 1993; Shaikh et al., 1993; Shaikh et al., 1994; Sommer, Lind, Heston, & Sobell, 1993; Van Tol et al., 1991, 1992), alcoholism (Chang et al., 1997), ADHD (e.g., La Hoste et al., 1996; Puumala et al., 1996; Tahir et al., 2000). The results of these studies have been mixed. To comprehend these findings, meta-analytic data-summarizing approaches have been recruited. Specifically, Faraone and colleagues (Faraone, Doyle, Mick, & Biederman, 2001) have carried out such a meta-analysis for ADHD and DRD4 allele 7 and have concluded that, although the association between ADHD and DRD4 is small, it is real.

In addition, a number of researchers have investigated the association between the 7-repeat allele and personality traits and have reported higher Novelty Seeking scores among unrelated individuals who were carriers of these alleles (Benjamin, Patterson, Greenberg, Murphy, & Hamer, 1996; Ebstein et al., 1996). Recently, Benjamin et al. (2000) have attempted to replicate this association in a sample of 455 adults, looking at polymorphisms within three different loci—DRD4, serotonin transported promoter regulatory region (5-HTTLPR; see later in this section), and catechol-O-methyltransferase (COMT; see later in this section). The findings suggest the presence of a functional pathway that links these various structures (DRD4, 5-HTTLPR, and COMT). Specifically, the researchers have concluded that the genotype–phenotype association between genetic polymorphisms and Novelty Seeking was observed in individuals lacking the 5-HTTLPR short allele and possessing long DRD4 alleles, with COMT playing a role of a modulator between 5-HTTLPR and DRD4.

Seeman et al. (1994) identified a substitution of valine by glycine—at amino acid position 194 at the beginning of exon 3. This substitution was reported to be present in U.S. individuals of African, but not European, ancestry.

Catalano, Nobile, Novelli, Nothen, and Smeraldi (1993) identified a 12-bp tandem duplication polymorphism in exon 1. The frequency of this polymorphism was reported only among Italians.

Nothen et al. (1994) identified a 13-bp deletion near the 3' end of the exon 1. This polymorphism causes a frameshift and premature termination of translation such that presumably no functional receptor is produced. This polymorphism has been studied among Germans.

A short poly-G tandem repeat polymorphism has been identified in the intron 1 (Petronis, O'Hara, et al., 1994).

A *Sma*I RFLP also exists in the 5' end of the noncoding region (Petronis, Van Tol, & Kennedy, 1994).

Thus the gene DRD4 appears to be rather variable and might serve as a candidate gene for many more molecular-genetic studies of behavior and personality.

DRD5 (Dopamine Receptor D5)

There has been some evidence that the DRD5 receptor exhibits association with ADHD (Daly, Hawi, Fitzgerald, & Gill, 1999; Tahir et al., 2000). There also have been reports of an association between DRD5 and schizophrenia (e.g., Muir et al., 2001). Results of studies attempting to find an association between DRD5 and bipolar disorders have been mixed (e.g., Asheron et al., 1998; Kirov, Jones, McCandless, Craddock, & Owen, 1999). The DRD5 gene has a number of variants in the coding region (e.g., Feng et al., 1998; Cravchik & Gejman, 1999) and a $[CA]_n$ repeat Barr et al., 2000).

DAT1 (Dopamine Transporter)

The dopamine transporter (DAT) is a member of the family of Na^+- and Cl^- (ion)-dependent neurotransmitter transporters (Giros & Caron, 1993). The human DAT protein consists of 620 amino acids; the gene maps to chromosome 5q15.3 and contains 15 exons. The DAT is believed to control the temporal and spatial activity of released dopamine by rapid reupdate (delivery) of the neurotransmitter into presynaptic terminals. Correspondingly, DAT plays an important role in regulating the action of dopamine on locomotion, cognition, affect, and neuroendocrine functions.

Due to the obvious importance of this gene in the dopaminergic pathway, researchers have attempted to establish associations between DAT and various neuropsychiatric conditions (e.g., bipolar affective disorder, Waldman, Robinson, & Feigon, 1997; schizoid/avoidant behavior, Blum et al., 1997; cocaine-induced paranoia, Gelernter, Kranzler, Satel, & Rao, 1994; and alcohol, Sander et al., 1997; Schmidt, Harms, Kuhn, Rommelspacher, & Sander, 1998). As a polymorphic marker of DAT, all these studies have utilized a variable number tandem repeat (VNTR) polymorphism in the 3' untranslated region of the gene (Vandenbergh et al., 1992). This polymorphism has been used so widely because it is highly informative (consists of eight different alleles) and because no other polymorphism had been readily available. However, the outcomes of these various studies are variable. Specifically, a number of authors (Cook et al., 1995; Gill, Daly, Heron, Hawi, & Fitzgerald, 1997) have found an association between DAT and ADHD, whereas others failed to find evidence for this association (Daly et al., 1999). In an attempt to consolidate these variable results, researchers (Grünhage et al., 2000; Vandenbergh et al.,

2000) have examined the gene structure, looking for unknown gene variants of importance for neuropsychiatric conditions; if they exist, such variants might explain why some of the previous results have failed to show linkage/association with the DAT1 VNTR. The research has demonstrated that the DAT gene is highly conserved—only two variants resulted in amino acid changes and the cosegregation with neuropsychiatric conditions. These investigations raise the possibility that level-of-expression variation, rather than variation in protein sequences, may be at least partially responsible for variation observed at the behavioral level (Vandenbergh et al., 2000).

COMT (*Catechol-O-Methyl Transferase Gene*)

Catechol-O-methyl transferase (COMT) is one of the enzymes that is important to the initial steps of metabolic transformation of catecholamines (specifically, dopamine and serotonin). COMT activity has been previously analyzed as a marker locus for schizophrenia, as well as for other psychiatric conditions. However, the results have been equivocal (Dunner, Levitt, Kumbaraci, & Fieve, 1977; Karege, Bovier, & Tissot, 1987; Philippu et al., 1985; Puzynski, Binzinsky, Mrozek, & Zaluska, 1983). Recently, COMT has been mapped to 22q11 (Grossman, Emanual, & Budarf, 1992). The genomic organization of the gene has been extensively studied and is mostly known, with only a few gaps left (Tenhunen et al., 1994).

The activity of the enzyme is determined by amino acid change in the protein, occurring as a result of a single-base pair change in exon 4 (G → A transition at codon 158 of membrane bound COMT, which corresponds to codon 108 of cytoplasmic COMT) of the COMT gene (Val → Met amino acid change) that has the effect of changing the otherwise thermostable, high-activity enzyme into a thermolabile, low-activity enzyme reducing enzyme activity to about 20% (Lachman et al., 1996; Karayiorgou et al., 1999).

A number of studies have suggested that COMT is associated with impulsivity and disinhibition (Kotler et al., 1999; Lachman, Nolan, Mohr, Saito, & Volavka, 1998; Strous, Bark, Parsia, Volavka, & Lachman, 1997). Researchers have also investigated associations between COMT and ADHD, although the results of these investigations have been controversial (Eisenberg et al., 1999; Hawi, Millar, Daly, Fitzgerald, & Gill, 2000). In addition, the homozygosity for the low-activity allele has been discovered to be a risk factor for obsessive–compulsive disorder (Karayiorgou et al., 1999). There have also been some failed attempts to find associations between the COMT and personality traits that confer vulnerability to anxiety, depression, and alcohol misuse (Henderson et al., 2000).

MAO (*Monoamine Oxidase*)

Monoamine oxidase (MAO) catalyzes the oxidative deamination of a number of biogenic amines, including the key neurotransmitters serotonin (5-HT), norepinephrine (NE), and dopamine, and the neuromodulator, phenylethylamine (PEA). On the basis of biochemical properties and functions, and, subsequently, by mapping and cloning independent genes, two forms of MAO (MAO A and MAO B) have been distinguished. The two forms have a number of general properties; most notably, dopamine is a substrate for both MAO A and MAO B. As for specific features, MAO A exhibits a higher affinity for 5-HT and NE, as well as for the inhibitor clorgyline (Johnston, 1968), whereas MAO B has a higher affinity for PEA, benzylamine, and the inhibitor deprenyl (Knoll & Magyar, 1972). In addition, although most tissues express both isoenzymes, human placenta and fibroblasts express predominantly MAO A, and platelets and lymphocytes express only MAO B (e.g., Shih, Chen, & Ridd, 1999).

The property of the MAOs to catabolize neurotransmitters has put these enzymes on the list of top candidates in studies of neurological diseases and psychiatric and behavior traits. Specifically, the role of MAO B in psychiatric disorders has been widely studied by utilizing platelets, which are easily obtained from whole blood and which lack MAO A expression. Low MAO activity in platelets has been shown to be associated with bipolar disorder, suicidal behavior, and alcoholism (Devor, Cloninger, Hoffman, & Tabakoff, 1993), as well as with personality traits such as sensation seeking, monotony avoidance, and impulsiveness, and thereby with an increased risk for drug abuse and psychiatric vulnerability (Oreland, 1993; Holschneider & Shih, 1998). Some recent results, however, demonstrated that smoking inhibits both MAO A and MAO B activity, challenging previous findings and positing the importance of revisiting earlier conclusions controlling for the effect of smoking (Fowler, Volkow, Wang, Pappas, Logan, McGregor, et al., 1996; Fowler, Volkow, Wang, Pappas, Logan, Shea, et al., 1996; Simpson et al., 1999).

Bach et al. (1998) demonstrated that MAO A and B are distinct, but closely related, X-linked genes. The MAO A and MAO B genomic sequences (Grimsby, Chen, Wang, Lan, & Shih, 1991; Chen, Powell, Hsu, Breakefield, & Craig, 1992) and promoters (Zhu, Grimsby, Chen, & Shih, 1992; Zhu & Shih, 1997) have been studied to generate polymorphisms with the aim of conducting genetic association and linkage studies of psychiatric disorders, behaviors, and personality traits.

A convincing demonstration of the MAO's involvement in the regulation of human behaviors has been obtained by Brunner and colleagues (Brunner, Nelen, Breakefield, Ropers, & Van Oost, 1993; Brunner, Nelen, Van Zandvoort, et al., 1993). These researchers studied a Dutch family in which eight males demonstrated a complex set of behaviors, including mild mental retardation and impulsive aggression. In the affected males, the molecular-genetic investigation revealed a single nucleotide mutation in the MAO A gene; the specimen analyses showed the suppressed levels of degradation products of 5-HT, dopamine, and norepinephrine. More studies are needed to establish the frequency of this mutation in humans and to verify the link between the mutation and impulsive aggression.

The MAO activity in the platelets is, at least to 75%, genetically controlled. However, details about this genetic control of the enzyme are, thus far, sparsely known. The biological role of platelet MAO is still unclear. However, it is not the activity in itself that affects the behavior—it is, for example, possible specifically to inhibit MAO B (the form in the platelets) without provoking any change in personality. The genetic regulation of thrombocyte MAO probably also regulates some property of the brain.

Moreover, a considerable amount of published evidence indicates that low levels of MAO may be associated with novelty seeking, substance use disorders, impulsive aggression, and other forms of behavior observed in the general population (for a review, see Volavka, 1999).

DβH (Dopamine-β-Hydroxylase)

DβH catalyzes the conversion of dopamine to norepinephrine, is released from sympathetic neurons in response to stimulation, and can be measured in human plasma. DβH plasma (or serum) activity levels vary widely among individuals (Weinshilboum Raymond, Elveback, & Weidman, 1973) but are stable within individuals over time (Fahndrich, Muller-Oerlinghausen, & Coper, 1982). According to a number of family and twin studies, the major portion of variability in plasma DβH activity is controlled by genes (Weinshilboum et al., 1973). Of special interest are those individuals who have very low levels of plasma DβH activity. The reason for this interest is that altered plasma DβH activity has been reported in a variety of psychiatric and neurological disorders (e.g., Matuzas, Meltzer, Uhlenhuth, Glass, & Tong, 1982; Nagatsu et al., 1982). Researchers have reported an association between ADHD and DβH (Daly et al., 1999) and maternal levels of DβH and children's autism (Robinson, Schulz, Macciardi, White, & Holden, 2001). The results of research on levels of plasma DβH activity in conduct disorder patients as compared with control individuals have indicated lower levels of plasma DβH in conduct disorder patients (Bowden, Deutsch, & Swanson, 1988; Rogeness, Hernandez, Macedo, & Mitchell, 1981; Rogeness, Hernandez, Macedo, Amrung, & Hoppe, 1986). Interestingly, a number of researchers have registered lower levels of plasma DβH activity in children who have grown up in abusive families and in families of parents with substance abuse (Gabel, Stadler, Bjorn, Shindledecker, & Bowden, 1995; Galvin et al., 1995), suggesting that the DβH gene can have various patterns of expression in different environments.

The DβH gene (DBH) was cloned and mapped to chromosome 9q34. This gene is the major quantitative-trait loci for plasma DβH activity, and polymorphic variation at the DβH gene is closely related to plasma DβH phenotypes. The DβH gene contains 12 exons. There are a number of polymorphisms reported at the DβH gene (e.g., Cubells et al., 1997, 1998, 2000; D'Amato et al., 1989; Wei, Ramchand, & Hemming, 1997). Recently, Zabetian et al. (2001) have reported a novel polymorphism (−1021C→T), in the 5' flanking region of the DβH gene that accounts for 35–52% of the variation in plasma DβH activity.

The Serotonergic System

Among the neurotransmitters, serotonin is undoubtedly the biogenic amine that gave rise to the greatest effort in understanding the genetic-based etiology of psychiatric disorders, human behaviors, and cognitive processes in the general population.

Serotonin, or 5-hydroxytryptamine (5-HT), is often referred to as the most pharmacologically versatile of all neurotransmitters, which, among other functions, induces activation and/or inhibition of smooth and cardiac muscle, exocrine and endocrine glands, central and peripheral neurons, and cells of the haematopoietic and immune systems. The basis of this versatility is the existence of multiple receptor sites. Moreover, serotonergic signaling appears to play a key role in the generation and modulation of a broad array of behaviors, including sleep, locomotion, feeding, vomiting, addiction, aggression, sexual activity, and affect (Wilkinson & Dourish, 1991). Serotonin has been implicated in a wide range of psychiatric conditions, including depression, anxiety disorders, obsessive–compulsive disorders, and substance abuse and dependence (for a review, see Lucki, 1998; Veenstra-VanderWeele, Anderson, & Cook, 2000).

Tryptophan Hydroxylase Gene (TPH)

The human tryptophan hydroxylase gene (TPH) is located on chromosome 11p14-15.3 and encodes the enzyme that catalyzes the rate-limiting step in the synthesis of 5-HT from tryptophan. Correspondingly, it is plausible that TPH variants can contribute to genetic variability of the serotonergic system in its relation to specific phenotypic variation. Researchers have detected a number of polymorphisms in the TPH gene, but no functional meaning has been assigned to these polymorphisms (Nielsen, Jenkins, Stefanisko, Jefferson, & Goldman, 1997). A few studies have established the connection between *TPH* polymorphisms and suicidality and antisocial alcoholism (Ishiguro, Saito, Shibuya, Toru, & Arinami, 1999; Mann et al., 1997; Nielsen et al., 1997; Rotondo et al., 1999; Tsai, Hong, & Wang, 1999).

5-HT Receptors

Among serotonin receptors, a few are of particular interest to studies of the genetic etiology of personality (see Table 2.2). Serotonergic pathways and receptors are essential components of higher mental functioning (Buhot, 1997; Meneses, 1999), although the specifics of the receptors' roles have not yet been established. However, available evidence, obtained by means of animal studies and analyses of the pharmacology of human disorders, strongly indicates that presynaptic 5-HT_{1A}, 5-HT_{1B}, $5\text{-HT}_{2A/2C}$, and 5-HT_3 receptors and postsynaptic $5\text{-HT}_{2A/2C}$ and 5-HT_4 receptors are involved in complex aspects of behavior and learning. An overview of the available literature suggests that the serotonergic system is a complex one, intimately connected with other neutransmitter systems, both in terms of the physical distribution of the receptors in the brain and in terms of overlapping functional tasks.

The genetic variability in 5-HT has been associated with or linked to hypertension, anxiety, depression, eating behaviors, sexual activity, and aggression. However, the majority of these links have been established on animal models. There have been relatively few studies investigating the role of genetic variability in 5-HT receptors for human behavior.

Specifically, genetic variants of 5-HT_{2A} have been studied in relation to schizophrenia, but the findings are inconsistent, with evidence both for (Spurlock et al., 1998) and against (Hawi et al., 1997) the presence of relationships. Similarly, there have been contradictory results with regard to the association between 5-HT_{2A} variants and alcoholism— Nakamura et al. (1999) found a significant association between alcoholism in a subset of patients with a genetic variant of the *HTR2A*, but Schuckit et al. (1999) were unable to confirm this association.

A number of various polymorphisms have been described in the *HTR2C* gene (Veenstra-VanderWeele et al., 2000). There have been a number of studies investigating the connections of these polymorphisms and alcoholism, but no associations have been reported (Himei et al., 2000; Lappalainen et al., 1999).

Finally, a number of researchers have investigated the role of *HTR1B* in various psychiatric and alcoholism phenotypes. Based on these studies, there is some evidence of the involvement of this gene in the etiology

TABLE 2.2. Serotonergic System

5-HT marker/receptor	Symbol	Location	Brain area in which 5-HT receptors and messenger RNA have been identified
5-HT$_{1A}$	HTR1A	5q11.2-13	Hippocampus, lateral septum, Raphé nucleus, amygdala
5-HT$_{1B}$	HTR1B	6q14.1	Globus pallidus, substantial nigra, olivary pretectal nucleus, dorsal subiculum, superior colliculi
5-HT$_{1D}$	HTR1D	1q36.12	Globus pallidus, substantial nigra, caudate-putamen, nucleus accumbens, frontal cortex
5-HT$_{1E}$	HTR1E	6q14-15	
5-HT$_{1F}$	HTR1F	3p12	
5-HT$_{2A}$	HTR2A	13q14.2	Claustrum, olfactory tuberle, frontal cortex, neocortex, Raphé nucleus
5-HT$_{2B}$	HT2B	2q37.1	Cortex, amygdala, caudate, hypothalamus
5-HT$_{2C}$	HTR2C	Xq23	Chorois plexus, substantial nigra, globus pallidus, neocortex, hippocampus
5-HT$_{3A/3B}$	HTR3A	11q23.2	
5-HT$_4$	HTR4	5q32	Hippocampus, caudate, amygdala, colliculi
5-HT$_5$	HTR5	7q34-36	Amygdala, hippocampus
5-HT$_6$	HTR6	1p36.13	Piriform and prefrontal cortex, striatum, hippocampus, amygdala
5-HT$_{7A}$	HTR7A	10q23.3-24.3	Hippocampus, amygdala, cortex, Raphé nucleus

of obsessive–compulsive disorder (Mundo, Richter, Sam, Macciardi, & Kennedy, 2000) and antisocial alcoholism (Lappalainen et al., 1998).

5-HT Transporter

Serotonin transporter (5-HTT) is involved in the presynaptic reuptake of serotonin to terminate and modulate serotonergic neurotransmission. A dysfunction of 5-HTT has been implicated in the etiology of psychiatric disorders such as mood, anxiety, obsessive–compulsive, and substance-abuse disorders. The human 5-HTT gene (SLC6A4) has been cloned and mapped on chromosome 17q11.1-12.

Heils et al. (1996) first identified an allele of 5-HTT with an insertion in the promoter region. The polymorphism (5-HTTLPR) consists of the repetitive sequence containing GC-rich repeat elements in the upstream regulatory region of the gene. The presence or absence of this insertion creates a short allele and a long allele. Studies of transfected cells in culture have shown differential transcriptional properties of the long and short variants (Lesch et al., 1996). Specifically, the basal transcriptional activity of the long variant is more than twice that of the short variant, which results in the short variant producing mRNA with substantially lower concentration of 5-HTT. These differences in 5-HTT mRNA synthesis lead to differences in 5-HTT expression and 5-HT cellular uptake (Lesch et al., 1996). Later researchers (Nakamura, Ueno, Sano, & Tanabe, 2000) have described 10 novel allele variants in the 5-HTTLPR polymorphism.

The 5-HTTLPR polymorphism has been studied in various psychiatric disorders, such as mood disorder (Kunugi et al., 1997), schizophrenia (Malhotra et al., 1998), panic disorder (Matsushita et al., 1997), autistic disorder (Cook et al., 1997; Klauck, Poustka, Benner, Lesch, & Poustka, 1997; Maestrini et al., 1999; Persico et al., 2000; Tordjman et al., 2001), and personality traits (Flory et al., 1999; Lesch et al., 1996). The findings have been controversial, with associations appearing and disappearing in various samples.

Of special interest is the research on the relation between the promoter polymorphism and neuroticism. The initial report associated the short allele and neuroticism in a case-controlled investigation and offered support to this finding by means of sib-pair analyses (Lesch et al., 1996). This report has been followed by a mixture of support and nonsupport (e.g., Hu et al., 2000; Mazzanti et al., 1998; Osher, Hamer, & Benjamin, 2000). An insight into this "collage" of replications and failures to replicate has been offered by the study of Gelernter, Cubells, Kidd, Pakstis, and Kidd (1999), which clearly demonstrated the need to take into account a complex pattern of frequencies of the short and long variants around the world. Specifically, this study has indicated dramatic differences in allele frequencies between two European populations, the Danes and the Adygei. This finding stresses the importance of taking into account the ethnic background of individuals involved in association studies due to the potential bias that can be introduced by the mere fact of variable genetic population background in frequencies of genetic variants of interest.

The second polymorphism has been described within intron 2 of *HTT*. This polymorphism consists of 9, 10, or 12 copies of a 16–17 repeat element and has been shown to have a potential transcription enhancer effect (Fiskerstrand, Lovejoy, & Quinee, 1999). This polymorphism has been studied in relation to bipolar disorder and schizophrenia, but the results have been contradictory (Esterling et al., 1998; Hranilovic et al., 2000).

Transcription Factor AP-2

The transcription factor AP-2 is one of the critical factors for neural gene expression and neural development. There are multiple isoforms of AP-2, of which two are the most abundant—α and β. However, the expression of AP-2β is higher than that of AP-2α. AP-2β is involved in the development of midbrain structures in the central nervous system (CNS; Mitchell, Timmons, Herbert, Rigby, & Tjian, 1991; Moser, Rüschoff, & Buettner, 1997). Because the Raphé serotonin nuclei are located within this area, Damberg et al. (2000) have speculated that this transcription factor might be involved in the development of personality and vulnerability for psychiatric disorders. Further support for the notion that this factor is of great biological importance is given by the fact that the levels of AP-2β in the brain stem of rats strongly correlates with levels of 5-HT in the frontal cortex and to a variety of behaviors of the animals. The question of importance is whether AP-2β is involved in the regulation of platelet MAO activity.

The AP-2β gene is located on chromosome 6p12-21.1 and includes a polymorphism region consisting of a variable number of [CAAA] repeats located in the second intron. The function of this polymorphism is unknown. Damberg et al. (2000) have linked the long-allele ([CAAA]$_5$) genotype of AP-2β to anxiety-related personality traits, indirect aggression, guilt, and binge-eating disorder. Moreover, homozygotes for the long allele have been found to have significantly lower levels of MAOB activity (Damberg et al., 2000).

The GABAergic System (γ-Aminobyturic Acid)

One of the major concepts in developmental science is that of "critical period"—a period in which sensory-driven activity patterns are able to induce long-lasting plasticity in specific neural circuits, thus causing functional changes that last throughout adulthood (Feldman, 2000). Although a holistic scientific picture of the emergence of critical periods is far from completion, major advancements in understanding critical periods have been made through methods of neuroscience and genetics (e.g., Fagiolini & Hensch, 2000). One of many remarkable discoveries in this area has been the work on the role of the process of inhibition in the critical period of plasticity. Based on a string of in vitro experiments, a developmental increase in inhibition has been proposed to function as a plasticity gate that suppresses long-term potentiation and closes the critical period (e.g., Feldman, Nicoll, Malenka, & Isaac, 1998). In contrast, a string of in vivo experiments has offered evidence in favor of the hypothesis that inhibition may actually promote, not restrict, plasticity during the critical period (Hensch et al., 1998). According to this hypothesis, the critical period onset is determined by maturation of the cortical circuit itself demonstrated by the very factor of increased inhibition. γ-aminobutyric acid (GABA) is the major neurotransmitter in the central nervous system of mammalian species that is, arguably, the conductor of the complex process of inhibition in the human brain.

GABA Receptors

At least three different receptor subtypes, the ionotropic $GABA_A$ and $GABA_C$ receptors and the metabotropic $GABA_B$ receptors, mediate inhibitory activations of GABA. These three types of GABA receptors can be distinguished pharmacologically by their selective responses to various receptor agonists and antagonists (Bormann, 2000). $GABA_A$ receptors are antagonized by the convulsant alkaloid bicuculline and are insensitive to the GABA analogue baclofen. $GABA_B$ receptors are insensitive to bicuculline and are activated stereo-selectively by baclofen. $GABA_C$ receptors are insensitive to both baclofen and bicuculline, but are responsive to cis-4-aminocrotonic acid, a structural analogue of GABA. However, some researchers (e.g., Barnard et al., 1998) argue that the $GABA_C$ receptors should be classified as a subset of $GABA_A$ receptors due to their ionotropic nature and phylogenetic proximity to $GABA_A$ receptors.

The GABA system constitutes the fundamental inhibitory system of the human brain. It has been shown (e.g., Redecker, Luhmann, Hagemann, Fritschy, & Witte, 2000) that experimentally induced cortical malformations result in a widespread dysregulation in the distribution of $GABA_A$ receptor subunits (i.e., a regionally differential reduction of $GABA_A$ receptor subunits in the damaged, as well as neighboring, areas), which, in turn, fundamentally challenges the patterns of signal transmission in the brain.

The $GABA_A$ receptor is a pentamer, assembled from a diversity of subunits, which gates a chloride conductance (e.g., Mehta & Ticku, 1999). So far, at least 20 different subunit subtypes of the pentameric $GABA_A$

receptors have been sequenced from the mammalian nervous system, comprising six α, four β, three γ, one δ, one ϵ, one θ, one π, and three ρ subunits, each with multiple isoforms, designated by numbers (Barnard et al., 1998; Bonnert et al., 1999). The majority of $GABA_A$ receptors contain variable combinations of α, β, and γ subunits, showing a specific regional and cellular distribution (Fritschy & Mohler, 1995). Generally, however, pentameric CNS $GABA_A$ receptors are combinations of at least one α and one β, with one or more γ, δ, or ϵ subunit (Sieghart, 1995). In turn, the subunit composition of a receptor determines its electrophysiological and pharmacological properties (Barnard et al., 1998; Narahashi, 1999). There is evidence obtained from comparative studies that $GABA_A$ receptor ϵ and θ subunits are evolving at a much faster rate than other known $GABA_A$ receptor subunits and that their expression patterns and functional properties may differ significantly between species (Sinkkonen, Hanna, Kirkness, & Korpi, 2000). The biological function that is acquired by each new gene family member appears to impose unique structural constraints. Correspondingly, the structural requirements for function of ϵ and θ subunits are more flexible than for other known $GABA_A$ receptor subunits. Consequently, they have evolved under less constraint and can tolerate more mutations. $GABA_A$ receptors share their fundamental structure and functional properties with an evolutionarily related superfamily of ligand-gated ion channels that also includes nicotine acetylcholine, 5-HT3, glycine, and $GABA_C$ (Ortells & Lunt, 1995). $GABA_A$ mRNA has been detected in the neocortex, amygdala, hippocampus, prefrontal cortex, thalamus, and dorsal/ventral lateral geniculate nucleus. Activation of the $GABA_A$ by GABA increases membrane conductance for anions, especially for chloride ions, usually resulting in hyperpolarization. It has been well established that the $GABA_A$/benzodiazepine ionophore receptor complex plays a major role in the pharmacology of several anziolytic and hypnotic drugs, as well as in the pathophysiology of stress, anxiety, and epilepsy (Mehta & Ticku, 1999; Ticku, 1991). Moreover, $GABA_A$ receptor-mediated neurotransmission has been implicated in the aggression-heightening effects of alcohol (Miczek, DeBold, van Erp, & Tornatzky, 1997). The cerebral cortical mantle, which includes the hippocampus and the neocortex, is an intricate network of neurons communicating via chemical and electrical synapses and using glutamate and GABA as the major neurotransmitters. Specifically, excitation is mediated mostly by glutamate[4] receptors of the NMDA[5] (ionotropic) or AMPA[6] subtypes, whereas GABA, acting via fast ($GABA_A$) and slow ($GABA_B$) receptors, is strongly inhibitory, as it profoundly decreases the excitability of individual neurons and suppresses the propensity of the network to generate synchronous discharges (Connors, Malenka, & Silva, 1988; Wells, Porter,

& Agmon, 2000). In other words, in both adult and neonate brains, $GABA_A$ receptors play the role of preventing runaway excitation leading to synchronous discharges. Blocking $GABA_A$ receptors unfailingly results in epileptiform events that consist of valleys of giant synaptic potentials and synchronous discharges of large populations of neurons. Thus researchers have realized the importance of GABAergic mechanisms for the limitation of excessive neuronal activity (Gloor, 1992).

$GABA_B$ receptors are relatively slow in their action and differ fundamentally from that of $GABA_A$ receptors. $GABA_B$ receptors are located in pre- and/or postsynaptic membranes and couple, respectively, to various Ca and K channels, presumably through both a membrane-delimited pathway and a pathway involving second messengers (Crunelli & Leresche, 1991; Misgeld, Bijak, & Jarolimek, 1995). The $GABA_B$ receptor gene has been cloned only recently (Kaupmann et al., 1997). Later, the structure of this gene was described (Goei et al., 1998). $GABA_B$ mRNA have been identified in the neocortex, amygdala, hippocampus, and dorsal/ventral lateral geniculate nucleus. Blocking $GABA_A$ receptors in the neocortex transforms cortical slow-wave oscillations into large-amplitude discharges consisting of a negative spike or multiple negative spikes riding on a positive wave. Further blocking of $GABA_B$ receptors in the neocortex slows the discharges and increments the number of negative spikes that form rhythmic neocortical oscillation (Castro-Alamancos, 2000).

There is some evidence that $GABA_C$ activation leads to an indirect, interneuron-mediated disinhibition (M. Schmidt, Boller, Özen, & Hall, 2001). $GABA_C$ mRNA have been registered in the retina, superior colliculus, dorsal/lateral geniculate nucleus, cerebellar Purkinje cells, and the stratum griseum superficiale. As of now, $GABA_C$ is the least studied GABA receptor.

The synaptic action of GABA is terminated by its high affinity reuptake transporters (GAT1, GAT2, GAT3, and GAT4).

A number of GABA receptors have been mapped in the human genome. Specifically, $GABA_A$ receptors are organized in a number of clusters—clusters on chromosomes 4, 5, 15, and X. Only one $GABA_B$ has been mapped so far (to short arm of chromosome 6).

Chromosome 4 $GABA_A$ Cluster (4p14)

This cluster contains β_1 subunit gene (*GABRB1*), α_2 and α_4 subunit genes (*GABRA2* and *GABRA4*, respectively), and γ_1 subunit gene (*GABG1*). There have been relatively few studies of the $GABA_A$ cluster on chromosome 4 with regard to human traits. Specifically, there have been some attempts to link genetic variability in *GABRA2* and *GABRA4* to panic disorder, but the researchers failed to establish linkage between these genes and panic disorder (Crowe et al., 1997).

Chromosome 5 GABA_A Cluster (5q31)

This cluster, located at 5q33, harbors the genes encoding the α_1, α_6, β_2, and γ_2 subunits of the GABA$_A$ (*GABR*). There are a number of genetic polymorphisms known for this GABA$_A$ cluster (Loh & Ball, 2000). Specifically, (1) GABA$_A$ subunit β_2 contains an *exonic* nucleotide substitution polymorphism; (2) subunit α_6 is characterized by two single-nucleotide polymorphisms, an *exonic* and a 3'-end of the gene polymorphisms; (3) subunit α_1 contains an *intronic* nucleotide substitution and a CA-repeat marker; (4) subunit γ_2 is characterized by a CA-repeat and two *intronic* single nucleotide polymorphisms (downstream and upstream of the 24bp exon).

A role for the GABA receptors in ethanol action has been suggested by animal studies that have demonstrated the development of cross-tolerance between alcohol and modulators of the GABA$_A$ receptor benzodiazepines and barbiturates (e.g., Khana, Le, Kalant, Chau, & Shah, 1997). In addition, benzodiazepines are used medically to treat alcohol withdrawal syndrome (for a review, see Holbrook, Growther, Lotter, Cheng, & King, 1999). Consequently, there have been a number of studies of the role of the selected GABA$_A$ receptor subunits in the development of alcohol dependence in humans (for a review, see Loh & Ball, 2000).

Several association studies of the GABA$_A$ receptor genes on 5q33-34 and alcohol dependence/alcohol-related physiological phenotypes have been conducted in different ethnic populations (for a review, see Loh & Ball, 2000), resulting in a set of findings that vary by gene, by the ethnic population examined, and by the specificity of the studied phenotype. For example, Loh et al. (1999) and Loh, Higuchi, et al. (2000) have described the presence of allelic association between *GABRB2* polymorphism and *GABRA6* polymorphism and alcohol dependence and Korsakoff's psychosis in a Scottish population. Sander et al. (1999) have found a significant allelic association of the investigated *GABRA6* polymorphism with dissocial alcoholism but no other subtype of alcoholism. Specifically, individuals carrying the common T-allele showed a sevenfold higher risk for alcohol dependence in the presence of a dissocial personality disorder than individuals lacking it. Correspondingly, it might be the case that the *GABRA6* polymorphism is associated with antisocial behavior rather than alcoholism. Similarly, there is some evidence supporting an association between the *GABRG2* polymorphism alcohol dependence and comorbid antisocial personality disorder (Loh et al., 2000), as well as linkage between the *GABRG2* polymorphism and alcohol dependence and criminal records (Radel, Vallejo, Long, & Goldman, 1999). However, Hsu et al. (1998) demonstrated no association between the marker in *GABRG2* and alcohol dependence. Parsian and Cloninger (1997) reported no association between alcohol dependence and the CA-repeat marker at the *GABRA1* but a suggestive association with *GABRA3*.

There also have been a number of studies of genetic variability in GABA$_A$ with regard to anxiety-related traits and conditions. However, the results of these searches have been contradictory.

Chromosome 15 GABA$_A$ Cluster (15q11)

This cluster of GABA genes contains genes for α_5, β_3, and γ_3 subunits (GABRA5, GABRB3, and GABRG3, respectively). Genes in this cluster have been reported to be rich in highly polymorphic $[CA]_n$ repeats (Glatt, Sinnett, & Lalande, 1994). The presence of genetic polymorphisms triggered a number of searches for links between genetic variation at this GABA cluster and behavioral/personality traits. There have been reports that associate polymorphisms in these genes with autism disorder (Cook et al., 1998; Martin et al., 1999), as well as reports that fail to replicate the association (e.g., Bass et al., 2000). Similarly, the results are contradictory for bipolar disorder, with evidence available for (Papadimitriou et al., 1998) and against (Duffy et al., 2000) links with this GABA cluster.

X Chromosome GABA$_A$ Cluster (Xq28)

This cluster includes three genes—genes for α_3, β_4, and ε_1. Similar to research with other *GABA$_A$* genes, researchers have investigated links between affective disorders and traits and variability in these genes. Similar to the situation with other *GABA$_A$* genes, the findings are contradictory: Some researchers have claimed the presence of connections (Debruyn, Raeymaekers, et al., 1994), whereas others have refuted them (e.g., Puertollano, Visedo, Saiz-Ruiz, Llinares, & Fernandez-Piqueras, 1995).

GABA$_B$

A number of mutations, functional and nonfunctional, have been reported in this gene (Hisama et al., 2001; Sander et al., 1999). However, none of these mutations have been linked to specific behavioral phenotypes.

Personality and Neurotransmitters: General Comments

The apparent confusing and inconsistent nature of the data presented in this section of the chapter seems discouraging. A few comments may be in order before the discussion proceeds.

First, review the publication dates for the majority of the reports discussed in the previous section. Virtually all work on the molecular basis of human behavior and personality has been completed since 1995, in a relatively short period of time. Thus the first and most obvious comment is that these studies represent only initial attempts at what we hope will turn out to be a rewarding enterprise. The future of this enterprise depends on a number of crucial factors. The first factor is our knowledge of the role and function of polymorphisms in coding and regulatory "zones" of genes and their impact on gene expression. Thus these polymorphisms should be identified, their physiology should be described, and the relationships between these polymorphisms and various human behaviors and traits should be investigated. The second factor is related to our ability to define variability in a behavior trait we are trying to link to variability on a genetic level. Specifically, what do we view as a dependent variable? Do we try to assess a spectrum of behaviors and come up with some "averaged" variable, which then will be associated with a polymorphic marker? Or do we try to preserve the variability of our observations and find associations between multivariate manifestations of human behavior across different situations (or in response to different stimuli)? The third factor here has to do with our increasing understanding of the importance of the developmental fluctuations both in psychological traits and gene expression. The more we know, the more obvious it becomes that human development at its multiple levels (from biochemical to spiritual) is more about transformation than stability. This brings up another question—how fair is our hope to discover stable consistent links between genes and human traits? All of this is just to make the point that the 6-year span of research into the molecular basis of personality is obviously not enough time to address these questions. In short, the field has just started working on them.

Second, what is obvious from the findings presented herein, is the need for a close collaboration between researchers who understand the biology of the genetic polymorphisms in the systems of neurotransmitters and researchers who understand the behavior that might be associated with these polymorphisms. No answers will come around from either of the sides. The answers are to be found at the intersection of theories, methods, and data.

With this said, the following section concludes the chapter by bringing into the discussion issues that *must* be dealt with to ensure the transition of the promising direction of molecular research on personality into a fruitful subfield of personality research.

GENES AND PERSONALITY: ANTICIPATING TOMORROW

Having provided a brief summary of the limits of our current understanding of the genetic basis of personality, I now comment on a number of issues crucial to guaranteeing progress in the future.

Why Neurotransmitters?

The majority of this chapter is devoted to the discussion of the research on the relationships between the genetic variability in selected systems of neurotransmitters and phenotypic variation in personality. This choice was driven by two considerations. The first has to do with the fact that the mere realization that genes matter is not enough—we need to understand to what extent and how. The systems of neurotransmitters appear to be good candidates for serving as the basis of personality-related genetic variation for the following reasons.

First, it has long been known from animal work that normal behavior is dependent on the normal functioning of systems of neurotransmitters. Within limits, a homeostasis prevails whereby hyperstimulation leads to downregulation and hypostimulation to upregulation of neurotransmitter systems. When such thresholds are violated, abnormal behaviors are observed. There are four major lines of research that have contributed to this summary. The first line assumes research involving selective breeding. It has been shown that rodent families can be selectively bred for differing neurotransmitter receptor populations and that behaviors of animals in different strains vary significantly in correlation with the receptor density characteristic of the inbred strain (e.g., Overstreet, Russell, Crocker, & Schiller, 1984). The second line of research assumes experimental manipulating of a receptor population by the administration of an irreversible agonist (compounds that are capable of directly activating the target receptor) or antagonist (compounds that prevent the transmitter's action, either directly, by competition with the transmitter for its receptor, or indirectly, by modification of the receptor and the receptor's environment) and by observing the recovery of an organism at different levels (physiological, sensory-perceptual, motoric, and cognitive) after such manipulation (e.g., Russell et al., 1989). The third line of research is engaged in studying the brains of aging animals. The assumption here is that, as aging processes progress, changes occur both functionally and structurally in neurotransmitter systems, and these effects can be understood through experimental work, both developmental and cross-sectional, with aging animals (e.g., Roth & Hess, 1982). The fourth line of research capitalizes on comparative approaches, mapping neurotransmitter networks to various brain regions and investigating both the location and density maps of various receptor maps (e.g., Russell, 1992).

Second, neurotransmitter systems appear to be perfect candidates because of their openness to the impact of the environment. Specifically, it has been shown by pharmacogenetics in both humans and animals that a very small change in a transmitter-receptor interaction may lead to substantial behavioral changes. One series of research studies has to do with manipulating the diet of rodents by substituting elements that are necessary for the synthesis of neurotransmitters with other elements (e.g., Russell et al., 1990). However, most of this research is carried out in the framework of experimental pharmacology, in which various substances are experimentally administered to animals or humans and their behavioral reactions registered after substance administration (e.g., Meller et al., 1986).

The "popularity" of neurotransmitter systems as possible candidates for the genetic substrate for personality does not, however, exclude a possibility that other genetic systems may be important as well. To my knowledge, the only genetic-research methodology utilized in the context of the search for the links between genetic variability and behavioral variability in "normal" personality was that of association studies—that is, studies assuming the presence of a candidate system rather than unfolding a systematic search for nonspecific (noncandidate) linkages between a trait of interest and a location in the genome. Both other genetic systems (e.g., systems of genes involved in hormonal regulation) and other genetic methodologies (e.g., systematic searches for nonspecific hot spots in the genome) might enhance our understanding of the genetic basis of personality. However, each of these strategies assumes the presence of knowledge, research rigor, and financial support that the field might not always (just yet) have.

GENETIC INTERACTIONS

The issue just discussed (why neurotransmitters?) brings up another point. So far, the overwhelming majority of the research has been conducted under the assumption that it is possible to find a strong relationship between a single deficiency (e.g., a specific functional mutation in a given region of a gene) and a complex behavior trait (e.g., novelty seeking). Yet one of the obvious observations that can be derived from the preceding discussion is that, although each gene in a neurotransmitter system plays its own role, each system works as a whole. Moreover, it is plausible to assume that various neurotransmitter systems interact with each other. Next I review a number of findings that allow us to assert that neurotransmitter systems work in close collaboration with each other, with the profile of a given system emerging as a function of the context of the other system with which the first system interacts.

I illustrate this point using the function of the GABA system as an example. GABA receptors show highly interactive properties, preserving the uniqueness of their operational mechanism and suggesting the high selectivity of GABA receptors.

GABA and Serotonin

There is evidence in the literature (Gervasoni et al., 2000) that suggests that an increase of GABAergic inhibitory tone present during wakefulness is likely responsible for the decrease in activity of the dorsal Raphé serotonergic cells during slow wave and paradoxical sleep. Researchers (Sibille, Pavlides, Benke, & Toth, 2000) have also shown that inactivation of the 5-HT$_{1A}$ receptor in mice results in alterations in the expression of GABA$_A$ receptor α subunits in amygdala, cerebral cortex, and hippocampus. The proposed mechanism is the following: Glutamatergic afferents impinge on projection neurons in the amygdala, and activation from these afferents is inhibited by GABA interneurons; 5-HT exerts an additional inhibitory input on projection neurons by directly activating the 5-HT$_{1A}$ receptor so that the lack of 5-HT$_{1A}$ receptors in these cells in the amygdala eliminates an important 5-HT input, which is otherwise necessary to maintain a proper expression of the GABA$_A$ receptor α subunits. In addition, 5-HT$_{1A}$ and GABA$_A$ receptors form a dual inhibitory mechanism that controls the activity of pyramidal cell axons in the human cortex (DeFelipe, Arellano, Gómez, Azmitia, & Muñoz, 2001).

GABA and Dopamine

There are multiple links between the dopaminergic system and the GABA by which dopamine might regulate GABA efflux by a variety of different means, orchestrating a pattern of activation and inhibition among neurons (e.g., striatal neurons; Schoffelmeer et al., 2000). Specifically, the dopamine pathway interacts with GABA and the GABA$_A$ receptor unit (Perez de la Mora, Ferre, & Fuxe, 1997). For example, an association study of alcohol dependence (Noble et al., 1998) has demonstrated that the risk of alcohol dependence was more robust when the genetic variants at the GABA$_A$β$_3$ receptor subunit gene on human chromosome 15 were combined with those at the DRD2 receptor gene.

GABA and Other Neurotransmitters

GABA has been shown to interact with the glutamate receptor (Kehoe & Vulfius, 2000; Oyama, Ikemoto, Kits, & Akaike, 1990), by which the activation mechanism is linked to the levels of GABA concentration. Researchers (Zilles, Wu, Crucio, & Schwegler, 2000) have investigated correlations between the densities of glutamate (excitatory receptor) and GABA$_A$ binding sites in the hippocampus of seven inbred mouse strains and strain-specific spatial learning capacities. Although significant correlations were found between the densities of glutamate binding sites and spatial learning indicators, the strongest receptor-behavioral correlations were obtained between the densities of $GABA_A$. This pattern of correlation suggests that there is a balance between the excitatory transmitter glutamate and the inhibitory transmitter GABA and that both systems are important for explaining the variation in spatial learning capacities between the inbred mice.

The medial septum/diagonal band of Broca (MSDB) sends cholinergic and GABAergic projections to the hippocampus. It has been shown that the cholinergic tone in the MSDB, which is critical to learning and memory in vivo, is, at least in part, GABA-dependent (Wu, Shanabrough, Leranth, & Alreja, 2000). Specifically, Alreja and colleagues (2000) have shown that, first, the muscarine tone in the MSDB is caused by a tonic release of the neurotransmitter acetylcholine that occurs from within the MSDB, presumably via axon collaterals of spontaneously firing septohippocampal cholinergic neurons. Second, the locally released acetylcholine in the MSDB provides a profound excitatory drive to the septohippocampal GABA neurons but has little or an opposing effect on the septohippocampal cholinergic neurons. Thus the memory-impairing effects of muscarine receptor antagonists can be attributed to the decrease in the septohippocampal GABA release. A muscarinic receptor antagonist-induced decrease in septohippocampal GABA release could, theoretically, disinhibit large numbers of hippocampal GABAergic neurons and increase both the feedback and feed-forward type of local hippocampal inhibition of pyramidal cells (Freund & Antal, 1988; Toth, Freund, & Miles, 1997) due to the fact that septohippocampal GABA neurons selectively innervate only the GABA interneurons in the hippocampus (Miettinen & Freund, 1992). In a long-term potentiation (LTP)-based model of learning and memory, such an effect would translate into a decreased likelihood for the induction of LTP, because LTP is preferentially induced when the pyramidal cells are maximally stimulated (Pavlides, Greenstein, Grudman, & Winson, 1988). In other words, the septohippocampal GABA in combination with the cholinergic pathway, rather than just the cholinergic pathway, as was assumed before, appears to be a key player in mediating the mnemonic effects.

Although these examples are intended to be only illustrations of possibilities, they do support the assertion that, most likely, the genetic variability related to variability in personality will be generated by both additive and nonadditive (interactive) factors descriptive of the diversity at the genetic level. This assertion brings us back to where we started— whatever genetic factors underlie personality, they are complex, they exhibit system interactions, and they are open to environmental impact (namely, this openness ensures the plasticity of personality!).

PERSONALITY: MULTIPLE LAYERS OF CONTEXT

To understand "behavioral signatures" (Shoda, 1999) of personality and the etiology of personality consistency and variability, we have to understand "behavioral imprints" of personality and the etiology of imprinting-imposed constraints. A helpful analogy here is that of main effects and interactions—to understand a variety of possible interactions, it is helpful to describe main effects that can form interactions.

Similar to constraint-imposing influences on personality carried out by cultures in which these personalities socialize (Kitayama & Markus, 1999), individual genotypes imprint genetic profiles of populations from which these genotypes originate (Cavalli-Sforza, 1998). Consider the following illustration.[7]

Two articles were published in the January 1999 issue of *Health Psychology* that purported to show that the dopamine transporter locus (*SLC6A3*) was associated with aspects of smoking (Lerman et al., 1999; Sabol et al., 1999). This conclusion should be challenged for a variety of reasons.

The first reason is related to the inadequate consideration of ethnic variation in the underlying frequencies of the alleles at the specific polymorphism (the 3' VNTR) at the dopamine transporter locus. Specifically, Lerman et al. (1999) indicted that their Caucasian sample consisted of 53.4% smokers and had an overall frequency of the 9-repeat allele of the *SLC6A3* 3' VNTR of 0.322; there was no significant association in that sample ($p = .08$). Their African American sample consisted of 66.7% smokers and had an overall frequency of the 9-repeat allele of 0.176; there was no significant association in that sample either ($p = .73$). The association became significant ($p = .04$) only when the two samples were combined, creating an illustration of a false positive generated by analyzing combined heterogeneous samples as though they were a single homogeneous sample. The roughly twofold difference in the allele frequency of the 9-repeat allele is almost certainly a correct reflection of the different ancestries of the two samples, based on the global sample of this polymorphism in 30 distinct ethnic groups done by Kang, Palmatier, and Kidd (1999); they found the frequencies of the 9-repeat allele to be only 13% in the West African Yoruba but 31% in the mixed European sample.

The result claimed in the Lerman et al. (1999) study is that "current smokers" (CS) have a lower frequency of 9-repeat-containing genotypes than individuals classified as "never smoked" (NS). As discussed previously, the very validity of this finding should be challenged. However, the claim was made that the copublished study by Sabol et al. (1999) had replicated that finding. Apparently, this statement is questionable as well. The Lerman et al. (1999) data for Caucasians are as follows: NS, A9/–

("–" stands for the absence of A9 allele), 130 (56%); NS, -/-, 103 (44%); CS, A9/-, 135 (47%); CS, -/-, 154 (53%). Sabol et al. (1999) present the following data for the same four groups: 258 (43%), 335 (56%), 119 (42%), 164 (58%). These numbers give a chi-square of 0.17 ($p = .68$), which, by all conventional assumption, should be considered as a nonsignificant finding. Thus, applying the same criteria that Lerman et al. (1999) applied in their study, this result should be classified as a failure to replicate, not as a replication. What is referred to as a replication result in the Sabol et al. (1999) study is significant only when former smokers (FS) were considered. Thus, somewhere along the line the hypothesis developed by Lerman et al. has been replaced by a different hypothesis. This new hypothesis, one of many that could have been and probably were tested, should be considered only with a significance level adjusted for multiple tests. However, such an adjustment makes the presented result not significant statistically.

Finally, another interesting detail about the two studies relates to the differences of frequencies of the 9-repeat allele in the different groups across the two samples. In the Sabol et al. (1999) study, frequencies of the 9-repeat allele in the three groups are NS = 0.248; CS = 0.238; FS = 0.307. In the Lerman et al. (1999) study, the frequencies in the four groups are: Caucasian NS = 0.355; Caucasian CS = 0.294; African Americans NS = 0.191; and African Americans CS = 0.168. Thus the frequency of the 9-repeat allele in the Lerman et al. (1999) Caucasian NS sample is higher than in any of the categories in the Sabol et al. (1999) study. This statement completes the argument and brings us back to its initial point—no conclusions originating from genetic association studies can be viewed as coherent without taking into account the multiple contexts in which personality exists, specifically the context of the genetic background of the population from which a given sample originates. (This is exactly the problem to which I referred earlier in discussing the 5-HTT findings).

SUMMARY

So what can be said to summarize the discussion in this chapter? In short, the story is complex. To paraphrase the famous words of Lashley (1964), I almost feel that in reviewing the evidence on the genetic engram of personality, the necessary conclusion is that personality is not possible—so far we have only disparate pieces of the puzzle, and nothing quite makes sense! And yet we all know that our current state of knowledge is only the beginning. Obviously, there is much to learn and much to discover, seeking the nature of dynamic events that occur within neuronal sites and looking for interactions between them in an attempt to understand the behavior of the complex, holistic systems that are personalities.

NOTES

1. The twin method makes a number of assumptions, among which is the assumption of equitability of MZ and DZ environments and the etiology of genetic similarities. (It is assumed that MZ twins share 100% of their genes, whereas DZ twins, on average, share only 50% of their genes; however, this assumption is made only with respect to main genetic effects, not interactive effects.)
2. Some of these descriptions might be somewhat technical. Although the complexity of the description is preserved with the aim of providing all necessary information for identification of specific polymorphisms (e.g., the location of a given polymorphism in a gene, the type of the polymorphism, the name of the restriction enzyme, the involved amino acids), general discussions that follow technical descriptions do not call for any specialized knowledge.
3. Genes are complex structures in their own right. To determine the direction of transcription, scientists label two ends of the gene as 5' (where the transcription starts) and 3' (where the transcription stops). Roughly, each gene consists of two main interrupted components: transcribed (also referred to as coding) region, made of exons, and untranscribed (also referred as noncoding), made of introns. Gene regulatory elements include promoter, response element, enhancer, and silencer.
4. Glutamate is the transmitter of the trisynaptic pathway from the entorhinal cortex via the dentate gyrus and CA3 to CA1 and the subiculum. Changes in the number and/or properties of glutamate receptors are thought to be one of the mechanisms underlying learning and memory.
5. N-methyl-D-aspartate receptor; mediates slow, voltage-dependent excitation and is of major importance for long-term potentiation. Long-term potentiation is the first step in a sequence of neuronal activities leading to memory formation.
6. D,L- α-amino-3-hydroxy-5-methyl-4-isoxalone propionate receptor; mediates fast excitation.
7. This example was developed and brought to my attention by Dr. Kenneth Kidd.

REFERENCES

Alreja, M., Wu, M., Liu, W., Atkins, J., Leranth, C., & Shanabrough, M. (2000). Muscrine tone sustains impulse flow in the septohippocampal GABA but not cholinergic pathway: Implications for learning and memory. *Journal of Neuroscience, 20,* 8103–8110.

Anthony, J. C. (2001). The promise of psychiatric enviromics. *British Journal of Psychiatry, 40*(Suppl.), S8–S11.

Arinami, T., Gao, M., Hamaguchi, H., & Toru, M. (1997). A functional polymorphism in the promoter region of the dopamine D2 receptor gene is associated with schizophrenia. *Human Molecular Genetics, 6,* 577–582.

Asherson, P., Mant, R., Halmans, P. O., Williams, J., Cardno, A., Murphy, K., Jones, L., Collier, D., McGuffin, P., & Owen, M. J. (1996). Lindage, association and mutational analysis of the dopamine D3 receptor gene in schizophrenia. *Molecular Psychiatry, 1,* 125–132.

Asherson, P., Mant, R., Williams, N., Cardno, A., Jones, L., Murphy, K., Collier, D. A., Nanko, S., Craddock, N., Morris, S., Muir, W., Blackwood, B., McGuffin, P., & Owen, M. J. (1998). A study of chromosome 4p markers and dopamine D5 receptor gene in schizophrenia and bipolar disorder. *Molecular Psychiatry, 3,* 310–320.

Ashford, J. R. (1981). General models for the joint action of mixtures of drugs. *Biometrics, 37,* 457–474.

Bach, A. W., Lan, N. C., Johnson, D. L., Abell, C.W., Bembenek, M. E., Kwan, S. W., Seeburg, P. H., & Shih, J. C. (1988). CDNA cloning of human liver monoamine oxidase A and B: Molecular basis of differences in enzymatic properties. *Proceedings of the National Academy of Sciences of the United States of America, 85,* 4934–4938.

Barnard, E. A., Skolnick, P., Olsom, R. W., Mohler, H., Sieghart, W., Biggio, G., Braestrup, C., Bateson, A. N., & Langer, S. Z. (1998). International Union of Pharmacology:15. Subtypes of gamma-aminobutyric acid A receptors: Classification on the basis of subunit structure and receptor function. *Pharmacological Review, 50,* 291–313.

Barr, C. L., Kennedy, J. L., Lichter, J. B., Van Tol, H. H. M., Wetterberg, L., Livak, K. J., & Kidd, K. K. (1993). Alleles at the dopamine D4 receptor locus do not contribute to the genetic susceptibility to schizophrenia in a large Swedish kindred. *American Journal of Medical Genetics. 48,* 218–222.

Barr, C. L., Wigg, K. G., Feng, Y., Zai, G., Malone, M., Roberts, W., Schachar, R., Tannock, R., & Kennedy, J. L. (2000). Attention-deficit hyperactivity disorder and the gene for the dopamine D5 receptor. *Molecular Psychiatry, 5,* 548–551.

Basile, V. S., Masellis, M., Badri, F., Paterson, A. D., Meltzer, H.Y., Lieberman, J. A., Potkin, S. G., Macciardi, F., & Kennedy, J. L. (1999). Association of the MscI polymorphism of the dopamine D3 receptor gene with tardive dyskinesia in schizophrenia. *Neuropsychopharmacology, 21,* 17–27.

Bass, M. P., Menold, M. M., Wolpert, C. M., Donnelly, S. L., Ravan, S. A., Hauser, E. R., Maddox, L. O., Vance, J. M., Abramson, R. K., Wright, H. H., Gilbert, J. R., Cuccaro, M. L., DeLong, G. R., & Pericak-Vance, M. A. (2000). Genetic studies in autistic disorder and chromosome 15. *Neurogenetics, 2,* 219–226.

Benjamin, J., Li, L., Patterson, C., Greenberg, R., Murphy, D., & Hamer, D. H. (1996). Population and familial association between the D4 dopamine receptor gene and measures of novelty seeking. *Nature Genetics, 12,* 81–84.

Benjamin, J., Osher, Y., Kotler, M., Gritsenko, I., Nemanov, L., Belmaker, R. H., & Ebstein, R. P. (2000). Association between tridimensional personality questionnaire (TPQ) traits and three functional polymorphisms: Dopamine receptor D4 (DRD4), serotonin transporter promoter region (5-HTTLPR) and catechol O-methyltransferase (COMT). *Molecular Psychiatry, 5,* 96–100.

Bergeman, C. S., Chipuer, H. M., Plomin, R., Pedersen, N. L., McClearn, G. E., Nesselroade, J. R., Costa, P. T. Jr., & McCrae, R. R. (1993). Genetics and environmental effects on openness to experience, agreeableness, and conscientiousness: An adoption/twin study. *Journal of Personality, 61,* 159–179.

Blum, K., Braverman, E. R., Wu, S., Cull, J .G., Chen, T. J. H., Gill, J., Wood, R., Eisenberg, A., Sherman M., Davis, K. R., Matthews, D., Fischer, L., Schnautz, N., Walsh, W., Pontius, A. A., Zedar, M., Kaats, G., & Comings, D. E. (1997). Association of polymorphisms of dopamine D2 receptor (DRD2), and dopamine transporter (DAT1) genes with schizoid/avoidant behaviors (SAB). *Molecular Psychiatry, 2,* 239–246.

Blum, K., Cull, J. G., Braverman, E. R., & Comings, D. E. (1996). Reward deficiency syndrome. *American Scientist, 84,* 132–145.

Blum, K., Sheridan, P. J., Wood, R. C., Braverman, E. R., Chen, T. J. H., Cull, J. G., & Comings, D.E. (1996). The D2 dopamine receptor gene as a predictor of "reward deficiency syndrome" (RDS) behavior: Bayes' Thoerem. *Journal of Royal Social Medicine, 87,* 396–400.

Bolos, A. M., Dean, M., Lucas-Derse, S., Ramsburg, M., Brown, G. L., & Goldman, D. (1990). Population and pedigree studies reveal a lack of association between the dopamine D2 receptor gene and alcoholism. *Journal of the American Medical Association, 264,* 3156–3160.

Bonnert, T. P., McKerman, R. M., Farrar, S., Le Bourdelles, B., Heavens, R. P., Smith, D. W., Hewson, L., Rigby, M. R., Sirinthsinghji, D. J., Brown, N., Wafford, K. A., & Whiting, P. J. (1999). Theta, a nolel gamma-aminobutyric acid type A receptor subunit. *Proceedings of the National Academy of Sciences of the United States of America, 96,* 9891–9896.

Bormann, J. (2000). The "ABC" of GABA receptors. *Trends in Pharmacological Science, 21,* 16–19.

Bouchard, T. J. (1994). Genes, environment, and personality. *Science Magazine, 264,* 1700–1701.

Bouchard, T. J., Lykken, D. T., McGue, M., Segal, N. L., & Tellegen, A. (1990). Sources of human psychological differences: The Minnesota study of twins reared apart. *Science, 250,* 223–228.

Bowden, C. L., Deutsch, C. K., & Swanson, J. M. (1988). Plasma dopamine-β-hydroxylase and monoamine oxidase in attention deficit disorder and conduct disorder. *Journal of American Academy of Child and Adolescent Psychiatry, 27,* 171–174.

Brunner, H. G., Nelen, M., Breakefield, X. O., Ropers, H. H., & Van Oost, B. A. (1993). Abnormal behavior associated with a point mutation in the structural gene for monoamine oxidase A. *Science, 262,* 578–580.

Brunner, H. G, Nelen, M. R, Van Zandvoort, P., Abeling, N. G. G. M., Van Gennip, A. H., Wolters, E. C., Kuiper, M. A., Ropers, H. H., & van Oost, B. A. (1993). X-linked borderline mental retardation with prominent behavioral disturbance: Phenotype, genetic localization, and evidence for disturbed monoamine metabolism. *American Journal of Human Genetics, 52,* 1032–1039.

Buhot, M.-C. (1997). Serotonin receptors in cognitive behaviors. *Current Opinions in Neurobiology, 7,* 243–254.

Castro-Alamancos, M. A. (2000). Origin of synchronized oscillations induced by neocortical disinhibition *in vivo. Journal of Neuroscience, 15,* 9195–9206.

Catalano, M., Nobile, M., Novelli, E., Nothen, M. M., & Smeraldi, E. (1993). Distribution of a novel mutation in the first exon of the human dopamine D4 receptor gene in psychotic patients. *Biological Psychiatry, 34,* 459–464.

Catalano, M., Sciuto, G., Dibella, D., Novelli, N., Nobile, M., & Bellodi, L. (1994). Lack of association between obsessive–compulsive disorder and the dopamine D-3 receptor gene: Some preliminary considerations. *American Journal of Medical Genetics, 54,* 253–255.

Cavalli-Sforza, L. L. (1998). The DNA revolution in population genetics. *Trends in Genetics, 14,* 60–65.

Cervone, D., & Shoda, Y. (Eds.). (1999). *The coherence of personality.* New York: Guilford Press.

Chang, F. M., & Kidd, K. K. (1997). Rapid molecular haplotyping of the first exon of the human dopamine D4 receptor gene by heteroduplex analysis. *American Journal of Medical Genetics, 74,* 91–94.

Chang, F.-M., Ko, H.-C., Lu, R.-B., Pakstis, A. J., & Kidd, K. K. (1997). The dopamine D4 receptor gene (DRD4) is not associated with alcoholism in three Taiwanese populations: Six polymorphisms tested separately and as haplotypes. *Biological Psychiatry, 41,* 394–405.

Chen, Z. Y., Powell, J. F., Hsu, Y. P., Breakefield, X. O., & Craig, I. W. (1992). Organization of the human monoamine oxidase genes and long-range physical mapping around them. *Genomics, 14,* 75–82.

Cilliers, P. (1998). *Complexity and postmodernism.* New York: Routledge.

Cloninger, C. R. (1994). The genetic structure of personality and learning: a phylogenetic model. *Clinical Genetics, 1994, 46,* 124–137.

Comings, D. E., Wu, H., Chiu, C., Ring, R. H., Dietz, G., & Muhleman, D. (1996). Polygenic inheritance of Tourette syndrome, stuttering, attention-deficit/hyperactivity, conduct and oppositional defiant disorder: The addictive and subtractive effect of the three dopaminergic genes DRD2, DβH and DAT$_1$. *American Journal of Medical Genetics, 67,* 264–268.

Connors, B. W., Malenka, R. C., & Silva, L. R. (1988). Two inhibitory post-synaptic potentials, and GABA$_A$ and GABA$_B$ receptor-mediated responses in neocortex of rat and cat. *Journal of Physiology, 406,* 443–468.

Cook, E. H., Courchesne, R. Y., Cox, N. J., Lord, C., Gonen, D., Guter, S. J., Lincoln, A., Nix, K., Haas, R., Leventhal, B. L., & Courchesne, E. (1998). Linkage-disequilibrium mapping of autistic disorder, with 15q11–13 markers. *American Journal of Human Genetics, 62,* 1077–1083.

Cook, J. E., Stein, M. A., Krasowski, M. D., Cox, N. J., Olkon, D. M., Kieffer, J. E., & Leventhal, B. L. (1995). Association of attention-deficit disorder and the dopamine transporter gene. *American Journal of Human Genetics, 56,* 993–998.

Cook, J. E., Jr., Courchesne, R., Lord, C., Cox, N. J., Yan, S., Lincoln, A., Haas, R., Courchesne, E., & Leventhal, B. L. (1997). Evidence of linkage between the serotonin transporter and autistic disorder. *Molecular Psychaitry, 2,* 247–250.

Cooper, J. R., Bloom, F. E., & Roth, R. H. (1996). *The biochemical basis of neuropharmacology.* New York: Oxford University Press.

Cravchik, A., & Gejman, P. V. (1999). Functional analysis of the human D5 dopamine receptor missense and nonsense variants: differences in dopamine binding affinities. *Pharmacogenetics, 9,* 199–206.

Cravchik, A., Sibley, D. R., & Gejman, P. V. (1996). Functional analysis of the human D2 dopamine receptor missense variants. *Journal of Biological Chemistry, 271,* 26013–26017.

Crowe, R. R., Wang, Z., Noyes, R., Jr., Albrecht, B. E., Darlison, M. G., Bailey, M. E., Johnson, K. J., & Zoega, T. (1997). Candidate gene study of eight GABA A receptor subunits in panic disorder. *American Journal of Psychiatry, 154,* 1096–1100.

Crunelli, V., & Leresche, N. (1991). A role of GABAb receptors in excitation and inhibition of thalamnocortical cells. *Trends in Neuroscience, 14,* 161–121.

Cubells, J. F., Kobayashi, K., Nagatsu, T., Kidd, K. K., Kidd, J. R., Calafell, F., Kranzler, H. R., Ichinose, H., & Gelertner, J. (1997). Population genetics of a functional variant of the dopamine b-hydroxylase gene (DBH). *American Journal of Medical Genetics, 74,* 374–379.

Cubells, J. F., Kranzler, H. R., McCance-Katz, E., Anderson, G. M., Malison, R. T., Price, L. H., & Gelertner, J. (2000). A haplotype at the DBH locus, associated with low plasma dopamine b-hydroxylase activity, also associates with cocaine-induced paranoia. *Molecular Psychiatry, 5,* 56–63.

Cubells, J. F., van Kammen, D. P., Kelley, M. E., Anderson, G. M., O'Connor, D. T., Price, L. H., Malison, R., Rao, P. A., Kobayashi, K., Nagatsu, T., & Gelertner, J. (1998). Dopamine b-hydroxylase: Two polymorphisms in linkage disequilibrium at the structural gene DBH associate with biochemical phenotypic variation. *Human Genetics, 102,* 533–540.

Daly, G., Hawi, Z., Fitzgerald, M., & Gill, M. (1999). Mapping susceptibility loci in attention deficit hyperactivity disorder: Preferential transmission of parental alleles at DAT1, DBH, and DRD5 to affected children. *Molecular Psychiatry, 4,* 192–196.

D'Amato, T., Leboyer, M., Malafosse, A., Samolyk, D., Lamouroux, A., Junien, C., & Mallet, J. (1989) Two *TaqI* dimorphic sites at the human beta-hydroxylase locus. *Nucleic Acids Research, 17,* 5871.

Damberg, M., Garpenstrand, H., Alfredsson, J., Ekblom, J., Forslund, K., Rylander, G., & Oreland, L. (2000). A polymorphic region in the human transcription factor AP-2b gene is associated with specific personality traits. *Molecular Psychiatry, 5,* 220–224.

Debruyn, A., Mendelbaum, K., Sandkuijl, L.A., Delvenne, V., Hirsch, D., Staner, L., Mendlewicz, J., Van Broeckhoven, C. (1994). Nonlinkage of bipolar illness to tyrosine hydroxylase, tyrosinase, and D2 and D4 dopamine receptor genes on chromosome 11. *American Journal of Psychiatry, 151,* 102–106.

Debruyn, A., Raeymaekers, P., Mendelbaum, K., Sandkuijl, L. A., Raes, G., Delvenne, V., Hirsch, D., Staner, L., Mendlewicz, J., & Van Broeckhoven, C. (1994). Linkage analysis of bipolar illness with X-chromosome DNA markers: A susceptibility gene in Xq27-q28 cannot be excluded. *American Journal of Medical Genetics, 54,* 411–419.

DeFelipe, J., Arellano, J. I., Gómez, A., Azmitia, E. C., & Muñoz, A. (2001). Pyramidal cell axons show a local specialization for GABA and 5-HT inputs in monkey and human cerebral cortex. *Journal of Comparative Neurology, 433,* 148–155.

Devor, E. J., Cloninger, C. R., Hoffman, P. L., & Tabakoff, B. (1993). Association of monoamine oxidase (MAO) activity with alcoholism and alcoholic subjects. *American Journal of Medical Genetics, 48,* 209–213.

Duffy, A., Turecki, G., Grof, P., Cavazzoni, P., Grof, E., Joober, R., Ahrens, B., Berghofer, A., Muller-Oerlinghausen, B., Dvorakova, M., Libigerova, E., Vojtechovsky, M., Zvolsky, P., Nilsson, A., Licht, R. W., Rasmussen, N. A., Schou, M., Vestergaard, P., Holzinger, A., Schumann, C., Thau, K., Robertson, C., Rouleau, G. A., & Alda, M. (2000). Association and linkage studies of candidate genes involved in GABAergic neurotransmission in lithium-responsive bipolar disorder. *Journal of Psychiatry and Neuroscience, 25,* 353–358.

Dunner, D. L., Levitt, M., Kumbaraci, T., & Fieve, R. R. (1977). Erythrocyte catechol-O-methyltransferase activity in primary affective disorde. *Biological Psychiatry, 12,* 237–244.

Eaves, L. J., Eysenck, H. J., & Martin, N. G. (1989). *Genes, culture and personality: An empirical approach,* San Diego, CA: Academic Press.

Eaves, L. J., Martin, N. G., Heath, A. C., Hewitt, J. K., & Neal, M. C. (1990). Personality and reproductive fitness. *Behavior Genetics, 20,* 563–568.

Ebstein, R., Novick, O., Umansky R., Priel, B., Osher Y., Blaine, D., Bennett, E. R., Nemanov, L., Katz, M., & Belmaker, R. H. (1996). Dopamine D4 receptor (*DRD4*) exon III polymorphism associated with the human personality trait of novelty seeking. *Nature Genetics, 12,* 78–80.

Ebstein, R. P., Segman, R., Benjamin, J., Osher, Y., & Belmaker, R. H. (1997). HT5-HT2C (HTR2C) serotonin receptor gene polymorphism associated with the human personality trait of reward dependence: Interaction with dopamine D4 receptor (D4DR) and dopamine D3 receptor (D3DR) polymorphisms. *American Journal of Medical Genetics, 74,* 65–72.

Eisenberg, J., Mei-Tal, G., Steinberg, A., Tartakovsky, E., Zohar, A., Gritsenko, I., Nemanov, L., & Ebstein, R. P. (1999). A haplotype relative risk study of catechol-O-methyltransferase (COMT) and attention deficit disorder (ADHD): Association of the high-enzyme activity val allele with ADHD impulsive-hyperactive phenotype. *American Journal of Medical Genetics (Neuropsychiatric Genetics), 88,* 497–502.

Esterling, L. E., Yoshikawa, T., Turner, G., Badner, J. A., Bengel, D., Gershon, E. S., Berrettini, W. H., & Detera-Wadleigh, S. D. (1998). Serotonin transporter (5-HTT) gene and bipolar affective disorder. *American Journal of Medical Genetics, 81,* 37–40.

Fagiolini, M., & Hensch, T. K. (2000). Inhibitory threshold for critical-period activation in primary visual cortex. *Nature, 404,* 183–186.

Fahndrich, M., Muller-Oerlinghausen, B., & Coper, H. (1982). Longitudinal assessment of MAO-, COMT-, and DBH- activity in patients with bipolar depression. *International Pharmacopsychiatry, 17,* 8–17.

Faraone, S. V., Doyle, A. E., Mick, E., & Biederman, J. (2001). Meta-analysis of the association between the 7-repeat allele of the dopamine D(4) receptor gene and ADHD. *American Journal of Psychiatry, 158,* 1052–1057.

Feldman, D. E. (2000). Inhibition and plasticity. *Nature Neuroscience, 3,* 303–304.

Feldman, D. E., Nicoll, R., Malenka, R. C., & Isaac, J. T. R. (1998). Long-term depression at thalamocortical synapses in developing rat somatosensory cortex. *Neuron, 21,* 347–357.

Feng, J., Sobell, J. L., Heston, L. L., Cook, E. H., Jr., Goldman, D., & Sommer, S. S. (1998). Scanning of the dopamine D1 and D5 receptor genes by REF in neuropsychiatric patients reveals a novel missense change at a highly conserved amino acid. *American Journal of Medical Genetics, 81,* 172–178.

Fiskerstrand, C. E., Lovejoy, E. A., & Quinee, J. P. (1999). An intronic polymorphic domain often associated with susceptibility to affective disorders has allele dependent differential enhancer activity in embryonic stem cells. *FEBS Letters, 458,* 171–174.

Flory, J. D., Manuck, S. B., Ferrell, R. E., Dent, K. M., Peters, D. G., & Muldoon, M. F. (1999). Neuroticism is not associated with the serotonin transporter (5-HTTLPR) polymorphism. *Molecular Psychiatry, 4,* 93–96.

Fowler, J. S., Volkow, N. D., Wang, G. J., Pappas, N., Logan, J., MacGregor, R., Alexoff, D., Shea, C., Schlyer, D., Wolf, A. P., Warner, D., Zezulkova, I., & Cilento, R. (1996). Inhibition of monoamine oxidase B in the brains of smokers. *Nature, 379,* 733–736.

Fowler, J. S., Volkow, N. D., Wang, G. J., Pappas, N., Logan, J., Shea, C., Alexoff, D., MacGregor, R. R., Schlyer, D. J., Zezulkova, I., & Wolf, A. P. (1996). Brain monoamine oxidase A inhibition in cigarette smokers. *Proceedings of the National Academy of Sciences of the United States of America, 93,* 14065–14069.

Freund, T. F., & Antal, M. (1988). GABA-containing neurons in the septum control inhibitory interneurons in the hippocampus. *Nature, 336,* 170–173.

Fritschy, J. M., & Mohler, H. (1995). GABA$_A$ receptor heterogeneity in the adult rat brain: Differential regional and cellular distribution of seven major subunits. *Journal of Comparative Neurology, 359,* 154–194.

Gabel, S., Stadler, J., Bjorn, J., Schindledecker, R., & Bowden, C. L. (1995). Homovanillic acid and monoamine oxidase in sons of substance-abusing fathers: Relationship to conduct disorder. *Journal of Studies on Alcohol, 56,* 135–139.

Galvin, M., Ten Eyck, R., Shekhar, A., Stilwell, B., Fineberg, N., Laite, G., & Karwisch, G. (1995). Serum dopamine beta hydroxylase and maltreatment in psychiatrically hospitalized boys. *Child Abuse and Neglect, 19,* 821–832.

Gelernter, J., Cubells, J. F., Kidd, J. R., Pakstis, A. J., & Kidd, K. K. (1999). Population studies of polymorphisms of the serotonin transporter protein gene. *American Journal of Medication Genetics, 88,* 61–66.

Gelernter, J., Kranzler, H. R., Satel, S. L., & Rao, P. A. (1994). Genetic association between dopamine transporter protein alleles and cocaine-induced paranoia. *Neuropsychopharmacology, 11,* 195–200.

Gelernter, J., O'Malley, S. O., Risch, N., Kranzler, R. R., Krystal, J., Merikangas, K., Kennedy, J. L., & Kidd, K. K. (1991). No association between an allele at the D2 dopamine receptor gene (DRD2) and alcoholism. *Journal of the American Medical Association, 47,* 1073–1077.

Gervasoni, D., Payron, C., Rampon, C., Barbagli, B., Chouvet, G., Urbain, N., Fort, P., & Luppi, P.-H. (2000). Role and origin of the GABAergic innervation of dorsal raphé serotonergic neurons. *Journal of Neuroscience, 20,* 4217–4225.

Gill, M., Daly, G., Heron, S., Hawi, Z., & Fitzgerald, M. (1997). Confirmation of association between attention deficit hyperactivity disorder and a dopamine transporter polymorphism. *Molecular Psychiatry, 2,* 311–313.

Giros, B., & Caron, M. G. (1993). Molecular characterization of the dopamine transporter. *Trends in Pharmacological Sciences, 14,* 43–49.

Glatt, K., Sinnett, D., & Lalande, M. (1994). The human gamma-aminobutyric acid receptor subunit beta 3 and alpha 5 gene cluster in chromosome 15q11-q13 is rich in highly polymorphic (CA)n repeats. *Genomics, 19,* 157–160.

Gloor, P. (1992). Role of the amygdala in temporal lobe epilepsy. In J. P. Aggleton (Ed.), *The amygdala: Neurobiological aspects of emotion, memory, and mental dysfunction* (pp. 505–538). New York: Wiley-Liss.

Goei, V. L., Choi, J., Ann, J., Bowlus, C. L., Raha-Chowdhury, R., & Gruen, J. (1998). Human gamma-aminobutyric acid B receptor gene: Complementary DNA cloning, expression, chromosomal location, and genomic organization. *Biological Psychiatry, 15,* 659–666.

Gomez-Casero, E., Perez de Castro, I., Saiz-Ruiz, J., Llinares, C., & Fernandez-Piqueras, J. (1996). No association between particular DRD3 and DAT gene polymorphism and manic-depression illness in a Spanish sample. *Psychiatric Genetics, 6,* 209–212.

Griffon, N., Crocq, M. A., Pilon, C., Martres, M. P., Mayerova, A., Uyanik, G., Burgert, E., Duvall, F., Macher, J. P., JavoyAgid, F., Tamminga, C. A., Schwartz, J. C., & Sokoloff, P. (1996). Dopamine D-3 receptor gene: Organization, transcript variants, and polymorphism associated with schizophrenia. *American Journal of Medical Genetics, 67,* 63–70.

Grigorenko, E. L. (2001). *Personality: The variability of heritability.* Unpublished manuscript.

Grimsby, J., Chen, K., Wang, L. J., Lan, N. C., & Shih, J. C. (1991). Human monoamine oxidase A and B genes exhibit identical exon-intron organization. *Proceedings of the National Academy of Sciences of the United States ofamerica, 88,* 3637–3641.

Grossman, M. H., Emanual, B. S., & Budarf, M. L. (1992). Chromosomal mapping of the human catechol-O-methyltransferase gene to 22q11-q11.2. *Genomics, 12,* 822–825.

Grünhage, F., Schulze, T. G., Müller, D. J., Lanczik, E., Albus, M., Borrmann-Hassenbach, M., Knapp, M., Cichon, S., Maier, W., Rietschel, M., Propping, P., & Nöthen, M. M. (2000). Systematic screening for DNA sequence variation in the coding region of the human dopamine transporter gene (DAT1). *Molecular Psychiatry, 5,* 275–282.

Gustavsson, J. P. (1997). *Stability and validity of self-reported personality traits.* Unpublished doctoral dissertation. Karolinska Institute, Stockholm, Sweden.

Hawi, Z., Millar, N., Daly, G., Fitgerald, M., & Gill, M. (2000). No association between cathecol-O-methyltransferase (*COMT*) gene polymorphism and attention deficit hyperactivity disorder (ADHD) in an Irish sample. *American Journal of Medical Genetics, 96,* 282–284.

Hawi, Z., Myakishev, M. V., Straub, R. E., O'Neil, A., Kendler, K. S., Walsh, D., & Gill, M. (1997). No association or linkage between the 5-HT2A/T102C polymorphism and schizophrenia in Irish families. *American Journal of Medical Genetics, 74,* 370–373.

Heath, A. C., Cloninger, C. R., & Martin, N. G. (1994). Testing a model for the genetic structure of personality: A comparison of the personality systems of Cloninger and Eysenck. *Journal of Personality and Social Psychology, 4,* 762–775.

Heath, A. C., Neale, M. C., Kessler, R. C., Eaves, L. J., & Kendler, K. (1992). Evidence for genetic influences on personality from self-reports and informant ratings. *Journal of Personality and Social Psychology, 63,* 85–96.

Heils, A., Teufel, A., Petri, S., Stoeber, G., Riederer, P., Bengel, D., & Lesch, K. P. (1996). Allelic variation of human serotonin transporter gene expressions. *Journal of Neurochemistry, 66,* 2621–2624.

Henderson, A. S., Korten, A. E., Jorm, A. F., Jacomb, P. A., Christensen, H., Rodgers, B., Tan, X., & Easteal, S. (2000). COMT and DRD3 polymorphisms, environmental exposures, and personality traits related to common mental disorders. *American Journal of Medical Genetics, 96,* 102–107.

Hensch, T. K., Fagiolini, M., Mataga, N., Stryker, M. P., Baekkeskov, S., & Kash, S. F. (1998). Local GABA circuit control of experience-dependent plasticity in developing visual cortex. *Science, 282,* 1504–1508.

Himei, A., Kono, Y., Yoneda, H., Sakai, T., Koh, J., Sakai, J., Inada, Y., & Immamichi, H. (2000). An association study between alcoholism and the serotonergic receptor gene. *Alcoholism: Clinical and Experimental Research, 24,* 341–342.

Hisama, F. M., Gruen, J. R., Choi, J. J., Husenovic, M., Grigorenko, E. L., Pauls, D., Mattson, R. H., Gelernter, J., Wood, F. B., & Goei, V. L. (2001). Human GABA B receptor 1 gene: Eight novel sequence variants. *Human Mutation, 17,* 349–350.

Holbrook, A. M., Growther, R., Lotter, A., Cheng, C., & King, D. (1999). Meta-analysis of benzodiazepine use in the treatment of acute alcohol withdrawal. *The Canadian Medical Association Journal, 160,* 649–655.

Holschneider, D. P., & Shih, J. C. (1998). Monoamine oxidase: Basic and clinical perspectives. In E. F. Bloom & D. Kupfer (Eds.), *Psychopharmacology: The fourth generation of progress* [CD-Rom]. New York: Lippincott Williams & Wilkins.

Hranilovic, D., Schwab, S. G., Jernej, B., Knapp, K., Borrmann, M., Lichtermann, D., Maier, W., & Wildenauer, D. B. (2000). Serotonin transporter gene and schizophrenia: Evidence for association/linkage disequilibrium in families with affected siblings. *Molecular Psychiatry, 5,* 91–95.

Hsu, Y. P., Seow, S. V., Loh, E. W., Wang, Y. C., Chen, C. C., Yu, J. M., & Cheng, A. T. (1998). Search for mutations near the alternatively spliced 8 amino-acid exon in the GABAA receptor γ_2 subunit gene and lack of allelic association with alcoholism among four aboriginal groups in Han Chinese in Taiwan. *Brain Research, Molecular Brain Research, 56,* 284–286.

Hu, S., Brody, C. L., Fisher, C., Gunzerath, L., Nelson, M. L., Sabol, S. Z., Sirota, L. A., Marcus, S. E., Greenberg, B. D., Murphy, D. L., & Hamer, D. H. (2000). Interaction between the serotonin transporter gene and neuroticism in cigarette smoking behavior. *Molecular Psychiatry, 5,* 181–188.

Johnston, J. P. (1968). Some observations upon a new inhibitor of monoamine oxidase in brain tissue. *Biochemical Pharmacology, 17,* 1285–1297.

Inada, T., Sugita, T., Dobasi, I., Inagaki, A., Kitao, Y., Matsuda, G., Kato, S., Takano, T., & Yagi, G. (1995). Dopamine D3 receptor gene polymorphism and the psychiatric symptoms seen in first-break schizophrenia patients. *Psychiatric Genetics, 5,* 113–116.

Ishiguro, H., Saito, T., Shibuya, H., Toru, M., & Arinami, T. (1999). The 5' region of the tryptophan hydroxylase gene: Mutation search and association study with alcoholism. *Journal of Neural Transmission, 106,* 1017–1025.

Iversen, D. S. (1984). Cortical monoamines and behavior. In L. Descarries, T. R. Reader, & H. H. Jasper (Eds.), *Monoamine innervation of cerebral cortex* (pp. 44–76). New York: Liss.

Iversen, L. L. (1993). The D4 and schizophrenia. *Nature Genetics, 365,* 393.

Kaessmann, H., Wiebe, V., Weiss, G., & Pääbo, S. (2001). Great ape DNA sequences reveal a reduced diversity and an expansion in humans. *Nature Genetics, 27,* 155–156.

Kamakura, S., Iwaki, A., Matsumoto, M., & Fukumaki, Y. (1997). Cloning and characterization of the 5'-flanking region of the human dopamine D4 receptor gene. *Biochemical and Biophysical Research Communications, 235,* 321–326.

Kang, A. M., Palmatier, M. A., & Kidd, K. K. (1999). Global variation of a 40-bp VNTR in the 3'-untranslated region of the dopamine transporter gene (SLC6A3). *Biological Psychiatry, 46,* 151–160.

Karayiorgou, M., Sobin, C., Blundell, M. L., Galke, B. L., Malinova, L., Goldberg, P., Ott, J., & Gogos, J. A. (1999). Family-based association studies support a sexually dimorphic effect of COMT and MAOA on genetic susceptibility to obsessive–compulsive disorder. *Biological Psychiatry, 45,* 1178–1189.

Karege, F., Bovier, J. M., & Tissot, R. (1987). The decrease of erythrocyte catechol-O-methyltransferase activity in depressed patients and its diagnostic significance. *Acta Psychiatrica Scandinavica, 76,* 303–308.

Kaupmann, K., Huggle, K., Heid, J., Flor, P. J., Bischoff, S., Mickel, S. J., McMaster, G., Angst, C., Bittiger, H., Froestl, W., & Bettler B. (1997). Expression cloning of GABA(B) receptors uncovers similarity to metabotrophic glutamate receptors. *Nature, 386,* 239–246.

Kehoe, J., & Vulfius, C. (2000). Independence of and interactions between GABA, glutamate-, and acetylcholine-activated CL conductances in *Aplysia* neurons. *Journal of Neuroscience, 20,* 8585–8596.

Khana, J. M., Le, A. D., Kalant, H., Chau, A., & Shah, G. (1997). Effect of lipid solubility on the development of chronic cross-tolerance between ethanol and different alcohols and barbiturates. *Pharmacological Biochemistry and Behavior, 57,* 101–110.

Kirov, G., Jones, I., McCandless, F., Craddock, N., & Owen, M. J. (1999). Family-based association studies of bipolar disorder with candidate genes involved in dopamine neurotransmission: DBH, DAT1, COMT, DRD2, DRD3, and DRD5. *Molecular Psychiatry, 4,* 558–565.

Kitayama, S., & Markus, H. R. (1999). *Yin* and *Yang* of the Japanese self: The cultural psychology of personality coherence. In D. Cervone & Y. Shoda (Eds.), *The coherence of personality* (pp. 242–302). New York: Guilford Press.

Klauck, S. M., Poustka, F., Benner, A., Lesch, K. P., & Poustka, A. (1997). Serotonin transporter (5-HTT) gene variants associated with autism? *Human Molecular Genetics, 6,* 2233–2238.

Knoll, J., & Magyar, K. (1972). Some puzzling pharmacological effects of monoamine oxidase inhibitors. *Advances in Biochemical Psychopharmacology, 5,* 393–408.

Kotler, M., Barak, P., Cohen, H., Averbuch, I. E., Grinshpoon, A., Gritsenko, I., Nemanov, L., & Ebstein, R. P. (1999). Homicidal behavior in schizophrenia associated with a genetic polymorphism determining low catechol O-methyltransferase (COMT) activity. *American Journal of Medical Genetics, 88,* 628–633.

Kunugi, H., Hattori, M., Kato, T., Tatsumi, M., Sakai, T., Sasaki, T., Hirose, T., & Nanko, S. (1997). Serotonin transporter gene polymorphisms: Ethnic difference and possible association with bipolar affective disorder. *Molecular Psychiatry, 2,* 457–462.

Lachman, H. M., Nolan, K. A., Mohr, P., Saito, T., & Volavka, J. (1998). Association between catechol O-methyltransferase genotype and violence in schizophrenia and schizoaffective disorder. *American Journal of Psychiatry, 155,* 835–837.

Lachman, H. M., Papolos, D. F., Saito, T., Yu, Y. M., Szumlanski, C. L., & Weinshilboum, R. M. (1996). Human catechol-O-methyltransferase pharmacogenetics: Description of a functional polymorphism and its potential application to neuropsychiatric disorders. *Pharmacogenetics, 6,* 243–250.

La Hoste, G. J., Swanson, J. M., Wigal, S., Glabe, C., Wigal, T., King, N., & Kennedy, J. (1996). Dopamine D4 receptor gene polymorphism is associated with attention-deficit hyperactivity disorder. *Molecular Psychiatry, 1,* 121–124.

Lannfelt, L., Sokoloff, P., Martres, M. P., Pilon, C., Giros, B., Jonsson, E., Sedvall, G., & Schwartz, J. C. (1992). Amino acid substitution in the dopamine D-sub-3 receptor as a useful polymorphism for investigating psychiatric disorders. *Psychiatric Genetics, 2,* 249–256.

Lappalainen, J., Long, J. C., Eggert, M., Ozaki, N., Robin, R. W., Brown, G. L., Naukkarinen, H., Virkkunen, M., Linnoila, M., & Goldman, D. (1998). Linkage of antisocial alcoholism to the serotonin 5-HT1B receptor gene in 2 populations. *Archives of General Psychiatry, 55,* 989–994.

Lappalainen, J., Long, J. C., Virkkunen, M., Ozaki, N., Goldman, D., & Linnoila, M. (1999). HTR2C Cys23Ser polymorphism in relation to CSF monoamine metabolic concentrations and DSM-II-R psychiatric diagnoses. *Biological Psychiatry, 46,* 821–826.

Lashley, K. S. (1964). *Brain mechanisms and intelligence: A quantitative study of injuries to the brain.* New York: Hafner.

Lerman, C., Caporaso, N. E., Audrain, J., Main, D., Bowman, E. D., Lockshin, B., Boyd, N. R., & Shields, P. G. (1999). Evidence suggesting the role of specific genetic factors in cigarette smoking. *Health Psychology, 18,* 14–20.

Lesch, K. P., Bengel, D., Heils, A., Sabol, S. Z., Greenberg, B. D., Petri, S., Benjamin, J., Muller, C. R., Hamer, D. H., & Murphy, D. L. (1996). Association of anxiety-related traits with a polymorphism in the serotonin transported gene regulatory region. *Science, 274,* 1527–1531.

Leve, L. D., Winebarger, A. A., Fagot, B. I., Reid, J. B., & Goldsmith, H. H. (1998). Environmental and genetic variance in children's observed and reported maladaptive behavior. *Child Development, 69,* 1286–1298.

Lichter, J. B., Barr, C. L., Kennedy, J. L., Van Tol, H. H. M., Kidd, K. K., & Livak, K. J. (1993). A hypervariable segment in the human dopamine receptor (DRD4) gene. *Human Molecular Genetics, 2,* 767–773.

Loehlin, J. C. (1992). *Genes and environment in personality development.* Thousand Oaks, CA: Sage.

Loehlin, J. C., Willerman, L., & Horn, J. M. (1982). Personality resemblances between unwed mothers and their adopted-away offspring. *Journal of Personality and Social Psychology, 42,* 1089–1099.

Loh, E.-W., & Ball, D. (2000). Role of the GABA(A)beta2, GABA(A)alpha6, GABA(A)alpha1 and GABA(A)gamma2 receptor subunit genes cluster in drug responses and the development of alcohol dependence. *Neurochemistry International, 37,* 413–423.

Loh, E.-W., Higuchi, S., Matsushita, S., Murray, R., Chen, C.-K., & Ball, D. (2000). Association analysis of the GABA$_A$ receptor subunit genes cluster on 5q33-34 and alcohol dependence in a Japanese population. *Molecular Psychiatry, 2000,* 301–307.

Loh, E.-W., Smith, I., Murray, R., McLaughlin, M., McNulty, S., & Ball, D. (1999). Association between variants at the GABA$_{Aβ2}$, GABA$_{Aα6}$ and GABA$_{Aγ2}$ gene cluster and alcohol dependence in a Scottish population. *Molecular Psychiatry, 4,* 539–544.

Lucki, L. (1998). The spectrum of behaviors influenced by serotonin. *Biological Spychiatry, 44,* 151–162.

Macciardi, F., Petronis, A., Van Tol, H. H. M., Marino, C., Cavallini, M. C., Smeraldi, E., & Kennedy, J. L. (1994). Analysis of the D4 dopamine receptor gene variant in an Italian schizophrenia kindred. *Archives of General Psychiatry, 51,* 288–293.

Maestrini, E., Lai, C., Marlow, A., Matthews, N., Wallace, S., Bailey, A., Cook, E. H., Weeks, D. E., & Monaco, A. P. (1999). Serotonin transporter (5-HTT) and gamma-aminobutyric acid receptor subunit beta3 (GABRB3) gene polymorphisms are not associated with autism in the IMGSA families. *American Journal of Medical Genetics, 88,* 492–496.

Malhotra, A. K., Goldman, D., Mazzanti, C., Clifton, A., Breier, A., & Pickar, D. (1998). A functional serotonin transporter (5-HTT) polymorphism is associated with psychosis in neuroleptic-free schizophrenics. *Molecular Psychiatry, 3,* 328–332.

Mann, J. J., Malone, K. M., Nielsen, D. A., Goldman, D., Erdos, J., & Gelernter, J. (1997). Possible association of a polymorphism of the tryptophan hydroxylase gene with suicidal behavior in depressed patients. *American Journal of Psychiatry, 154,* 1451–1453.

Martin, R. E., Menold, M. M., Wolpert, C. M., Bass, M. P., Donnelly, S. L., Ravan, S. A., Zimmerman, A., Gilbert, J. R., Vance, J. M., Maddox, L. O., Wright, H. H., Abramson, R. K., DeLong, G. R., Cuccaro, M. L., & Pericak-Vance, M. A. (1999). Analysis of linkage disequilibrium in γ-aminobutyric acid receptor subunit genes in autistic disorder. *American Journal of Medical Genetics, 96,* 43–48.

Matsushita, S., Muramatsu, T., Kimura, M., Shirakawa, O., Mita, T., Nakai, T., & Higuchi, S. (1997). Serotonin transporter gene regulatory region polymorphism and panic disorder. *Molecular Psychiatry, 2,* 390–392.

Matuzas, W., Meltzer, N. Y., Uhlenhuth, E. H., Glass, R. M., & Tong, C. (1982). Plasma dopamine-beta-hydroxylase activity in depressed patients. *Biological Psychiatry, 17,* 1415–1424.

Mazzanti, C. M., Lappalainen, J., Long, J. C., Bengel, D., Naukkarinen, H., Eggert, M., Virkkunen, M., Linnoila, M., & Goldman, D. (1998). Role of the serotonin transporter promoter polymorphism in anxiety-related traits. *Archives of General Psychiatry, 55,* 936–940.

Mehta, A. K., & Ticku, M. K. (1999). An update on GABA$_A$ receptors. *Brain Research Review, 29,* 196–217.

Meller, E., Helmer-Matyjek, E., Bohmaker, K., Adler, C. H., Friedhoff, A. J., & Goldstein, M. (1986). Receptor reserve at striatal dopamine autoreceptors: Implications for selectivity of dopamine agonists. *European Journal of Pharmacology, 123,* 311–314.

Meneses, A. (1999). 5-HT system and cognition. *Neuroscience and Biobehavioral Reviews, 23,* 1111–1125.

Miczek, K. A., DeBold, J. F., van Erp, A. M., & Tornatzky, W. (1997). GABA$_A$-benzodiazepine receptor complex and aggression. *Recent Developments in Alcoholism, 13,* 137–171.

Miettinen, R., & Freund, T. F., (1992). Convergence and segregation of septal and median raphe inputs onto different subsets of hippocampal inhibitory interneurons. *Brain Research, 594,* 263–272.

Miles, D. R., & Carey, G. (1997). Genetic and environmental architecture on human aggression. *Journal of Personality and Social Psychology, 72,* 207–217.

Misgeld, U., Bijak, M., & Jarolimek, W. A. (1995). A physiological role for

GABAb receptors and the effects of baclofen in the mammalian central nervous system. *Progress in Neurobiology, 46,* 432–462.

Mitchell, P., Waters, B., Vivero, C., Le, F., Donald, J., Tully, M., Campedelli, K. L., Sokoloff, P., & Shine, J. (1993). Exclusion of close linkage of bipolar disorder to the dopamine D3 receptor gene in nine Australian pedigrees. *Journal of Affective Disorders, 27,* 213–224.

Mitchell, P. J., Timmons, P. M., Herbert, J.M., Rigby, P. W., & Tjian, R. (1991). Transcription factor AP-2 is expressed in neural crest lineages during mouse embryogenesis. *Genes and Development, 5,* 105–119.

Moser, M., Rüschoff, J., & Buettner, R. (1997). Comparative analysis of AP-2α and AP-2β gene expression during murine embryogenesis. *Developmental Dynamics, 208,* 115–124.

Muir, W. J., Thomson, M. L., McKeon, P., Mynett-Johnson, L., Whitton, C., Evans, K. L., Porteous, D. J., & Blackwood, D. H. (2001). Markers close to the dopamine D5 receptor gene (DRD5) show significant association with schizophrenia but not bipolar disorder. *American Journal of Medical Genetics, 105,* 152–158.

Mundo, E., Richter, M. A., Sam, F., Macciardi, F., & Kennedy, J. L. (2000). Is the 5-HT(1 Dbeta) receptor gene implicated in the pathogenesis of obsessive–compulsive disorder? *American Journal of Psychiatry, 157,* 1160–1161.

Nagatsu, T., Wakui, Y., Kato, T., Fujita, K., Kondo, T., Yokochi, F., & Narabayashi, H. (1982). Dopamine-beta-hydroxylase activity in cerebrospinal fluid of Parkinsonian patients. *Biomedical Research, 3,* 95–98.

Nakamura, N., Ueno, S., Sano, A., & Tanabe, H. (2000). The human serotonin transporter gene linked polymorphism (5-HTTLPR) shows ten novel allelic variants. *Molecular Psychiatry, 3,* 32–38.

Nakamura, T., Matsushita, S., Nishiguchi, N., Kimura, M., Yoshiona, A., & Higuchi, S. (1999). Association of a polymorphism of the 5HT2A receptor gene promoter region with alcohol dependence. *Molecular Psychiatry, 4,* 85–88.

Nanko, S., Fukuda, R., Hattori, M., Sasaki, T., Dai, X. Y., Yamaguchi, K., & Kazamatsuri, H. (1994). Further evidence of no linkage between schizophrenia and the dopamine D3 receptor gene, *American Journal of Medical Genetics, 54,* 264–267.

Nanko, S., Hattori, M., Ikeda, K., Sasaki, T., Kazamatsuri, H., & Kuwata, S., (1993b). Dopamine D4 receptor polymorphism and schizophrenia. *Lancet, 341,* 689–690.

Nanko, S., Hattori, M., Ueki, A. & Ikeda, K. (1993). Dopamine D3 and D4 receptor gene polymorphisms and Parkinson's disease. *Lancet, 342*(8865), 250.

Narahashi, T. (1999). Chemical modulation of sodium channels and $GABA_A$ receptor channel. *Advances in Neurology, 79,* 457–480.

Neiswanger, K., Hill, S. Y., & Kaplan, B. B. (1993). Association between alcoholism and the *Taq* 1 A RFLP of the dopamine D2 receptor gene in the absence of linkage. *Psychiatric Genetics, 3,* 130.

Netter, P., Henning, J., & Roed, I. S. (1996). Serotonin and dopamine as mediators of sensation seeking behavior. *Neuropsychobiology, 34,* 155–165.

Nielsen, D. A., Jenkins, G. L., Stefanisko, K. M., Jefferson, K. K., & Goldman, D. (1997). Sequence, splice site, and population frequency distribution analyses of the polymorphic human tryptophan hydroxylase intron 7. *Molecular Brain Research, 45,* 145–148.

Noble, E. P. (1993). The D2 dopamine receptor gene: A review of association studies in alcoholism. *Behavior Genetics, 23,* 117–127.

Noble, E. P., Zhang, X., Ritchie, T., Lawford, B. R., Grosse, S. C., Young, R. M., & Sparkes, R. S. (1998). D2 dopamine receptor and GABA$_A$ receptor β_3 subunit genes and alcoholism. *Psychiatry Research, 81,* 133–147.

Nothen, M. M., Cichon, S., Hemmer, S., Hebebrand, J., Remschmidt, H., Lehmkuhl, G., Poustka, F., Schmidt, M., Catalano, M., Fimmers, R., Korner, J., Rietschel, M., & Propping, P. (1994). Human dopamine D4 receptor gene: Frequent occurrence of a null allele and observation of homozygosity. *Human Molecular Genetics, 3,* 2207–2212.

Oreland, L. (1993). Monoamine oxidase in neuropsychiatric disorders. In P. Yasuhara, S. H. Parves, M. Sandler, K. Oguchi, & E. Nagatsu (Eds.). *Monoamine oxidase: Basic and clinical aspects* (pp. 219–247). Utrecht, Germany: VSP Press.

Ortells, M. O., & Lunt, G. G. (1995). Evolutionary history of the ligand-gated ion-channel superfamily of receptors. *Trends in Neuroscience, 18,* 121–127.

Osher, Y., Hamer, D., & Benjamin, J. (2000). Association and linkage of anxiety-related traits with a functional polymorphism of the serotonin transporter gene regulatory region in Israeli sibling pairs. *Molecular Psychiatry, 5,* 216–219.

Overstreet, D. H., Russell, R. W., Crocker, A. D., & Schiller, G. D. (1984). Selective breeding for differences in cholinergic function: Pre- and post-synaptic mechanisms involved in sensitivity to the anticholinesterase, DFP. *Brain Research, 294,* 327–332.

Oyama, Y., Ikemoto, Y., Kits, K. S., & Akaike, N. (1990). GABA affects the glutamate receptor-chloride channel complex in mechanically isolated and internally perfused *Aplysia* neurons. *European Journal of Pharmacology, 185,* 43–52.

Papadimitriou, G. N., Dikeos, D. G., Karadima, G., Avramopoulos, D., Daskalopoulou, E. G., Vassilopoulos, D., & Stefanis, C. N. (1998). Association between the GABA(A) receptor alpha5 subunit gene locus (GABRA5) and bipolar affective disorder. *American Journal of Medical Genetics, 81,* 73–80.

Parsian, A., & Cloninger, C. R. (1997). Human GABA$_A$ receptor α_1 and α_3 subunits genes and alcoholism. *Alcoholism, Clinical and Experimental Research, 21,* 430–433.

Pavlides, C., Greenstein, Y. J., Grudman, M., & Winson, J. (1988). Long-term potentiation in the dentate gyrus is induced preferentially on the positive phase of theta-rhythm. *Brain Research, 439,* 383–387.

Pedersen, N. L., Plomin, R., McClearn, G. E., & Friberg, L. (1988). Neuroticism, extraversion, and related traits in adult twins reared apart and reared together. *Journal of Personality and Social Psychology, 55,* 950–957.

Perez de la Mora, M., Ferre, S., & Fuxe, K. (1997). GABA-dopamine receptor-receptor interactions in neostriatal membranes of the rate. *Neurochemical Research, 22,* 1051–1054.

Persico, A. M., Militerni, R., Bravaccio, C., Schneider, C., Melmed, R., Conciatori, M., Damiani, V., Baldi, A., & Keller, F. (2000). Lack of association between serotonin transporter gene promoter variants and autistic disorder in two ethnically distinct samples. *American Journal of Medical Genetics, 96,* 123–127.

Petronis, A., O'Hara, K., Barr, C. L., Kennedy, J. L., & Van Tol, H. H. M. (1994). (G)n-mononucleotide polymorphism in the human D4 dopamine receptor (DRD4) gene. *Human Genetics, 93,* 719.

Petronis, A., Van Tol, H. H. M., & Kennedy, J. L. (1994). A *SmaI* PCR-RFLP in the 5' noncoding region of the human D4 dopamine receptor gene (DRD4). *Human Heredity, 44,* 58–60.

Philippu, C., Hoo, J. J., Milech, U., Argarwall, D. P., Schrappe, O., & Goedde, H. W. (1985). Cathecol-O-methyltransferase activity of erythrocytes in patients with endogenous psychosis. *Psychiatry Research, 4,* 139–146.

Previc, F. H. (1999). Dopamine and the origins of human intelligence. *Brain and Cognition, 41,* 299–350.

Puertollano, R., Visedo, G., Saiz-Ruiz, J., Llinares, C., & Fernandez-Piqueras, J. (1995). Lack of association between manic-depressive illness and a highly polymorphic marker from GABRA3 gene. *American Journal of Medical Genetics, 60,* 434–435.

Puumala, T., Ruotsalainen, S., Jakala, P., Koivisto, E., Riekkinen, P., Jr., & Sirvio, J. (1996). Behavioral and pharmacological studies on the validation of a new animal model for attention deficit hyperactivity disorder. *Neurobiology of Learning and Memory, 66,* 198–211.

Puzynski, S., Binzinsky, A., Mrozek, S., & Zaluska, M. (1983). Studies on biogenic amine metabolizing enzyme (DBH, COMT, MAO) and pathogenesis of affective illness: II. Erythrocyte catechol-O-methyltransferase activity in endogeneous depression. *Acta Psychiatrica Scandinavica, 67,* 96–100.

Radel, M., Vallejo, R. J., Long, J. C., & Goldman, D. (1999). Sib-pair linkage analysis of GABRG2 to alcohol dependence. *Alcoholism: Clinical and Experimental Research, 23,* 59A.

Redecker, C., Luhmann, H. J., Hagemann, G., Fritschy, J.-M., & Witte, O. W. (2000). Differential downregulation of $GABA_A$ receptor subunits in widespread brain regions in the freeze-lesion model of focal cortical malformations. *Journal of Neuroscience, 20,* 5045–5053.

Ren, R., Mayer, B. J., Cichetti, P., & Baltimore, D. (1993). Identification of a ten-amino acid proline-rich SH3 binding site. *Science, 259,* 1157–1161.

Rietschel, M., Nothen, M. M., Albus, M., Maier, W., Minges, J., Bondy, B., Korner, J., Hemmer, S., Fimmers, R., Moller, H. J., Wildenauer, D., & Propping, P. (1996). Dopamine D-3 receptor Gly9/Ser9 polymorphism and schizophrenia: No increased frequency of homozygosity in German familial cases. *Schizophrenia Research, 20,* 181–186.

Robinson, P. D., Schulz, C. K., Macciardi, F., White, B. N., & Holden, J. J. A. (2001). *Genetically determined low maternal serum dopamine β-hydroxylase levels and the etiology of autism spectrum disorders.* Unpublished manuscript.

Rogeness, G. A., Hernandez, J. M., Macedo, C. A., Amrung, S. A., & Hoppe, S. K. (1986). Near-zero plasma dopamine-β-hydroxylase and conduct disorder in emotionally disturbed boys. *Journal of the American Academy of Child Psychiatry, 25*, 521–527.

Rogeness, G. A., Hernandez, J. M., Macedo, C. A., & Mitchell, E. L. (1981). Biochemical differences in children with conduct disorder socialized and undersocialized. *American Journal of Psychiatry, 139*, 307–311.

Rose, R. J., & Kaprio, J. (1988). Frequency of social contact and intrapair resemblance of adult monozygotic cotwins: Or does shared experience influence personality after all? *Behavior Genetics, 18*, 309–328.

Rose, R. J., Koskenvuo, M., Kaprio, J., Sarna, S., & Langinvainio, H. (1988). Shared genes, shared experiences, and similarity of personality: Data from 14,288 adult Finnish co-twins. *Journal of Personality and Social Psychology, 54*, 161–171.

Rotondo, A., Schuebel, K., Bergen, A., Aragon, R., Virkkunen, M., Linnoila, M., Goldman, D., & Nielsen, D. (1999). Identification of four variants in the tryptophan hydroxylase promoter and association to behavior. *Molecular Psychiatry, 4*, 360–368.

Roth, G. S., & Hess, G. D. (1982). Changes in the mechanisms of hormone and neurotransmitter action during aging: Current status of the roles of receptor and post-receptor alterations. *Mechanics of Aging Development, 20*, 175–194.

Rothman, K. J., Greenland, S., & Walker, A. M. (1980). Concepts of interaction. *American Journal of Epidemiology, 112*, 467–470.

Rothschild, L. G., Badner, J., Cravchik, A., Gershon, E. S., & Gejman, P. V. (1996). No association detected between a D-3 receptor gene-expressed variant and schizophrenia. *American Journal of Medical Genetics, 67*, 232–234.

Russell, R. W. (1992). Interactions among neurotransmitters: Their importance to the "integrated organism". In E. D. Levin, M. W. Decker, & L. L. Butcher (Eds.), *Neurotransmitter interactions and cognitive function* (pp. 1–14). Boston, MA: Birkhäuser.

Russell, R. W., Booth, R. A., Smith, C. A., Jenden, D. J., Roch, M., Rice, K. M., & Lauretz, S. D. (1989). Roles of neurotransmitter receptors in behavior: Recovery of function following decreases in muscarine sensitivity induced by cholinesterase inhibition. *Behavior Neuroscience, 103*, 881–892.

Russell, R. W., Jenden, D. J., Booth, R. A., Lauretz, S. D., Roch, M., & Rice, K. M. (1990). Global *in vivo* replacement of choline by N-aminodeanal: Testing a hypothesis about progressive degenerative dementia: II. Physiological and behavioral effects. *Pharmacological Biochemistry and Behavior, 103*, 881–892.

Sabate, O., Campione, D., d'Amato, T., Martres, M. P., Sokoloff, P., Giros, B., Leboyer, M., Jay, M., Guedj, F., & Thibaut, F. (1994). Failure to find evidence for linkage or association between the dopamine D3 receptor gene and schizophrenia. *American Journal of Psychiatry, 151*, 107–111.

Sabol, S. Z., Nelson, M. L., Fisher, C., Gunzerath, L., Brody, C. L., Hu, S., Sirota, L. A., Marcus, S. E., Greenberg, B. D., Lucas, F. R., IV, Benjamin, J., Murphy, D. L., & Hamer, D. H. (1999). A genetic association for cigarette smoking behavior. *Health Psychology, 18*, 7–13.

Sander, T., Harms, H., Podschus, J., Finckh, U., et al. (1995). Dopamine D1, D2 and D3 receptor genes in alcohol dependence. *Psychiatric Genetics, 5*(4), 171–176.

Sander, T., Harms, H., Podschus, J., Finckh, U., Nickel, B., Rolfs, A., Rommelspacher, H., & Schmidt, L. G. (1997). Allelic association of a dopamine transporter gene polymorphism in alcohol dependence with withdrawal seizures or delirium. *Biological Psychiatry, 41,* 299–304.

Sander, T., Peters, C., Kämmer, G., Samochowiec, J., Zirra, M., Mischke, D., Ziegler, A., Kaupmann, K., Bettler, B., Epplen, J. T., & Riess, O. (1999). Association analysis of exonic variants of the gene encoding the GABA_B receptor and idiopathic generalized epilepsy. *American Journal of Medical Genetics, 88,* 305–310.

Scarr, S., Webber, P. L., Weinberg, R. A., & Wittig, M. A. (1981). Personality resemblance among adolescents and their parents in biologically related and adoptive families. *Journal of Personality and Social Psychology, 40,* 885–898.

Schmidt, L. G., Harms, H., Kuhn, S., Rommelspacher, H., & Sander, T. (1998). Modification of alcohol withdrawal by the A9 allele of the dopamine transporter gene. *American Journal of Psychiatry, 155,* 474–478.

Schmidt, M., Boller, M., Özen, G., & Hall, W. (2001). Disinhibition in rat colliculus mediated by GABA_C receptors. *Journal of Neuroscience, 15,* 691–699.

Schoffelmeer, A. N. M., Vanderschuren, L. J. M. J., De Vries, T. J., Hogenboom, F., Warden, G., & Mulder, A. (2000). Synergistically interacting dopamine D1 and NMDA receptors mediate nonvesicular transporter-dependent GABA release from rat striatal medium spiny neurons. *Journal of Neuroscience, 20,* 3496–3505.

Schuckit, M. A., Mazzanti, C., Smith, T. L., Ahmed, U., Radel, M., Iwata, N., Goldman, D. (1999). Selective genotyping for the role of 5-HT2A, 5-HT2C, and GABA alpha 6 receptors and the serotonin transporter in the level of response to alcohol: A pilot study. *Biological Psychiatry, 45,* 647–651.

Seaman, M. I., Fisher, J. B., Chang, F., & Kidd, K. K. (1999). Tandem duplication polymorphism upstream of the dopamine D4 receptor gene (DRD4). *American Journal of Medical Genetics, 88,* 705–709.

Seeman, P., Guan, H. C., & Van Tol, H. H M. (1993). Dopamine D4 receptors elevated in schizophrenia. *Nature, 365,* 441–445.

Seeman, P., Ulpian, C., Chouinard, G., Van Tol, H. H., Dwosh, H., Lieberman, J. A., Siminovitch, K., Liu, I. S., Waye, J., & Voruganti, P. (1994). Dopamine D4 receptor variant, D4GLYCINE194, in Africans, but not in Caucasians: No association with schizophrenia. *American Journal of Medical Genetics, 54,* 384–390.

Shaikh, S., Collier, D. A. Kerwin, R. W., Pilowsky, L. S., Gill, M., Xu, W. M., & Thornton, A. (1993). Dopamine D4 receptor subtypes and response to clozapine. *Lancet, 341,* 116.

Shaikh, S., Gill, M., Owen, M., Asherson, P., McGuffin, P., Nanko, S., Murray, R. M., & Collier, D. A. (1994). Failure to find linkage between a functional polymorphism in the dopamine D4 receptor gene and schizophrenia. *American Journal of Medical Genetics, 54,* 8–11.

Shih, J. C., Chen, K., & Ridd, M. J. (1999). Monoamine oxidase: From genes to behavior. *Annual Review of Neuroscience, 22,* 197–217.

Shoda, Y. (1999). Behavioral expressions of a personality system: Generation and perception of behavioral signatures. In D. Cevrone & Y. Shoda (Eds.), *The coherence of personality* (pp. 155–181). New York: Guilford Press.

Sibille, E., Pavlides, C., Benke, D., & Toth, M. (2000). Genetic inactivation of the serotonin$_{1A}$ receptor in mice results in downregulation of major GABA$_A$ receptor a subunits, reduction of GABA$_A$ receptor binding, and benzodiazepine-resistant anxiety. *Journal of Neuroscience, 20,* 2758–2765.

Sieghart, W. (1995). Structure and pharmacology of gamma-aminobutyric acid A receptor subtypes. *Pharmacological Review, 47,* 181–234.

Simpson, G. M., Shih, J. C., Chen, K., Flowers, C., Kumazawa, T., & Spring, B. (1999). Schizophrenia, monoamine oxidase activity, and cigarette smoking. *Neuropsychopharmacology, 20,* 392–394.

Sinkkonen, S. T., Hanna, M. C., Kirkness, E. F., & Korpi, E. R. (2000). GABA$_A$ receptor ε and θ subunits display unusual structural variation between species and are enriched in the rat locus ceruleus. *Journal of Neuroscience, 20,* 3588–3595.

Sommer, S. S., Lind, T. J., Heston, L. L., & Sobell, J. L. (1993). Dopamine D4 receptor variants in unrelated schizophrenic cases and controls. *American Journal of Medical Genetics, 48,* 90–93.

Souery, D., Lipp, O., Mahieu, B., Mendelbaum, K., De Martelaer, V., Van Broeckhoven, C., & Mendlewicz, J. (1996). Association study of bipolar disorder with candidate genes involved in catecholamine neurotransmission: *DRD2, DRD3, DAT1,* and *TH* genes. *American Journal of Medical Genetics, 67,* 366–368.

Spurlock, G., Heils, A., Holmans, P., Williams, J., D'Souza, U. M., Cardno, A., Murphy, K. C., Jones, L., Buckland, P. R., McGuffin, P., Lesch, K. P., & Owen, M. J. (1998). A family based association study of T102C polymorphism in 5HT2A and schizophrenia plus identification of new polymorphisms in the promoter. *Molecular Psychiatry, 3,* 42–49.

Strous, R. D., Bark, N., Parsia, S. S., Volavka, J., & Lachman, H. M. (1997). Analysis of a functional catechol-O-methyltransferase gene polymorphism in schizophrenia: Evidence for association with aggressive and anti-social behavior. *Psychiatry Research, 69,* 71–77.

Suarez, B. K., Parsian, A., Hampe, C. L., Todd, R. D., Reich, T., & Cloninger, C. R. (1994). Linkage disequilibria at the D2 dopamine receptor locus (DRD2) in alcoholics and controls. *Genomics, 19,* 12–20.

Szathmáry, E., Jordán, F., & Pál, C. (2001). Can genes explain biological complexity? *Science, 292,* 1315–1316.

Tahir, E., Yazgan, Y., Cirakoglu, B., Ozbay, F., Waldman, I., & Asherson, P. J. (2000). Association and linkage of DRD4 and DRD5 with attention deficit hyperactivity disorder (ADHD) in a sample of Turkish children. *Molecular Psychiatry, 5,* 396–404.

Tanaka, T., Igarashi, S., Onodera, O., Tanaka, H., Takahashi, M., Maeda, M., Kameda, K., Tsuji, S., & Ihda, S. (1996). Association study between schizophrenia and dopamine D3 receptor gene polymorphism. *American Journal of Medical Genetics, 67,* 366–368.

Tellegen, A., Lykken, D. T., Bouchard, T. J., Wilcox, K. J., Rich, S., & Segal, N. L. (1988). Personality similarity in twins reared apart and together. *Journal of Personality and Social Psychology, 54,* 1031–1039.

Tenhunen, J., Salminen, M., Lundstrom, K., Kiviluoto, T., Savolainen, R., & Ulmanen, I. (1994). Genomic organization of the human catechol O-methyltransferase gene and its expression from two distinct promoters. *European Journal of Biochemistry, 223,* 1049–1059.

Ticku, M. K. (1991). Drug modulation of GABA$_A$-mediated transmission. *Seminars in Neuroscience, 3,* 211–218.

Tordjman, S., Gutneckt, L., Carlier, M., Spitz, E., Antoine, C., Slama, F., Cohen, D. J., Ferrari, P., Roubertoux, P. L. & Anderson, G. M. (2001). Role of the serotonin transporter in the behavioral expression of autism. *Molecular Psychiatry, 6,* 434–439.

Toth, K., Freund, T. F., & Miles, R. (1997). Disinhibition of rat hippocampal pyramidal cells by GABAergic afferents from the septum. *Journal of Physiology, 500,* 463–474.

Tsai, S. J., Hong, C. J., & Wang, Y. C. (1999). Tryptophan hydroxylase gene polymorphism (A218C) and suicidal behaviors. *NeuroReport, 10,* 3773–3775.

Vandenbergh, D. J., Persico, A. M., Hawkins, A. L., Griffin, G. A., Li, X., Jabs, E. W., & Uhl, G. R. (1992). Human dopamine transporter gene (DAT$_1$) maps to chromosome 5p15.3 and displays a VNTR. *Geonomics, 14,* 1866–1868.

Vandenbergh, D. J., Thompson, M. D., Cook, E. H., Bendahhou, E., Nguyen, T., Krasowski, M. D., Zarribian, D., Comings, D., Sellers, E. M., Tyndale, R. F., George, S. R., O'Dowd, B. F., & Uhl, G. R. (2000). Human dopamine transporter gene: Coding regions conservation among normal, Tourette's disorder, alcohol dependence, and attention-deficit hyperactivity disorder populations. *Molecular Psychiatry, 5,* 283–292.

Van Tol, H. H. M., Bunzow, J. R., Guan, H. C., Sunahara, R. K., Seeman, P., Niznik, H. B., & Civelli, O. (1991). Cloning of the gene for a human dopamine D4 receptor with high affinity for the antipsychotic clozapine. *Nature, 350,* 610–614.

Van Tol, H. H. M., Wu, C. M., Guan, H. C., Ohara, K., Bunzow, J. R., Civelli, O., Kennedy, J., Seeman, P., Niznik, H. B., & Jovanovic, V. (1992). Multiple dopamine D4 receptor variants in the human population. *Nature, 358,* 149–152.

Veenstra-VanderWeele, J., Anderson, G., & Cook, E. H. (2000). Pharmacogenetics and the serotonin system: Initial studies and future directions. *European Journal of Pharmacology, 410,* 165–181.

Viken, R. J., Rose, R. J., Kaprio, J., & Koskenvuo, M. (1994). A developmental genetic analysis of adult personality: Extraversion and neuroticism from 18 to 59 years of age. *Journal of Personality and Social Psychology, 66,* 722–730.

Volavka, J. (1999). The neurobiology of violence: An update. *Journal of Neuropsychiatry and Clinical Neurosciences, 11,* 307–314.

Waldman, I. D., Robinson, B. F., & Feigon, S. A. (1997). Linkage disequilibrium between the dopamine transporter gene (DAT1) and bipolar affective disorder: Extending the transmission disequilibrium test (TDT) to examine genetic heterogeneity. *Genetic Epidemiology, 14,* 699–704.

Wei, J., Ramchand, C. N., & Hemming, G. P. (1997). Possible control of dopamine-beta-hydroxylase via a docominant mechanism associated with the polymorphic $(GT)_n$ repeat in its gene locus in healthy individuals. *Human Genetics, 99,* 52–55.

Weinshilboum, R. M., Raymond, F. A., Elveback, L. R., & Weidman, W. H. (1973). Serum dopamine-beta-hydroxylase activity: Sibling–sibling correlation. *Science, 181,* 943–945.

Wells, J. E., Porter, J. T., & Agmon, A. (2000). GABAergic inhibition suppresses paroxysmal network activity in the neonatal rodent hippocampus and neocortex. *Journal of Neuroscience, 20,* 8822–8830.

Wiese, C., Lannfeld, L., Kristbjarnarson, H., Yang, L., Zoega, T., Sokoloff, P., Ivarsson, O., Schwartz, J. C., Moises, H. W., & Helgarson, T. (1993). No evidence of linkage between schizophrenia and D3 dopamine receptor gene locus in Icelandic pedigree. *Psychiatric Research, 46,* 69–78.

Wilkinson, L. O., & Dourish, C. T. (1991). *Serotonin and animal behavior: Basic and clinical aspects.* New York: Wiley-Liss.

Wu, M., Shanabrough, M., Leranth, C., & Alreja, M. (2000). Cholinergic excitation of septohippocampal GABA but not cholinergic neurons: Implications for learning and memory. *Journal of Neuroscience, 20,* 3900–3908.

Zabetian, C. P., Anderson, G. M., Buxbaum, S. G., Elston, R. C., Ichinose, H., Nagatsu, T., Kim, K.-S., Kim, C.-H., Malison, R. T., Gelernter, J., & Cubells, J. F. (2001). A quantitative-trait analysis of human plasma-dopamine-β-hydroxylase activity: Evidence for a major functional polymorphism at the *DBH* locus. *American Journal of Human Genetics, 68,* 515–522.

Zhu, Q. S., Grimbsy, J., Chen, K., & Shih, J. C. (1992). Promoter organizations and activity of human monoamine oxidase (MAO) A and B genes. *Journal of Neuroscience, 12,* 4437–4446.

Zhu, Q. S., & Shih, J. C. (1997). An extensive repeat structure down-regulates human monoamine oxidase A promoter activity independent of an initiator-like sequence. *Journal of Neurochemistry, 69,* 1368–1373.

Zilles, K., Wu, J., Crucio, W. E., & Schwegler, H. (2000). Water maze and radizl maze learning and the density of binding sites of glutamate, GABA, and serotonin receptors in the hippocampus of inbred mouse strains. *Hippocampus, 10,* 213–225.

CHAPTER 3

Individual Differences in Childhood Shyness
Origins, Malleability, and Developmental Course

LOUIS A. SCHMIDT
NATHAN A. FOX

The adult personality literature has a long and rich history in its references to (Allport, 1937; Murray, 1938) and its search for (see, e.g., Eysenck, 1947, 1953, 1967, 1990) psychophysiological correlates of individual differences in personality. Allport (1937) called personality traits, "neuropsychic dispositions" and seemed to hope for more "aid from neurophysiology" (p. 319), whereas Murray (1938) emphasized that personality processes are "dominant configurations in the brain" and regretted "at present . . . they must be inferred" (p. 45). Eysenck (1947), following the lead of the promissory note suggested by Allport and Murray almost a decade earlier, was among the first contemporary personality theorists to examine the psychophysiological basis of personality traits and to establish in a systematic body of empirical research that there were significant physiological correlates of individual differences in personality. Unfortunately, the developmental psychology community during this time was slow to embrace the notion of a biological influence on individual differences in personality. This was due largely to the fact that the zeitgeist in child development reflected that of mainstream psychology in the 1940s and for the next four decades. During this period, behaviorism was firmly in place, and the idea that internal processes may influence behavior was viewed disparagingly. The following 30 years or so witnessed the impact of cognitive psychology, in which rules, abstractions, and categories became the common lexicon. Biology was again relegated to the side as psychology dealt solely with the "mind." Within the past two decades, however, we have seen a shift in the prevailing mood in how behavior is viewed. This shift has been due largely to theoretical and methodological advances in the field of neuroscience. The 1990s ushered in the "decade of the brain," and brain mechanisms involved in regulating and motivating behavior in animals and humans were reliably identified. Indeed, the idea that internal processes such as emotion and physiology may influence behavior is no longer foreign today due primarily to the work with animals by LeDoux (1996) and Panksepp (1998) and the work with humans by Damasio (1999) and Davidson (2000). The field of personality development, similar to many facets of psychology today, has not been immune to these rapid developments and advances in the neurosciences.

In this chapter, we discuss one temperamental trait that has been the focus of our respective research programs and that of much research over the past two decades in the field of personality development. We have come to know this trait as "behavioral inhibition" or temperamental shyness. The study of the biological basis of childhood shyness, which has been the focus of our research, provides a model example to examine and address some of the popular issues in developmental research today. These questions inform both developmentalists and adult personality theorists and concern questions such as: Are there neural mechanisms underlying personality? Are these brain systems open to change? and What factors influence change?

We address five overarching questions in this chapter, specifically:

1. What is shyness and why study it?
2. Are there neural substrates of temperamental shyness?
3. Are changes in phenotypic expression of temperamental shyness coincident with physiological changes?
4. Are there individual differences in temperamental shyness?
5. What are the origins of different types of temperamental shyness in children?

We conclude by providing some suggestions for future research in this area.

WHAT IS SHYNESS AND WHY STUDY IT?

Shyness reflects a preoccupation of the self in response to, or anticipation of, novel social encounters. Although shyness is a ubiquitous phenomenon that a large percentage of adults have reported experiencing at some point in their lives (Zimbardo, 1977), a smaller percentage of adults and children (around 10–15%) are consistently anxious, quiet, and behaviorally inhibited during social situations, particularly unfamiliar social situations (see Cheek & Buss, 1981; Kagan, 1994). As is discussed later, many of these shy children exhibit a distinct pattern of behavioral and physiological responses during baseline conditions and in response to social challenge in infancy and through the early school-age years (see Calkins, Fox, & Marshall, 1996; Fox, Henderson, Rubin, Calkins, & Schmidt, 2001; Fox et al., 1995; Fox, Schmidt, Calkins, Rubin, & Coplan, 1996; Kagan, Reznick, & Snidman, 1987, 1988; Schmidt & Fox, 1998; Schmidt, et al., 1997; Schmidt, Fox, Schulkin, & Gold, 1999). Moreover, some of these children may be at risk for anxiety and internalizing-related (e.g., depression, social withdrawal) problems during early development (see, e.g., Hirshfeld et al., 1992; Rubin, Stewart, & Coplan, 1995) and problems during later years (Bell et al., 1993; Caspi, Elder, & Bem, 1988; Schmidt & Fox, 1995; Zimbardo, 1977). These children we describe as temperamentally shy.

ARE THERE NEURAL SUBSTRATES OF TEMPERAMENTAL SHYNESS?

Neural Circuitry of the Fear System

Current thinking suggests that the origins of shy behavior may be linked to the dysregulation of some components of the fear system (LeDoux, 1996; Nader & LeDoux, 1999). Fear is a highly conserved emotion that is seen across mammals. It is the study of fear that has produced the most reliable evidence to date concerning the neuroanatomical circuitry of emotion. There is a rich and growing literature from studies of conditioned fear in animals that suggests that the frontal cortex and forebrain limbic areas are important components of the fear system. The frontal cortex is known to play a key role in the regulation of fear and other emotions. This region is involved in the motor facilitation of emotion expression, the organization and integration of cognitive processes that underlie emotion, and the ability to regulate emotions (see Fox, 1991, 1994). The frontal region also appears to regulate forebrain sites involved in the expression of emotion. The amygdala (and central nucleus) is one such forebrain/limbic site. There are demonstrated functional anatomical connections between the amygdala and the frontal region. The amygdala (and the central nucleus) receives input from neocortical sites, in particular, the frontal cortex. There are also links between the amygdala (and the central nucleus) and lower brain stem nuclei that are used in the regulation of autonomic output. The central nucleus of the amygdala receives visceral projections from the solitary and parabrachial nuclei in the lower brain stem, projecting directly to these regions in addition to other areas of the brain stem that are intimately involved in arousal (see Rosen & Schulkin, 1998, and Schulkin, McEwen, & Gold, 1994, for reviews of the neuroanatomical connections of the amygdala and neural circuitry of the fear system).

The amygdala (particularly the central nucleus) is known to play a significant role in the autonomic and behavioral aspects of conditioned fear (LeDoux, Iwata, Cicchetti, & Reis, 1988). For example, electrical stimulation of the central nucleus facilitates fear-potentiated startle responses (Rosen & Davis, 1988), whereas lesions to the amygdala and the central nucleus disrupt conditioned fear (Gallagher, Graham, & Holland, 1990; Hitchcock & Davis, 1986; Kapp, Frysinger, Gallagher, & Haselton, 1979; LeDoux, Sakaguchi, Iwata, & Reis, 1986). Still others have shown that electrically kindling the amygdala, but not the dorsal hippocampus, facilitates fear responses in rats (Rosen, Hamerman, Sitcoske, Glowa, & Schulkin, 1996). The amygdala also appears to be involved in the attentional aspects related to the recognition of changes in negatively valenced environmental stimuli (Gallagher & Holland, 1994). Interestingly, the amygdala is known to be more reactive in defensive rather than nondefensive cats (Adamec, 1991). These behaviors may be analogous to those seen in temperamentally shy children.

Temperamental Antecedents of Shyness

The focus of our research programs has been on understanding the biological basis of childhood shyness and identifying early infant predictors of shyness using a multimeasure, multimethod approach (see Schmidt & Fox, 1999). Much of this work was influenced by the research of Jerome Kagan and his colleagues at Harvard. Kagan and his colleagues (Kagan & Snidman, 1991a, 1991b) have argued that the origins of shyness in some children may be linked to individual differences in early infant reactivity. For example, infants who exhibit a high degree of motor activity and distress in response to the presentation of novel auditory and visual stimuli during the first 4 months of life exhibit a high degree of behavioral inhibition and shyness during the preschool and early school-age years. There is, in addition, evidence to suggest that there may be a genetic etiology to inhibited behavior. Kagan and colleagues (DiLalla, Kagan, & Reznick, 1994) noted in a behavior study of 157 twin pairs aged 24 months that monozygotic twins showed stronger intraclass correlations of inhibited behavior to unfamiliar stimuli than dizygotic twins and nontwin siblings. Kagan (1994, 1999) speculated that individual differences in infant reactivity to novelty may be linked to sensitivity in forebrain circuits involved in the processing and regulation of emotion. Kagan (1994, 1999) has argued that children who become easily distressed and subdued during the presentation of novel stimuli may have a lower threshold for arousal in forebrain areas, particularly the central nucleus of the amygdala. This hypothesis is based largely on findings from studies of animals in which the amygdala plays an important role in the regulation and maintenance of conditioned fear.

We have used measures of frontal electroencephalographic (EEG) activity and the startle eyeblink response to test Kagan's speculation (see Schmidt & Fox, 1999, for a review). These two measures are thought to index forebrain limbic and frontal cortical areas involved in the regulation of emotion. The choice to use frontal EEG measures comes from two lines of research. First, the pattern of frontal EEG activity is known to be related to the processing of emotion. In a series of studies with human infants, Fox and his colleagues (see Fox, 1991, for a review) have noted that the pattern of frontal EEG activity distinguishes different types of emotion. Infants exhibit greater relative right frontal EEG activity during the processing of negative emotion (e.g., fear, disgust, sadness) and greater relative left frontal EEG activity during the processing of positive emotions (e.g., happiness, joy, interest). In a series of studies with human adults, Davidson and his colleagues (see Davidson, 1993; Davidson & Rickman, 1999, for a review; see also Schmidt & Trainor, 2001) have noted similar relations between the pattern of asymmetrical frontal brain activity and the processing of emotion.

A second line of research suggests that individual differences in the pattern of resting frontal brain electrical activity (EEG) may reflect a predisposition (i.e., trait) to experience and express positive and negative emotion, both in infants (see, e.g., Fox, 1991, 1994) and adults (see, e.g., Davidson, 1993). For example, Fox and his colleagues have noted a relationship between individual differences in resting frontal EEG activity and affective or temperamental style. Infants who displayed greater relative resting right frontal EEG activity were more likely to cry and exhibit distress to an approaching stranger during the 2nd half of the 1st year of life than infants who exhibit greater relative left resting frontal EEG activity (Davidson & Fox, 1989; Fox, Bell, & Jones, 1992). A similar relation between the pattern of resting frontal EEG asymmetry and affective style has been noted in adults.

In a series of studies with adults, Davidson and his colleagues have noted a relationship between the pattern of resting frontal EEG activity and affective style. Adults who exhibit a pattern of greater relative resting right frontal EEG activity are known to rate affective film clips more negatively (Tomarken, Davidson, & Henriques, 1990) and are likely to be more depressed (Henriques & Davidson, 1990, 1991) than adults who exhibit greater relative resting left frontal EEG activity. In addition, adults who exhibited a stable pattern of right frontal asymmetry across a 3-week time period reported more intense negative emotion in response to negative affective film clips compared with individuals who displayed stable left frontal EEG asymmetry (Wheeler, Davidson, & Tomarken, 1993).

The other measure of choice that we have used to index forebrain contributions to shyness has been the startle eyeblink response. The startle response is a brain-stem- and forebrain-mediated behavioral response that occurs to the presentation of a sudden and intense stimulus, and its neural circuitry is well mapped (Davis, Hitchcock, & Rosen, 1987). Although the startle paradigm has been used extensively in studies of conditioned fear in animals, this measure has been adapted for studies concerning the etiology of anxiety in humans. Similar to frontal EEG measures, there are two lines of research that have implicated the startle response in emotion regulation.

The first line has demonstrated that the magnitude of the startle response varies linearly with the valence of emotion. Lang and his colleagues (see Lang, Bradley, & Cuthbert, 1990, for a review) have shown that adults exhibit exaggerated startle responses during the processing of highly arousing negatively valenced stimuli (e.g., accident scenes) and attenuated startle responses during the processing of highly arousing positively valenced stimuli (e.g., opposite sex nudes), compared with their reactions to neutral stimuli (e.g., light bulb). A second line of research has found that individual differences in the startle response are linked to affective style. For example, adults who score high on trait measures of anxiety (Grillon, Ameli, Foot, & Davis, 1993) and children who are behaviorally inhibited (Snidman & Kagan, 1994) are known to exhibit a heightened baseline startle response.

Using a design identical to that reported by Kagan and Snidman (1991b), Fox and his colleagues (Calkins et al., 1996) examined the behavioral and psychophysiological antecedents of shyness in a group of infants selected at age 4 months for temperamental constellations thought to predict behavioral inhibition and shyness in early childhood. Eighty-one healthy infants were selected at age 4 months from a larger sample of 207 infants. The infants were observed in their homes at age 4 months and videotaped as they responded to novel auditory and visual stimuli. The 81 infants were selected based on their frequency of motor activity and the degree of positive and negative affect they displayed in response to these novel stimuli. Three reactivity groups were formed: *Negative reactive* (*n* = 31) comprised infants who displayed both high amounts of motor activity and negative affect and low amounts of positive affect;

positive reactive (n = 19) comprised infants who displayed both high amounts of motor activity and positive affect and low amounts of negative affect; and *low reactive* (n = 31) comprised infants who displayed low amounts of motor activity and low amounts of both positive affect and negative affect. The infants were then seen in the laboratory at 9, 14, and 24 months, at which time regional brain electrical activity (EEG) was recorded using a Lycra stretch cap while the infant was seated, alert, and attentive. EEG was recorded from the left and right anterior and posterior brain regions. The startle eyeblink response was recorded during a stranger-approach situation at 9 months of age. Startle eyeblink responses were measured from two miniature electrodes placed around the infant's right eye. Infants were presented with a 95 dB burst of white noise for 50 ms and during the approach of an unfamiliar adult. In addition, behavioral responses to the presentation of unfamiliar social and nonsocial stimuli were indexed at 14 and 24 months. We (Schmidt & Fox, 1998) found that infants classified as *negative reactive* at 4 months exhibited a significantly greater startle amplitude to an approaching stranger at 9 months than did infants in the other two 4-month reactivity groups. The negative reactive infants were also more likely to exhibit greater relative right frontal EEG activity at 9 months (Calkins et al., 1996) and 24 months (Fox, Calkins, & Bell, 1994) and more inhibition to novel stimuli at ages 14 and 24 months (Calkins et al., 1996; Fox et al., 1994) than the other two 4-month reactivity groups. These findings were consistent with Kagan's prediction. It seems plausible, then, to speculate that the frontal EEG and startle measures may be indexing individual differences in forebrain and limbic sensitivity.

Behavioral and Physiological Correlates in Temperamentally Shy Children

The pattern of physiological and behavioral responses seen in temperamentally reactive infants appears to be preserved into the preschool and early school-age years and is predictive of shyness. In a series of studies of preschoolers and early school-aged children, Fox and Schmidt and their colleagues noted that preschoolers who displayed a high proportion of shy behavior during peer play groups at age 4 exhibited significantly greater relative resting right frontal EEG asymmetry (Fox et al., 1995; Fox et al., 1996) and higher morning basal salivary cortisol levels (Schmidt et al., 1997) than did children displaying relatively less shy behavior at age 4. Also, children displaying a high degree of observed shy behavior during peer play were rated as contemporaneously shy at age 4 by their mothers, and a significant proportion of them were likely to have been in the *negative reactive* temperamental group at age 4 months (Schmidt et al.,

1997). Kagan and his colleagues (Kagan et al., 1987, 1988; Snidman & Kagan, 1994) had also noted earlier that temperamentally shy children were characterized by elevated morning basal cortisol levels, a high and stable heart rate, and exaggerated startle responses compared with their nonshy counterparts. More recently, Schmidt, Fox, Schulkin, et al. (1999) found that temperamentally shy children exhibited a distinct pattern of physiological responses across different physiological measures in response to stress. Schmidt, Fox, Schulkin, et al. (1999) noted that, compared with their nonshy counterparts, temperamentally shy 7-year-olds exhibited a significantly greater increase in right, but not left, frontal EEG activity and a significantly greater increase in heart rate during a self-presentation task as the task became more demanding. These physiological responses were paralleled by an increase in overt signs of behavioral anxiety. We also noted that children who were classified as low in social competence (a feature of shyness) exhibited a significantly greater change in salivary cortisol reactivity in response to the self-presentation task than did socially competent children (Schmidt, Fox, Sternberg, et al., 1999). These data suggest that children who are classified as temperamentally shy during the preschool and early school-age years exhibit a distinct pattern of frontal brain activity, heart rate, and salivary cortisol levels during baseline conditions and in response to stress.

Behavioral and Physiological Correlates of Temperamentally Shy Young Adults

One of the goals of our research program on shyness has been to examine the developmental course and outcomes of temperamental shyness beyond the early childhood years, given that temperamental shyness appears to remain stable and predictive of developmental outcomes (Caspi et al., 1988). Overall, the behavioral and physiological correlates and outcomes associated with temperamentally shy children are comparable with those seen in adults who score high on trait measures of shyness. For example, adults who report a high degree of trait shyness are likely to report concurrent feelings of negative self-worth and problems with depression in both elderly (Bell et al., 1993) and young (Schmidt & Fox, 1995) adult populations and to display a distinct pattern of central and autonomic activity during resting conditions and in response to social stressors (see Schmidt & Fox, 1999, for a review).

In two separate studies (Schmidt, 1999; Schmidt & Fox, 1994), we examined the behavioral and physiological correlates of shyness in a group of young adults who scored high on self-report measures of trait shyness (Cheek & Buss, 1981). We recorded regional brain electrical activity

(EEG) and heart rate during baseline conditions and during a socially challenging situation. We found that, compared with their nonshy counterparts, adults reporting a high degree of trait shyness exhibited greater relative baseline right frontal EEG activity and a higher and more stable heart rate in anticipation of a social encounter with an unfamiliar same-sex peer. (High heart rate and low heart rate variability are thought to reflect markers of an ability to regulate stress [Porges, 1991].) The findings for adults extended our prior work with temperamentally shy children. That is, during baseline and socially challenging situations, a pattern of physiological activity was observed on frontal brain activity and heart rate in adults who scored high on a self-report measure of trait shyness that was similar to that in temperamentally shy children and high-reactive infants. Regardless of age, temperamental shyness was related to greater relative right frontal EEG activity during baseline conditions and to an increase in autonomic and frontal brain activity during social stress. Given the similarities in physiological activity between temperamentally shy children and young adults during baseline and emotionally challenging conditions, these data, taken together, raise the possibility that the origins of shyness for some people may be rooted in early temperamental constellations that may be inherited and preserved over the lifespan.

ARE CHANGES IN PHENOTYPIC EXPRESSION OF TEMPERAMENTAL SHYNESS COINCIDENT WITH PHYSIOLOGICAL CHANGES?

Although historical accounts, such as Freud's writings and Spitz's work with children who were orphaned, suggested that personality was fixed at an early age, recent behavioral and neuroscience data seriously question this view. Indeed, the idea that the affective system is open to change appears to be more the rule than the exception. Brain systems involved in affective processes are highly plastic during early postnatal life and beyond, and the brain is highly susceptible to environmental input during the early years of life. The socialization processes that form personality are not immune to these influences. In fact, our research demonstrates that some of the infants classified as highly reactive and easily distressed by novelty in early infancy do not go on to develop shyness, suggesting that children in this category are open to change (Fox et al., 2001). What are the experiential factors that may be influential in affecting this change?

   To date, comparatively few studies have examined the stability of infant behavioral and physiological predictors that underlie childhood shyness. Kagan (1991) noted that there was a fair degree of discontinuity in behavioral inhibition during the first 7 years of life. However, these sets of observations were based on behavioral and physiological measures collected at or after the 2nd year of life. The lack of attention directed toward the stability of infant predictors of childhood shyness has been due in large part to the small number of existing longitudinal studies that could answer such questions.

We have attempted to make inroads into rectifying this apparent void in the literature in at least three ways: (1) by examining the short-term stability within age group of infant behavioral and physiological measures that are known to correlate with and to be predictive of childhood shyness, (2) by examining the stability of behavioral and physiological measures within the infant temperament category that Kagan describes as predictive of behavioral inhibition and childhood shyness, and (3) by identifying factors from our longitudinal data that appear to influence change in the phenotypic expression of shyness.

Stability of Frontal EEG Asymmetry Measure within Age Group

We (Schmidt, 2000) have examined the short-term stability of frontal EEG asymmetry by studying second-by-second stability for 90 seconds in the pattern of frontal EEG activity in relation to temperament and autonomic patterning in 9-month-old human infants. We computed a traditional frontal EEG asymmetry score using right frontal EEG power *minus* left frontal EEG power for each of the 1-second periods. Positive scores on this metric are thought to reflect greater relative left frontal EEG activity (Davidson & Tomarken, 1989). We then formed three groups of infants based on the psychometric properties of the individual asymmetry scores. *Group 1* comprised infants whose mean value was negative across the individual asymmetry scores and whose variability was low; *Group 2* comprised infants whose mean value was positive across the individual asymmetry scores and whose variability was low; and *Group 3* comprised infants whose mean value was around zero across the individual asymmetry scores and whose variability was high. In other words, Groups 1 and 2 exhibited a stable pattern of either right or left frontal EEG activity, whereas infants in Group 3 exhibited a pattern of frontal EEG activity that was highly variable and changing. We were able to distinguish the three groups based on measures of maternal report of infant temperament and heart rate. Group 1 infants were, overall, reported to be more easily distressed by novelty and exhibited a higher resting heart rate than infants in the other two asymmetry groups. These findings suggest that infants exhibiting a stable pattern of greater relative right frontal EEG activity are more likely to be temperamentally distressed by novelty as reported by their mothers at age 9 months. This temperamental distress is analogous to the temperamental reactions that Kagan (Kagan & Snidman, 1991b) describes as being predictive of childhood shyness.

Stability of Behavioral and Physiological Measures across Ages

We (Fox et al., 2001) have examined the stability of behavioral and physiological measures within the infant temperament group that Kagan has found to be predictive of behavioral inhibition and shyness with the hope of understanding why some of these infants do not go on to develop shyness. As noted earlier, we selected three temperamentally reactive groups at age 4 months (i.e., *negative, positive,* and *low reactive*). Infants in the negative reactive group have been found to display behavioral inhibition in the 2nd year. We examined the stability of behavior and frontal EEG asymmetry from 9 to 24 months and noted the following: (1) as predicted, a significant percentage of infants within the high-reactive group exhibited a stable pattern of right frontal EEG activity from 9 to 24 months of age; (2) those who exhibited this pattern across this time period were likely to be behaviorally inhibited at 24 months; and (3) within the high-reactive-temperament category, those infants whose behavior patterns changed over age also displayed a change in frontal EEG asymmetry. Both biology and behavior were linked, remaining constant over time for those infants who displayed continuity of shyness and change over time for those who changed from shy to nonshy in their behavior.

Influence of Gender and Day Care

A third area of interest is to look for variables that may be related to or influence change. We (Fox et al., 2001) noted that the children who remained continuously shy across the first 4 years of life were more likely to be boys than girls and more likely to be in home care than day-care. In other words, girls were more likely than boys to change in the expression of temperamental shyness (to display less shy behavior over time). This pattern also was true for children who entered day care more than for those who stayed at home. Although we did not have any direct measures of mother–infant interaction, these two findings suggest that patterns of early socialization may influence the expression of temperamental shyness. In our data, boys who displayed behavioral inhibition were more likely to remain inhibited and shy over time. A number of researchers have commented on the differential salience of shyness for boys versus girls (Stevenson-Hinde & Glover, 1996). Boys who are shy are more of a source of concern for parents than are girls, because in U.S. culture boys are not expected to be fearful or nonexploratory in novel environments. This increased salience could possibly bring with it increased concern on the part of parents and overprotectiveness toward the child. Rather than moderating the child's fear and shyness, such maternal overprotectiveness might actually serve to exacerbate the shy behavior. In a study with 4-year old inhibited children, we (Rubin, Cheah, & Fox, 2001) found that those shy children with overprotective mothers were more likely to display social withdrawal when confronted with unfamiliar peers than were inhibited children whose mothers were not overprotective. The day care finding might lend further support to this explanation. Temperamentally inhibited infants placed in day care were less likely to remain inhibited over time. Although we did not observe caregiving behavior within the different day care contexts, it is reasonable to assume that young children in day care are less likely to be given oversolicitous and overindulgent responsive caregiving, the type of caregiving behavior that may support shyness. In this sense, the day care experience may serve to moderate the temperament in much the same way that nonindulgent, nonoverprotective mothers may do with their children. These speculations await further intensive observation of the mother–infant interaction among temperamentally shy infants and young children.

ARE THERE INDIVIDUAL DIFFERENCES IN TEMPERAMENTAL SHYNESS?

Another goal of our research program is to understand individual differences in temperamental shyness. Not all temperamentally shy adults or children are alike. Our research suggests that different etiologies, correlates, and developmental outcomes are associated with individual differences in temperamental shyness (see, e.g., Rubin & Asendorpf, 1993).

The notion that there may be different types of shyness is not new (see, e.g., Cheek & Krasnoperova, 1999). This idea stems from empirical work derived from the adult personality literature nearly two decades ago (Cheek & Buss, 1981), as well as from theoretical work by Buss (1986) almost 15 years ago. Cheek and Buss (1981) described at least two types of shyness in undergraduates: individuals who are shy and low in sociability and individuals who are shy and high in sociability. (Interestingly, Eysenck, 1956, postulated a similar argument some 25 years earlier by examining the intersection of extraversion and neuroticism.) Cheek and Buss (1981) then proceeded to distinguish these two subtypes on behavioral measures. The shy–high-sociable undergraduates exhibited more overt behavioral anxiety during an unfamiliar social situation than the shy–low-sociable undergraduates.

Buss (1986) presented a theory in which he argued that there may be at least two types of shyness: an early-developing fearful shyness that is linked to stranger fear and wariness (perhaps analogous to the behaviorally inhibited children described by Kagan, 1994) and a later-developing self-conscious shyness that is linked to concerns with self-presentation. Little empirical research, however, has been done to substantiate Buss's theoretical model. Two studies that do exist in the literature have found support for Buss's claim in young adults. For example, Bruch, Giordano, and Pearl (1986) noted differences between fearful and self-consciously shy undergraduates in background and current adjustment. Bruch et al. (1986) noted that fearfully shy adults exhibited significantly lower scores on a test measuring how to deal with hypothetical problematic social situations than did nonshy and self-consciously shy counterparts; the nonshy and self-consciously shy groups were not distinguishable. Schmidt and Robinson (1992) found differences in self-esteem between the two shyness subtypes; the fearfully shy group reported significantly lower self-esteem than the self-consciously shy and nonshy groups.

We have used an approach–avoidance framework analogous to that of Cheek and Buss (1981) to conceptualize different types of shyness. Asendorpf and Meier (1993) have used a similar approach to conceptualize different types of shyness in children. As mentioned early, Cheek and Buss (1981) examined the relation between shyness and sociability. Cheek and Buss argued that people avoid social situations for different reasons. Some people avoid social situations because they experience fear and anxiety in such situations (i.e., they are shy); others avoid social situations because they prefer to be alone rather than with others (i.e., they are introverted). Cheek and Buss (1981) then noted that if shyness is nothing more than low sociability, then the two traits should be highly related such that being high on one trait means being low on the other. The extent to which they might be orthogonal was an empirical question. Cheek and Buss (1981) noted that the two traits were only modestly related, and they were able to distinguish them on a behavioral level. High shy–high social undergraduates exhibited significantly more behavioral anxiety than did undergraduates who reported other combinations of shyness and sociability.

We (Schmidt, 1999; Schmidt & Fox, 1994) examined the extent to which shyness and sociability were distinguishable on electrocortical and autonomic measures. Using a design identical to that reported by Cheek and Buss (1981), we attempted to distinguish shyness and sociability on regional EEG, heart rate, and heart rate variability measures collected during baseline and during a social stressor. We found that high shy–high social (i.e., the *conflicted* subtype) undergraduates exhibited a significantly faster and more stable heart rate than high shy–low social (i.e., the *avoidant* subtype) participants in response to an anticipated unfamiliar social situation (Schmidt & Fox, 1994). We also noted that both the high shy–high social (i.e., the conflicted subtype) and the high shy–low social (i.e., the avoidant subtype) undergraduates exhibited a pattern of greater relative right frontal EEG activity during baseline. However, the two subtypes were distinguishable based on the pattern of activity in the left, but not the right, frontal area. High shy–high social (the conflicted subtype) participants exhibited significantly greater activity in the left frontal EEG lead than did high shy–low social (the avoidant subtype) participants. A similar pattern of resting frontal EEG activity has been found in high shy–high social and high shy–low social 6-year-olds (Schmidt & Sniderman, 2001) similar to those noted in the young adults. These sets of findings, taken together, suggest that different types of shyness are distinguishable on behavioral, cortical, and autonomic levels during baseline conditions and in response to social challenge.

WHAT ARE THE ORIGINS OF DIFFERENT TYPES OF TEMPERAMENTAL SHYNESS IN CHILDREN?

The Model

We have been developing a frontal activation–neuroendocrine–experiential model that may account for different types of temperament shyness. This model includes a complex interaction among the environment, frontal cortex, and the hypothalamic–pituitary–adrenocortical (HPA) and serotonergic systems. We believe that the frontal cortex plays a regulatory role in mediating forebrain areas such as the amygdala and HPA system in maintaining fear triggered by genes that code for the transportation of serotonin. It may be at the level of the frontal cortex that individual differences in temperamental shyness emerge.

We speculate that genes that code for the transportation of serotonin may play an important role in the regulation of some components of the fear system, which includes the frontal cortex, forebrain limbic area, and HPA system. Serotonin has been implicated as a major neurotransmitter involved in anxiety and withdrawal (Westernberg, Murphy, & Den Boer, 1996). Some temperamentally shy individuals may possess a genetic polymorphism that contributes to a reduced efficiency of the transportation of serotonin. Such a genetic polymorphism has been noted in adults who score high on measures of neuroticism (Lesch et al., 1996). The action of this reduced serotonin expression may be particularly evident in the forebrain limbic and frontal cortex, where there are dense concentrations of serotonin receptors. The reduction of serotonin may play an important role in regulating the amygdala and HPA system: Serotonin may serve to inhibit (or regulate) the action of amygdaloid firing and activation of the HPA system. The reduction of serotonin contributes to overactivation of the amygdala and the HPA system in some individuals. The overactive amygdala stimulates the HPA system and the release of increased cortisol. This increase in cortisol may contribute to the pattern of frontal EEG activity noted early between shyness subtypes.

For example, it is possible that there is differential lateralization of glucocorticoid receptors in the frontal cortex. The frontal cortex is rich in corticosteroid receptors and has been implicated in regulating the HPA system in animals (Diorio, Viau, & Meaney, 1993). Cortisol (corticosterone in animals) is known to facilitate fear-related behaviors and responses in animals and humans, including heightened corticotropin-releasing hormone startle responses (Lee, Schulkin, & Davis, 1994) and freezing behavior (Takahashi & Rubin, 1994) in rats. Moreover, exogenous administration of synthetic cortisol is known to increase right frontal EEG activity (a marker of stress) and anxious mood in healthy human adults (Schmidt, Fox, Goldberg, Smith, & Schulkin, 1999), and adults with agitated depression (i.e., comorbidity of depression and anxiety) are known to exhibit elevated endogenous cortisol levels (Gold, Goodwin, & Chrousos, 1988).

The overactive amygdala and dysregulated HPA system perhaps lead to the increased activity noted on resting psychophysiological and neuroendocrine measures that index forebrain and frontal cortical functioning. (Interestingly, the startle response, autonomic, and frontal EEG measures are all known to be sensitive to the manipulation of cortisol and have been linked to emotion dysregulation). With this in mind, it may not be a coincidence that some temperamentally shy children are characterized by elevated basal cortisol levels, high and stable resting heart rate, exaggerated baseline startle, and greater relative resting right frontal EEG activity. Resting EEG and heart rate measures may be by-products, not casual agents, of a dysregulated fear system. The left frontal area may have a more dense collection of glucocorticoid receptors or a greater binding affinity for cortisol in high shy–high social (the conflicted subtype) people than is found in high shy–low social (the avoidant subtype) people; hence the pattern of greater activity in the left than right frontal area for the former group. Thus it is at the level of the frontal cortex that we observe individual differences in shyness. When the two shy subtypes encounter actual or perceived social stress, there is an increase in heart rate, cortisol, and frontal EEG activity. The two subtypes will differ, however, in the pattern of behavior and left frontal EEG activity. The shy–social subtype will experience an approach–avoidance conflict and a greater increase in left frontal EEG activity; the shy–low-social subtype will not experience the same conflict, as they do not have the same need to affiliate. Thus this subtype will tend to avoid social situations and will not present with the same pattern of left frontal EEG activity, although they may evidence an increase in cortisol and heart rate. It is important to point out that a number of environmental factors contribute to social stress, including parenting style, peer relations, school environment, and familial and extrafamilial variables, among many others that can trigger social inhibition in this model. Moreover, we believe that the conflicted and avoidant subtypes may be on different pathways of developmental problems. Conflicted children are likely to be highly reticent, desiring to be a part of the peer group but having problems doing so and, we think, might be on a pathway to social anxiety; the avoidant child, on the other hand, may have problems simply engaging in any social situations and may avoid them all together, desiring instead to be alone, and, we think, on a pathway to social withdrawal and depression.

Testing the Model: Future Directions

We are currently conducting a number of studies that test the frontal activation–neuroendocrine–experiential model either directly or indirectly. A number of questions have been framed regarding the issue that test: (1) different levels of the model; (2) directionality of the model; and (3) generalizability of the model to other types of children in normal and atypical development. These questions are discussed next.

First, *Is there a molecular genetic basis to different types of shyness?* We are beginning to examine the model on a genetic level (Schmidt, Fox, Perez-Edgar, Hu, & Hamer, 2001; Schmidt, Fox, Rubin, Hu, & Hamer, in press). We are currently analyzing DNA data collected from the children whom we have been following longitudinally to examine the molecular genetics and genetic variation in behavioral and physiological measures implicated by the model.

Second, *Do environmental factors influence the model prenatally and postnatally?* We are examining the influence of behavioral, cognitive-affective, and physiological functioning in infants who have been exposed prenatally to synthetic steroids. Synthetic steroids are routinely given to mothers at risk for preterm delivery and are used to facilitate fetal maturation. Little is known, however, in terms of how they influence the developing brain. Because these steroids interact with the adrenocortical system, it is possible that children treated with them may develop shyness that mimics temperamental shyness in the normally developing child.

We are also examining the model in children of parents clinically diagnosed with social phobia to see to what extent parental psychopathology influences the model.

Third, *Are there differences in cognitive processes (i.e., automatic and controlled processes) in temperamentally shy children?* We are currently examining direct and indirect responses to facial expressions of emotion and eye gaze in temperamentally shy children. Behavior and physiology are being measured concurrently in order to see if we can differentiate individual differences in shyness and different cognitive levels.

Fourth, *Are the patterns of resting physiology implicated in the model present in other states of consciousness?* In collaboration with members of the Brock University Sleep Laboratory, we are examining measures of frontal EEG activation and asymmetry during sleep in relation to temperamental shyness. If the pattern of frontal EEG reflects a trait, it should be present in other states of consciousness. Findings from these studies may shed some light on the issue of directionality. That is, if the pattern of frontal EEG asymmetry is present during sleep, it might suggest that the frontal EEG measure is reflecting processes that are perhaps not cortical. In sleep, we are in some sense turning off the cortex and possible contributions to the frontal EEG asymmetry measure. If the asymmetries exist during sleep, it may suggest that contributions from subcortical systems play an important role and that subcortical systems are playing a critical role (i.e., "bottom up" vs. "top-down").

Fifth, *Are brain-based measures of emotion spared in atypical development?* We have begun to examine the model in children and adults and the processing of emotion in children with Down syndrome, autism, selective mutism, and conduct disorders in normal development and adults with schizophrenia (Goldberg & Schmidt, 2001) and social phobia in order to see to what extent the model generalizes to these other populations.

CONCLUSIONS

Almost seven decades ago, Allport (1937) and Murray (1938) left a promissory note, and in this note there was a call to future researchers to consider the role of neural processes in personality. Since that time, mainstream psychology has seen many changes and has been influenced and dominated by different schools of thought. These early ideas were not lost, however. We agree with Walter Mischel's recent comment in the *APA Monitor* (January, 2000, pp. 82–83) that researchers should not try "to re-invent the wheel, but to build-on, create and go beyond theories that have already been developed." The issues addressed in this chapter can be traced to the early ideas and work of several adult personality theorists such as Allport, Murray, and Eysenck and their influence. We hope that the keen reader will also appreciate how far we have come since these early notions in our understanding and appreciation of complex personality traits and phenomena such as human shyness.

ACKNOWLEDGMENTS

The writing of this chapter and some of the work reported herein was supported by grants from the National Institutes of Health (HD 17899) and the John D. and Catherine T. MacArthur Foundation's Network on the Transition from Infancy to Childhood awarded to Nathan Fox and the Natural Sciences and Engineering Research Council of Canada (NSERC: 203710-00) and the Social Sciences and Humanities Research Council of Canada (SSHRC: 410-99-1206) awarded to Louis Schmidt.

REFERENCES

Adamec, R. E. (1991). Individual differences in temporal lobe sensory processing of threatening stimuli in the cat. *Physiology and Behavior, 49*, 445–464.

Allport, G. W. (1937). *Personality: A psychological interpretation.* London: Constable.

Asendorpf, J. B., & Meier, G. H. (1993). Personality effects on children's speech in everyday life: Sociability mediated exposure and shyness-mediated reactivity to social situations. *Journal of Personality and Social Psychology, 64*, 1072–1083.

Bell, I. R., Martino, G. M., Meredith, K. E., Schwartz, G. E., Siani, M. W., & Morrow, F. D. (1993). Vascular disease risk factors, urinary free cortisol, and health histories in older adults: Shyness and gender interactions. *Biological Psychology, 35*, 37–49.

Bruch, M. A., Giordano, S., & Pearl, L. (1986). Differences between fearful and self-conscious shy subtypes in background and current adjustment. *Journal of Research in Personality, 20*, 172–186.

Buss, A.H. (1986). A theory of shyness. In W. H. Jones, J. M. Cheek, & S. R. Briggs (Eds.), *Shyness: Perspectives on research and treatment* (pp. 39–46). New York: Plenum Press.

Calkins, S. D., Fox, N. A., & Marshall, T. R. (1996). Behavioral and physiological antecedents of inhibited and uninhibited behavior. *Child Development, 67*, 523–540.

Caspi, A., Elder, G. H., & Bem, D. J. (1988). Moving away from the world: Life-course patterns of shy children. *Developmental Psychology, 24*, 824–831.

Cheek, J. M., & Buss, A. H. (1981). Shyness and sociability. *Journal of Personality and Social Psychology, 41*, 330–339.

Cheek, J. M., & Krasnoperova, E. N. (1999). Varieties of shyness in adolescence and adulthood. In L.A. Schmidt & J. Schulkin (Eds.), *Extreme fear, shyness, and social phobia: Origins, biological mechanisms, and clinical outcomes* (pp. 224–250). New York: Oxford University Press.

Damasio, A. R. (1999). *The feeling of what happens: Body and emotion in the making of consciousness.* New York: Harcourt Brace.

Davidson, R. J. (1993). The neuropsychology of emotion and affective style. In M. Lewis & J. M. Haviland (Eds.), *Handbook of emotions* (pp.143–154). New York: Guilford Press.

Davidson, R. J. (2000). Affective style, psychopathology, and resilience: Brain mechanisms and plasticity. *American Psychologist, 55,* 1196–1214.

Davidson, R. J., & Fox, N. A. (1989). The relation between tonic EEG asymmetry and ten-month-olds' emotional response to separation. *Journal of Abnormal Psychology, 98,* 127–131.

Davidson, R. J., & Rickman, M. (1999). Behavioral inhibition and the emotional circuitry of the brain: Stability and plasticity during the early childhood years. In L. A. Schmidt & J. Schulkin (Eds.), *Extreme fear, shyness, and social phobia: Origins, biological mechanisms, and clinical outcomes* (pp. 67–87). New York: Oxford University Press.

Davidson, R. J., & Tomarken, A. J. (1989). Laterality and emotion: An electrophysiological approach. In F. Boller & J. Grafman (Eds.), *Handbook of neuropsychology* (pp. 419–441). Amsterdam: Elsevier Science.

Davis, M., Hitchcock, J. M., & Rosen, J. B. (1987). Anxiety and the amygdala: Pharmacological and anatomical analysis of the fear-potentiated startle paradigm. In G. Bower (Ed.), *The psychology of learning and motivation* (Vol. 21, pp. 263–305). San Diego, CA: Academic Press.

DiLalla, L. F., Kagan, J., & Reznick, J. S. (1994). Genetic etiology of behavioral inhibition among 2-year-old children. *Infant Behavior and Development, 17,* 405–412.

Diorio, D., Viau, V., & Meaney, M. J. (1993). The role of the medial prefrontal cortex (cingulate gyrus) in the regulation of hypothalamic-pituitary-adrenal responses to stress. *Journal of Neuroscience, 13,* 3839–3847.

Eysenck, H. J. (1947). *Dimensions of personality.* London: Routledge & Kegan Paul.

Eysenck, H. J. (1953). *The structure of human personality.* London: Methuen.

Eysenck, H. J. (1956). The questionnaire measurement of neuroticism and extraversion. *Revista Psicologia, 50,* 113–140.

Eysenck, H. J. (1967). *The biological basis of personality.* Springfield, IL: Thomas.

Eysenck, H. J. (1990). Biological dimensions of personality. In L. A. Pervin (Ed.), *Handbook of personality: Theory and research* (pp. 244–276). New York: Guilford Press.

Fox, N. A. (1991). If it's not left, it's right: Electroencephalogram asymmetry and the development of emotion. *American Psychologist, 46,* 863–872.

Fox, N. A. (1994). Dynamic cerebral processes underlying emotion regulation. In N. A. Fox (Ed.), The development of emotion regulation: Behavioral and biological considerations. *Monographs of the Society for Research in Child Development, 59*(2–3, Serial No. 240), 152–166.

Fox, N. A., Bell, M. A., & Jones, N. A. (1992). Individual differences in response to stress and cerebral asymmetry. *Developmental Neuropsychology, 8*, 161–184.

Fox, N. A., Calkins, S. D., & Bell, M. A. (1994). Neural plasticity and development in the first two years of life: Evidence from cognitive and socioemotional domains of research. *Development and Psychopathology, 6*, 677–696.

Fox, N. A., Henderson, H. A., Rubin, K. H., Calkins, S. D., & Schmidt, L. A. (2001). Continuity and discontinuity of behavioral inhibition and exuberance: Psychophysiological and behavioral influences across the first four years of life. *Child Development, 72*, 1–21.

Fox, N. A., Rubin, K. H., Calkins, S. D., Marshall, T. R., Coplan, R. J., Porges, S. W., Long, J. M., & Stewart, S. (1995). Frontal activation asymmetry and social competence at four years of age. *Child Development, 66*, 1770–1784.

Fox, N. A., Schmidt, L. A., Calkins, S. D., Rubin, K. H., & Coplan, R. J. (1996). The role of frontal activation in the regulation and dysregulation of social behavior during the preschool years. *Development and Psychopathology, 8*, 89–102.

Gallagher, M., Graham, P. W. A., & Holland, P. C. (1990). The amygdala central nucleus and appetitive Pavlovian conditioning: Lesions impair one class of conditioned behavior. *Journal of Neuroscience, 10*, 1906–1911.

Gallagher, M., & Holland, P. C. (1994). The amygdala complex: Multiple roles in associative learning and attention. *Proceedings of the National Academy of Sciences, 91*, 11771–11776.

Gold, P. W., Goodwin, F. K., & Chrousos, G. P. (1988). Clinical and biochemical manifestations of depression (Pts. 1–2). *New England Journal of Medicine, 319*, 348–353; 413–420.

Goldberg, J. O., & Schmidt, L. A. (2001). Shyness, sociability, and social dysfunction in schizophrenia. *Schizophrenia Research, 48*, 343–349.

Grillon, C., Ameli, R., Foot, M., & Davis, M. (1993). Fear-potentiated startle: Relationship to state/trait anxiety in healthy subjects. *Biological Psychiatry, 33*, 566–574.

Henriques, J. B., & Davidson, R. J. (1990). Regional brain electrical asymmetries discriminate between previously depressed subjects and healthy controls. *Journal of Abnormal Psychology, 99*, 22–31.

Henriques, J. B., & Davidson, R. J. (1991). Left frontal hypoactivation in depression. *Journal of Abnormal Psychology, 100*, 535–545.

Hirshfeld, D. R., Rosenbaum, J. F., Biederman, J., Bolduc, E. A., Faraone, S. V., Snidman, N., Reznick, J. S., & Kagan, J. (1992). Stable behavioral inhibition and its association with anxiety disorder. *Journal of the American Academy of Child and Adolescent Psychiatry, 31*, 103–111.

Hitchcock, J., & Davis, M. (1986). Lesion of the amygdala, but not the cerebellum or the red nucleus, block conditioned fear as measured with potentiated startle paradigm. *Behavioral Neuroscience, 100*, 11–22.

Kagan, J. (1991). Continuity and discontinuity in development. In S. E. Brauth, W. S. Hall, R. J. Dooling (Eds.), *Plasticity of development* (pp. 11–26). Cambridge, MA: MIT Press.

Kagan, J. (1994). *Galen's prophecy: Temperament in human nature.* New York: Basic Books.

Kagan, J. (1999). The concept of behavioral inhibition. In L. A. Schmidt & J. Schulkin (Eds.), *Extreme fear, shyness, and social phobia: Origins, biological mechanisms, and clinical outcomes* (pp. 3–13). New York: Oxford University Press.

Kagan, J., Reznick, J. S., & Snidman, N. (1987). The physiology and psychology of behavioral inhibition in children. *Child Development, 58,* 1459–1473.

Kagan, J., Reznick, J. S., & Snidman, N. (1988). Biological basis of childhood shyness. *Science, 240,* 167–171.

Kagan, J., & Snidman, N. (1991a). Temperamental factors in human development. *American Psychologist, 46,* 856–862.

Kagan, J., & Snidman, N. (1991b). Infant predictors of inhibited and uninhibited profiles. *Psychological Science, 2,* 40–44.

Kapp, B. S., Frysinger, R. C., Gallagher, M., & Haselton, J. R. (1979). Amygdala central nucleus lesions: Effects on heart rate conditioning in the rabbit. *Physiology and Behavior, 23,* 1109–1117.

Lang, P. J., Bradley, M. M., & Cuthbert, B. N. (1990). Emotion, attention, and the startle reflex. *Psychological Review, 97,* 377–395.

LeDoux, J. E. (1996). *The emotional brain.* New York: Simon & Schuster.

LeDoux, J. E., Iwata, J., Cicchetti, P., & Reis, D. J. (1988). Different projections of the central amygdaloid nucleus mediate autonomic and behavioral correlates of conditioned fear. *Journal of Neuroscience, 8,* 2517–2519.

LeDoux, J. E., Sakaguchi, A., Iwata, J., & Reis, D. J. (1986). Interruption of projections from the medial geniculate body to an archi-neo-striatal field disrupts the classical conditioning of emotional responses to acoustic stimuli in the rat. *Neuroscience, 17,* 615–627.

Lee, Y., Schulkin, J., & Davis, M. (1994). Effect of corticosterone on the enhancement of the acoustic startle reflex by corticotropin releasing factor (CRF). *Brain Research, 666,* 93–98.

Lesch, K. P., Bengel, D., Heils, A., Sabol, S. Z., Greenberg, B. D., Petri, S., Benjamin, J., Muller, C. R., Hamer, D. H., & Murphy, D. L. (1996). Association of anxiety-related traits with a polymorphism in the serotonin transporter gene regulatory region. *Science, 274,* 1527–1531.

Murray, H. A. (1938). *Explorations in personality.* New York: Oxford University Press.

Nader, K., & LeDoux, J. (1999). The neural circuits that underlie fear. In L. A. Schmidt & J. Schulkin (Eds.), *Extreme fear, shyness, and social phobia: Origins, biological mechanisms, and clinical outcomes* (pp. 119–139). New York: Oxford University Press.

Panksepp, J. (1998). *Affective neuroscience: The foundations of human and animal emotions.* New York: Oxford University Press.

Porges, S. W. (1991). Vagal tone: An autonomic mediator of affect. In J. Garber & K.A. Dodge (Eds.), *The development of emotion regulation and dysregulation* (pp. 111–128). Cambridge, UK: Cambridge University Press.

Rosen, J. B., & Davis, M. (1988). Enhancement of acoustic startle by electrical stimulation of the amygdala. *Behavioral Neuroscience, 102,* 195–202.

Rosen, J. B., Hamerman, E., Sitcoske, M., Glowa, J. R., & Schulkin, J. (1996). Hyperexcitability: Exaggerated fear-potentiated startle produced by partial amygdala kindling. *Behavioral Neuroscience, 110,* 43–50.

Rosen, J. B., & Schulkin, J. (1998). From normal fear to pathological anxiety. *Psychological Review, 105,* 325–350.

Rubin, K. H., & Asendorpf, J. (1993). *Social withdrawal, inhibition, and shyness in childhood.* Hillsdale, NJ: Erlbaum.

Rubin, K. H., Cheah, C., & Fox, N. A. (2001). Emotion regulation, parenting, and display of social reticence in preschoolers. *Early Education and Development, 12,* 97–115.

Rubin, K. H., Stewart, S. L., & Coplan, R. J. (1995). Social withdrawal in childhood: Conceptual and empirical perspectives. In T. Ollendick & R. Prinz (Eds.), *Advances in clinical child psychology* (Vol. 17, pp. 157–196). New York: Plenum Press.

Schmidt, L. A. (1999). Frontal brain electrical activity in shyness and sociability. *Psychological Science, 10,* 316–320.

Schmidt, L. A. (2000). *Psychometric properties of resting frontal brain electrical activity (EEG) and temperament in 9 month-old human infants.* Manuscript submitted for publication.

Schmidt, L. A., & Fox, N. A. (1994). Patterns of cortical electrophysiology and autonomic activity in adults' shyness and sociability. *Biological Psychology, 38,* 183–198.

Schmidt, L. A., & Fox, N. A. (1995). Individual differences in young adults' shyness and sociability: Personality and health correlates. *Personality and Individual Differences, 19,* 455–462.

Schmidt, L. A., & Fox, N. A. (1998). Fear-potentiated startle responses in temperamentally different human infants. *Developmental Psychobiology, 32,* 113–120.

Schmidt, L. A., & Fox, N. A. (1999). Conceptual, biological, and behavioral distinctions among different categories of shy children. In L. A. Schmidt & J. Schulkin (Eds.), *Extreme fear, shyness, and social phobia: Origins, biological mechanisms, and clinical outcomes* (pp. 47–66). New York: Oxford University Press.

Schmidt, L. A., Fox, N. A., Goldberg, M. C., Smith, C. C., & Schulkin, J. (1999). Effects of acute prednisone administration on memory, attention, and emotion in healthy human adults. *Psychoneuroendocrinology, 24,* 461–483.

Schmidt, L. A., Fox, N. A., Perez-Edgar, K., Hu, S., & Hamer, D. H. (2001). Association of DRD4 with attention problems in normal childhood development. *Psychiatric Genetics, 11,* 25–29.

Schmidt, L. A., Fox, N. A., Rubin, K. H., Hu, S., & Hamer, D. H. (in press). Molecular genetics of shyness and aggression in preschoolers. *Personality and Individual Differences.*

Schmidt, L. A., Fox, N. A., Rubin, K. H., Sternberg, E. M., Gold, P. W., Smith, C., & Schulkin, J. (1997). Behavioral and neuroendocrine responses in shy children. *Developmental Psychobiology, 30,* 127–140.

Schmidt, L. A., Fox, N. A., Schulkin, J., & Gold, P. W. (1999). Behavioral and psychophysiological correlates of self-presentation in temperamentally shy children. *Developmental Psychobiology, 35,* 119–135.

Schmidt, L. A., Fox, N. A., Sternberg, E. M., Gold, P. W., Smith, C., & Schulkin, J. (1999). Adrenocortical reactivity and social competence in seven-year-olds. *Personality and Individual Differences, 26,* 977–985.

Schmidt, L. A., & Robinson, T. R., Jr. (1992). Low self-esteem in differentiating fearful and self-conscious forms of shyness. *Psychological Reports, 70,* 255–257.

Schmidt, L. A., & Sniderman, C. E. (2001, April). Frontal brain activation in distinguishing childhood shyness and sociability. In R. J. Coplan & C. H. Hart (Chairs), *Multiple forms of shyness/withdrawal/inhibition: Conceptualizations, assessments, and outcomes.* Symposium conducted at the meeting of the Society for Research in Child Development, Minneapolis, MN.

Schmidt, L. A., & Trainor, L. J. (2001). Frontal brain electrical activity (EEG) distinguishes *valence* and *intensity* of musical emotions. *Cognition and Emotion, 15,* 487–500.

Schulkin, J., McEwen, B. S., & Gold, P. W. (1994). Allostasis, amygdala, and anticipatory angst. *Neuroscience and Biobehavioral Reviews, 18,* 385–396.

Snidman, N., & Kagan, J. (1994). The contribution of infant temperamental differences to acoustic startle response [Abstract]. *Psychophysiology, 31,* S92.

Stevenson-Hinde, J., & Glover, A. (1996). Shy girls and boys: A new look. *Journal of Child Psychology and Psychiatry, 37,* 181–187.

Takahashi, L. K., & Rubin, W. W. (1994). Corticosteroid induction of threat-induced behavioral inhibition in preweanling rats. *Behavioral Neuroscience, 107,* 860–868.

Tomarken, A. J., Davidson, R. J., & Henriques, J. B. (1990). Resting frontal brain asymmetry predicts affective responses to films. *Journal of Personality and Social Psychology, 59,* 791–801.

Westernberg, H. G., Murphy, D. L., & Den Boer, J. A. (Eds.). (1996). *Advances in the neurobiology of anxiety disorders.* New York: Wiley.

Wheeler, R. W., Davidson, R. J., & Tomarken, A. J. (1993). Frontal brain asymmetry and emotional reactivity: A biological substrate of affective style. *Psychophysiology, 30,* 82–89.

Zimbardo, P. G. (1977). *Shyness: What is it and what to do about it.* New York: Symphony Press.

CHAPTER 4

States, Traits, and Symptoms
Investigating the Neural Correlates of Emotion, Personality, and Psychopathology

WENDY HELLER
JENNIFER I. SCHMIDTKE
JACK B. NITSCHKE
NANCY S. KOVEN
GREGORY A. MILLER

Human emotion has not been easy to define in a way that has achieved broad consensus. It is perhaps best conceptualized as a complex set of processes, including subjective experiences, functional states, self-reports, physiological events, and behavioral expressions. Emotions are accompanied by cognitive processes that involve attention, memory, and other aspects of information processing. Most of these components can unfold both within or outside of conscious awareness, with effort or automatically. Because this broad range of processes involves just about everything humans do (e.g., thinking, feeling, acting, communicating, digesting), we can assume that, broadly defined, emotion recruits neural circuitry in most parts of the brain. One of our long-term goals is to understand the way in which each of these brain regions contributes to emotion, how they interact, and the implications for individual differences in affect, personality, and clinical syndromes. One strategy we have used to investigate the role of different brain regions in emotion is to decompose affective states into more fundamental dimensions.

As we review in this chapter, we have used the circumplex model of emotion to map valence and arousal onto specific brain regions. We have also used personality and clinical constructs as a way to further deconstruct complex emotional states and to investigate the relations between affect, personality, and clinical symptoms. For example, we have shown that, if we distinguish between two different types of anxiety, we can account for conflicting findings regarding patterns of regional brain activity in anxiety.

Our approach to research on emotion, personality, and psychopathology rests on a neuropsychological model developed by Heller (1990, 1993) in which psychological theories of emotion are used to decompose emotional states into two components, valence and arousal, with direct parallels to specific brain regions (see Figure 4.1).

Heller's model integrates the dimensional circumplex model of emotion (based primarily on self-report measures; for review, see Larsen & Diener, 1992) with neuropsychological data on cognitive, emotional, and autonomic functioning during different affective states. The model has

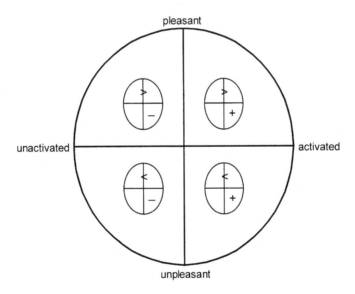

FIGURE 4.1. Valence and arousal or activation dimensions of the circumplex model of emotion mapped onto patterns of brain activity. The small circles represent a schematic brain divided into four quadrants, with top being the front of the brain and bottom the back, and the plus, minus, and greater-than signs representing the hypothesized patterns of activity that would be associated with different emotions on the circumplex.

made a variety of contributions to this area of research by providing testable predictions about the activity and function of different brain regions associated with various emotions, personality traits, and clinical symptoms. In the course of testing these predictions, we and others have garnered important data not only with regard to specific brain regions involved in emotion and personality but also about psychological phenomena that play a critical role in understanding psychopathology, particularly anxiety and depression (e.g., types of anxiety, comorbidity between depression and anxiety). In the process, the original model has been refined and, with our recent and continuing incursion into functional magnetic resonance imaging (fMRI) research, to some extent replaced by a more specific focus on individual brain regions.

As an initial heuristic, the model divided the brain into four quadrants and mapped emotional dimensions onto broad regions. It predicted that different patterns of brain activity would be associated with each of the four different quadrants delineated by the valence and arousal, or activation (as per Larsen & Diener, 1992), dimensions of the emotion circumplex. Activated pleasant affect, such as elation or euphoria, should be associated with increased left, relative to right, frontal as well as increased right posterior activity. Activated unpleasant affect, such as anxiety or fear, should be associated with increased right, relative to left, frontal as well as increased right posterior activity. Unactivated pleasant affect, such as calmness or relaxation, should be associated with increased left, relative to right, frontal combined with decreased right posterior activity. Finally, unactivated unpleasant affect, such as boredom or depression, should be associated with increased right, relative to left, frontal and decreased right posterior activity. An important implication of the model was that, if depression and anxiety co-occur (as is very common), it is possible that the effects on right posterior activity would cancel each other out. Furthermore, comparing groups or studies with different amounts of depression and anxiety represented in the sample could lead to spurious inconsistencies.

STATES AND SYMPTOMS: BRAIN ACTIVITY IN DEPRESSION AND ANXIETY

The data have generally supported this model. Electroencephalogram (EEG) and blood-flow measures of brain activity have demonstrated that depressed individuals, who are hypothesized to experience a nonactivated form of unpleasant affect, show reduced right parietotemporal activity. Behavioral studies have also provided support for the idea that activity in the posterior right hemisphere is reduced during depressed states; depressed individuals display poorer performance on tasks that are assumed to be processed by the posterior right hemisphere, such as dichotic listening and dot enumeration, as well as the Chimeric Faces Task (Levy, Heller, Banich, & Burton, 1983), which is believed to measure asymmetries in posterior activity (for review, see Heller, 1990; Heller, 1993; Heller & Nitschke, 1998).

Research has also shown that normal controls in induced negative (unactivated unpleasant) mood states demonstrate predicted effects on posterior right hemisphere activity. Negative mood inductions have been shown to be related to slower reaction times for right hemisphere lateralized visual stimuli (Ladavas, Nicoletti, Umilta, & Rizzolatti, 1984) and for a digit-matching task for stimuli presented to the left visual field and hence the right hemisphere (Banich, Stolar, Heller, & Goldman, 1992). These effects were not found for stimuli presented to the left hemisphere, suggesting that observed differences were a result of decreased activity in the posterior right hemisphere.

It has also been shown that the Chimeric Faces Task, which correlates very well with hemispheric nonemotional task performance asymmetry (processing nonemotional facial, pictorial, and language stimuli—tasks that are presumed to be localized to the parietotemporal regions of the brain), also correlates with self-reported measures of behavioral arousal (Heller, Nitschke, & Lindsay, 1997). A very reliable correlation resulted between scores on the Chimeric Faces Task and self-reported behavioral arousal; as self-reported arousal increased, relative right hemisphere processing also increased.

In another approach, we examined asymmetric hemispheric activity using the Chimeric Faces Test in college students reporting high levels of depression and anxiety (Heller, Etienne, & Miller, 1995). We screened more than 1,000 undergraduates to obtain an appropriate sample of 68 individuals who had specific combinations of depression and anxiety levels. Confirming previous results, we found depression to be associated with reduced right hemisphere activity. In contrast, anxiety was associated with increased right hemisphere activity.

We replicated these findings in two more recent studies: One involved a sample of inpatients and outpatients diagnosed with major depression, and the other a new group of 80 undergraduates selected for scores on measures of psychopathology. Participants were given the State–Trait Anxiety Inventory (STAI; Spielberger, Gorsuch, Lushene, Vagg, & Jacobs, 1983) to measure anxiety and the Beck Depression Inventory (BDI; Beck, Rush, Shaw, & Emery, 1979) to measure depression. In simultaneous regressions, the STAI, the BDI, and their interaction accounted for significant variance in hemispheric asymmetry in each sample. Furthermore, in a series of hierarchical regressions, each predictor accounted for unique variance in asymmetry. Most important, higher scores on the STAI were associated with more right hemisphere activity, whereas higher scores on the BDI were associated with less right hemisphere activity (Keller et al., 2000).

In summary, depression has been associated with evidence for reduced activity in posterior regions of the right hemisphere and anxiety with increased activity in these regions in all of our studies to date. Importantly, these effects typically emerge only when the variance associated with depression is removed from a measure of anxiety and vice versa. Thus, our findings confirm our assertion that it is crucial to separate depression and anxiety, either statistically or via experimental design, in efforts to examine brain function in psychopathology.

TRAITS AND SYMPTOMS: ANXIOUS AROUSAL, ANXIOUS APPREHENSION, AND BRAIN ACTIVITY

The results of these studies also led us to make a distinction between two aspects of anxiety, specifically, anxious apprehension and anxious arousal, in a refinement of our original model. Psychological theories have distinguished anxious apprehension (worry), which involves verbal rumination about possible negative outcomes of events and is focused on the future, from anxious arousal (panic), a more immediate fear response that involves autonomic hyperarousal. Because our model argued that right posterior regions of the brain are particularly involved in the arousal aspect of emotion, failure to specify which type of anxiety is involved in a given study could contribute to inconsistent results in the literature on brain activity in anxiety and depression. In past studies of anxiety, some investigators reported increased right hemisphere activity, whereas others reported increased left hemisphere activity. Extensive review of these studies (e.g., Heller & Nitschke, 1998; Heller, Nitschke, Etienne, & Miller, 1997; Nitschke, Heller, & Miller, 2000) supported the conclusion that increased right hemisphere activity was most likely to be indicated when the type of anxiety being investigated was anxious arousal, as would be expected in studies of people with panic disorder or in stress-inducing experimental conditions. In contrast, increased left hemisphere activity was more often reported when anxious apprehension was being studied, as defined by trait anxiety, worry, or verbal rumination.

A series of studies in our lab showed that this distinction between types of anxiety can be quite important. In one study, we selected participants based on a measure of anxious apprehension and subjected them to a mildly stressful experimental paradigm in which they listened to emotional narratives having high fear or sadness ratings (Heller, Nitschke,

Etienne, et al., 1997). Electroencephalographic activity was examined for the four brain regions of interest (right and left anterior and posterior) during rest and during emotional narrative presentation. During both conditions, trait apprehensive participants differed from nonanxious, nondepressed controls in showing higher left than right frontal activity (consistent with predictions for anxious apprehension). In contrast, during emotional narrative presentation, trait apprehensive participants differed from controls in showing a selective increase in right posterior activity. These results confirmed our prediction that participants who were selected on the basis of anxious apprehension would be more likely to respond to a stressful task with anxious arousal, which we anticipated would be associated with increased right posterior activity. Furthermore, this confirmation and clarification of our model would not have emerged had we not been careful to take into account the high comorbidity of depression and anxiety. A group of participants who were both depressed and anxious did not differ from the control group, confirming our model's prediction that effects can cancel in right posterior regions.

We followed up that within-subject manipulation of anxious arousal using a between-groups design to compare types of anxiety (Nitschke, Heller, Palmieri, & Miller, 1999). We selected people using questionnaires that focused on anxious apprehension or anxious arousal and measured regional EEG activity at rest. An interaction for group and region showed a differential hemispheric asymmetry, with the anxious arousal group showing more right than left hemisphere activity.

Taken together, these findings are exciting because they help to explain inconsistencies in the scientific literature. They may also prove to be helpful in the discrimination of different anxiety disorders, as the two types of anxiety differ in the degree to which they are present in various diagnoses. For example, anxious apprehension is particularly salient in generalized anxiety disorder, whereas anxious arousal predominates in panic disorder. To investigate this issue further in a specific disorder, we examined these two types of anxiety in posttraumatic stress disorder (PTSD). We found that anxious arousal was most strongly associated with posttraumatic stress disorder symptoms, although anxious apprehension also accounted for unique variance (Palmieri, Heller, & Miller, 2001).

We have also examined the psychometric properties of measures of anxious apprehension and anxious arousal in more depth with a variety of the most commonly used questionnaires (Nitschke, Heller, Imig, McDonald, & Miller, 2001). In this research, correlational and confirmatory factor analyses indicated that anxious apprehension and anxious arousal were clearly distinguishable from each other and from depression, negative affect, and positive affect. These findings are important because they provide the first conclusive evidence that anxious apprehension is not merely a feature or subcategory of depression or negative affect.

The fact that these two types of anxiety are distinguished in regional EEG extends the psychological and autonomic evidence that suggests they are distinct constructs and highlights the need to consider the presence of both in diagnostic, treatment, and research procedures. Our findings also suggest that anxious arousal and anxious apprehension are associated with very different neural networks (Nitschke et al., 2000; Nitschke et al., 1999). We have recently hypothesized that anxious arousal is associated with an "emotion surveillance" system supported by the right hemisphere. In behavioral studies, the right hemisphere has been shown to be primed by ambiguous and threatening stimuli and has been hypothesized to play a role in orienting to such stimuli. In addition, samples characterized by anxious arousal consistently show increased right hemisphere activity at rest (for review, see Nitschke et al., 2000), suggesting that anxious arousal is associated with the engagement of the emotional surveillance system even in the absence of an emotional stimulus. This right hemisphere system may correspond to the cortical processes that McNally (1998) postulated to accompany a subcortical circuit involved in attentional biases toward threat. Thus, anxious arousal can be hypothesized to produce a set of behaviors that includes attentional and other cognitive responses designed to evaluate the presence of a threat.

In contrast to anxious arousal, we have argued that deficits in the performance of anxious people during attentionally demanding tasks are due to interference effects of anxious apprehension and that their neural loci include areas involved in working memory, such as the dorsolateral prefrontal cortex, Broca's area in the left anterior hemisphere, and left posterior areas around the angular and supramarginal gyrus (Nitschke et al., 2000).

Traits and States: Neuroticism, Extraversion, and Brain Activity

The research described above has obvious implications for individual differences in emotional dispositions, personality traits, and susceptibility to symptoms of psychopathology. In an attempt to integrate our model of affect-related regional brain activity specifically with research in personality, we applied it to theory and research that has empirically derived an orthogonal two-dimensional model representing personality dimensions.

As previously described, research in emotion and mood generally supports the idea that affective experience can be broadly represented in a two-dimensional structure. A separate tradition in theoretical and empirical personality scholarship has also sought to identify major dimensions or traits that can adequately describe and predict behavior, with less emphasis on emotion per se. Two major dimensions of personality, extraversion and neuroticism, have been repeatedly identified across different methodologies. Eysenck (1987) placed these two bipolar dimensions at a 90-degree angle to each other and used this organization to explicate the personality types proposed by Galen and Hippocrates (see Figure 4.2). Subsequent research has suggested that personality can be more thoroughly captured using an expanded five-factor model (Digman & Inouye, 1986; Digman & Takemoto-Chock, 1981; McCrae & Costa, 1987; McCrae & Costa, 1989; McCrae, Costa, & Busch, 1986; Peabody, 1984; Peabody & Goldberg, 1989). These five factors are generally agreed to be Extraversion, Agreeableness, Conscientiousness, Neuroticism, and Openness to Experience. Factors 1 and 4 of this five-factor model closely resemble the constructs proposed by Eysenck and others. Although Almagor, Tellegen, and Waller (1995) argued that seven dimensions provide an even more accurate representation by including mood-dispositional descriptors, Extraversion and Neuroticism nonetheless emerge and are identified by Almagor et al. as two of the seven factors.

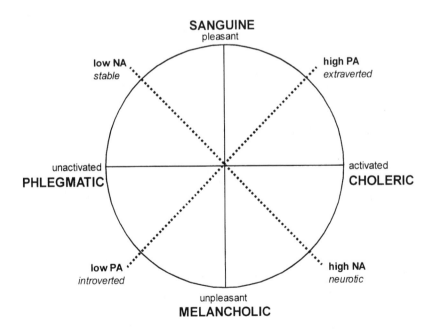

FIGURE 4.2. The relationship of the dimensions of positive and negative affect, valence and arousal or activation, personality dimensions of extraversion and neuroticism, and the temperament types.

Just as positive and negative affect have been proposed as a rotated alternative to the valence–arousal model, the alternative to the Eysenck model that Gray (1987) proposed, with dimensions of anxiety and impulsivity, can be shown to be rotational variants of extraversion and neuroticism. In sum, diverse methodological approaches have provided strong support for the idea that the personality traits of extraversion and neuroticism are reliable and fundamental aspects of human behavior.

Furthermore, there is evidence that the emotion-focused (valence–arousal or activation, or positive–negative affect) circumplex structure and the personality-focused (extraversion–neuroticism or anxiety–impulsivity) circumplex structure are systematically related (Diener, Larsen, Levine, & Emmons, 1985; Larsen & Diener, 1985). Relating the valence (pleasant–unpleasant) and arousal or activation (activated–unactivated) dimensions to Galen's temperament types, Diener and colleagues were able to demonstrate that these basic dimensions of affect are systematically related to Galen's typologies. The relation of the basic dimensions of affect with the temperament types also allows an association of affective dimensions with Eysenck's basic dimensions of personality, extraversion and neuroticism. Based on the relations among these factors, it can be argued that both sets of dimensions are simply alternative ways of describing the same phenomena, possibly implemented by the same underlying brain structures.

Watson and Tellegen's (1985) positive and negative affect dimensions can similarly be mapped onto extraversion and neuroticism. Because positive and negative affect are argued to be located at a 45-degree rotation to Russell's (1980) pleasantness and arousal or activation dimensions (Watson & Tellegen, 1985), it follows that they occupy the same rotation as Eysenck's extraversion and neuroticism traits (see Figure 4.2). In fact, a great deal of research supports the idea that Eysenck's basic personality traits are related to Watson and Tellegen's positive and negative affect dimensions (e.g., Meyer & Shack, 1989), suggesting that the two-dimensional models of mood and personality share a structural identity and a common core source of variation.

Costa and McCrae (1980) investigated the relations between extraversion, neuroticism, and positive and negative affect and found that negative affect was strongly related to neuroticism, not extraversion, whereas positive affect was more strongly related to extraversion. Trait measures of extraversion and neuroticism were also found to be predictive of levels of positive and negative affect 10 years later. Similarly, Tellegen (1985), investigating the relations between self-reported current mood and personality measured by his Multidimensional Personality Questionnaire (MPQ), found evidence relating extraversion to positive affect and neuroticism to negative affect. Using the Positive and Negative Affect Schedule

(Watson, Clark, & Tellegen,1988), Fujita, Diener, and Sandvik (1991) also found that extraversion was highly correlated with positive affect and that neuroticism was highly correlated with negative affect.

In a direct test of the fit of the circumplex model of affect with a circumplex model of personality, Larsen (1989) found that activated pleasant affect was related to a cluster of extraversion traits and that activated unpleasant affect was related to a cluster of neuroticism traits. Many other studies have demonstrated significant relations between the experience of pleasant and unpleasant affect and extraversion and neuroticism (Diener & Emmons, 1984; Hotard, McFatter, McWhirter, & Stegall, 1989; Kendell, MacKenzie, West, McGuire, & Cox, 1984; Kirkcaldy, 1984; Larsen & Ketelaar, 1989, 1991; O'Malley & Gillette, 1984; Thayer, Takahashi, & Pauli, 1988; Warr, Barter, & Brownbridge, 1983; Watson, 1988; Williams, 1981).

In summary, converging evidence suggests that these two "separate" two-dimensional models may actually be different conceptualizations of the same underlying substrates that contribute to both affective states and the traits of extraversion and neuroticism. Because Heller's neuropsychological model of emotion uses the emotion circumplex to represent the relations between affective states and brain activity, it provides a framework for making predictions for patterns of brain activity that should correspond to the personality traits of extraversion and neuroticism. Accordingly, we hypothesized that patterns of brain activity associated with pleasant and unpleasant affective states on the circumplex would also be strongly associated with extraversion and neuroticism.

Four predictions were made for activity in the four brain regions related to extraversion and neuroticism based on the placement of each in the circumplex model (see Figure 4.3).

Extraversion should be associated with greater relative left frontal activity, as well as increased right posterior region activity, and introversion should be associated with greater relative right frontal activity, as well as decreased right posterior region activity. Neuroticism should be associated with greater relative right frontal and increased right posterior region activity. Finally, emotional stability (the opposite pole of neuroticism) should be associated with greater relative left frontal and decreased right posterior activity.

To test these predictions, reports of extraversion and neuroticism (NEO-Personality Inventory—Revised; Costa & McCrae, 1992), and current mood were collected, and resting EEG was recorded for male and female right-handed participants on one occasion for eight 60-second resting baseline periods (Schmidtke & Heller, 2001). Mean log-transformed alpha power was extracted from the EEG for each electrode site, and asymmetry scores were computed across homologous electrode sites by sub-

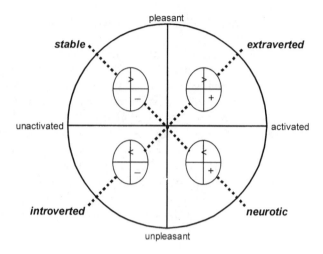

FIGURE 4.3. The dimensions of personality mapped onto the hypothesized patterns of brain activity associated with emotions as represented on the circumplex model.

tracting left from right hemisphere mean log-transformed power. As predicted, results indicated that greater relative right posterior activity was associated with higher neuroticism, and this finding remained unchanged when the effect of current mood was included in the hierarchical regression model. In contrast, predicted effects for extraversion and neuroticism associated with frontal activity emerged when the effect of current mood was included in the statistical model.

Despite evidence that extraversion has been related to increased right hemisphere activity (for a review, see Heller, 1993) and the prediction that it would be related, specifically, to greater relative right posterior activity, it was found to be related to frontal activity, and only after the effects of current mood were included in the model. A potential explanation for the lack of findings for extraversion in the posterior regions is the power associated with the predicted effects for extraversion; observed power for the effects in the posterior regions was very small (< .15). Additional research with a larger number of participants, ideally those defined as stable in their patterns of EEG activity across multiple recording sessions, is necessary to further investigate predictions for activity in the posterior regions regarding extraversion.

In general, however, these findings indicate that personality traits can predict patterns of resting regional brain activity, as indexed by baseline scalp EEG alpha over frontal and posterior regions. Resting posterior EEG activity was related to higher neuroticism scores in the predicted direction, even after the effects of current mood were included in the statistical model. Resting frontal EEG activity was found to be related to extraversion and neuroticism in the predicted direction after the effect of current mood was considered.

Given the finding of greater relative left frontal activation for anxious apprehension discussed previously, one might wonder why similar predictions were not made for neuroticism with relative left frontal EEG activity, as the construct of neuroticism would presumably encompass anxiety associated with worry and rumination. Although these components of anxiety have often traditionally been included in measures of neuroticism, our research supports the idea that they may actually be related to separate neural networks as a result of the working memory and language processes involved (Nitschke et al., 2000).

In addition, although the construct of worry is closely related to neuroticism, it has recently been considered to be a completely separate construct (Keogh, French, & Reidy, 1998). Our study of the psychometric properties of anxious apprehension mentioned previously, which found anxious apprehension to be clearly distinguished from negative affect, a construct highly related to neuroticism, supports this assertion. Rather than viewing anxious apprehension as a facet of the trait of neuroticism, it may be more accurate to conceptualize it as a separate but related construct.

It is conceivable that neuroticism is more closely related to our concept of anxious arousal. However, items associated with anxious arousal are intermingled with items associated with anxious apprehension on personality inventories commonly used to assess neuroticism, such as the NEO-PI-R, so it is difficult to disentangle the relative contribution of the two constructs. More research is needed to examine the psychometric relationships among anxious apprehension, anxious arousal, negative affect and neuroticism, and their respective associations with different neural circuits and substrates.

Traits, States, and Symptoms: Influences on Individual Differences in Cognition and Attention

Perhaps one of the most useful contributions of understanding the patterns of regional brain activity that characterize personality traits and clinical syndromes is the potential insight it provides into individual differences in cognitive capabilities and styles. Numerous studies have shown that activity in regions of the cortex specialized for particular modes of information processing predicts performance on tasks that benefit from that type of computation. In the vast majority of studies (see Heller, Nitschke, & Lindsay, 1997, for discussion), increased activity is associated with better performance, whereas deficient activity is associated with decrements in performance. For example, reduced activity in right posterior regions, reflected in reduced left hemispatial biases on a face judgment task and in left ear deficits on dichotic listening tasks (e.g., Bruder, 1995), is also manifested in poor performance on paper-and-pencil tasks that depend on visuospatial information processing (for review, see Heller & Nitschke, 1997). Similar deficits appear on a variety of tasks that draw on other specialized capacities of the right hemisphere, including important aspects of language (e.g., pragmatics such as turn-taking in a conversation).

Both anxious apprehension and anxious arousal types of anxiety, as well as depression, are characterized by specific cognitive biases and impairments (for reviews, see Heller & Nitschke, 1997; McNally, 1998; Nitschke et al., 2000). Anxiety in general has been strongly associated with an attentional bias to threatening stimuli (for review, see Compton, Heller, Banich, Palmieri, & Miller, 2000; McNally, 1998). In various paradigms, attention is captured by ambiguous, emotional, or threatening information; this phenomenon has been documented in trait and state anxiety and in every anxiety disorder category in the *Diagnostic and Statistical Manual of Mental Disorders* (DSM-IV; American Psychiatric Association, 1994) including generalized anxiety disorder (e.g., Mathews & MacLeod, 1985), panic disorder (e.g., Ehlers, Margraf, Davies, & Roth, 1988), specific phobia (e.g., Watts, McKenna, Sharrock, & Trezise, 1986), PTSD (e.g., McNally, Kaspi, Riemann, & Zeitlin, 1990), social phobia (e.g., Hope, Rapee, Heimberg, & Dombeck, 1990), and obsessive–compulsive disorder (e.g., Foa, Ilai, McCarthy, Shoyer, & Murdock, 1993). We have argued that these attentional biases toward threat-related stimuli dovetail with specializations of the right posterior region for visual and spatial attention, vigilance, and autonomic arousal, reflecting the activity of an emotional surveillance system (Nitschke et al., 2000). Our recent fMRI research suggests that this area may include temporal, parietal, and occipital regions of the right hemisphere (Compton et al., 2001; Miller, 2000).

Anxiety can impair performance on many tasks, particularly when the tasks are difficult or the conditions are stressful. We have argued that these deficits reflect anxious apprehension, which interferes with performance on attentionally demanding tasks due to the impact of worrisome thoughts on attention to task-relevant information. As mentioned previously, we have posited that the neural mechanisms involved in anxious apprehension include areas involved in working memory, among them dorsolateral prefrontal cortex, Broca's area in left anterior cortex, and left posterior areas around the angular and supramarginal gyrus (Nitschke et al., 2000).

In depression, deficits have been described for explicit memory, executive functions, and visuospatial skills (for review, see Heller & Nitschke, 1997). DSM-IV identifies difficulties in thinking and concentrating as fundamental components of major depressive episodes and dysthymia. Biases in attention, memory, and judgment have also been documented, with depressed people more likely to attend to unpleasant than pleasant stimuli, to show better recall of unpleasant than pleasant information, and to make more negative judgments about hypothetical and actual life events (Heller & Nitschke, 1997). We have argued that decreased activity in prefrontal brain regions can account for many of the cognitive impairments in depression, including memory for material on tasks that require or benefit from information-organizing strategies, the ability to access errors accurately, problem solving, and cognitive flexibility. Depression has also been consistently associated with impairments on tasks associated with right posterior regions of the brain (e.g., Deldin, Keller, Gergen, & Miller, 2000; Keller et al., 2000; for review of earlier studies, see Heller & Nitschke, 1997). These findings are consistent with evidence that there is decreased activity in these brain regions (Banich et al., 1992; Liotti & Tucker, 1992; Otto, Yeo, & Dougher, 1987).

In recent research, we have been examining the implications of these patterns of brain activity for cognition and attention. We developed a procedure for use with nonclinical samples that is sensitive to a wide range of individual differences in the degree to which emotion information interferes with performance. We used a variant of the Stroop task that is sometimes called the emotional Stroop (which we prefer to call an emotional interference paradigm). The stimuli are either neutral, appetitive, or threat words that are printed in different colors. One word is presented at a time. The participants are told to ignore the words and to identify the color by pushing a button. As predicted, behavioral results indicated that the right hemisphere was differentially activated by emotional stimuli in this task, particularly by threatening words (Compton et al., 2000).

We have extended this research by using the emotional interference paradigm in two fMRI studies (Compton et al., 2001; Heller et al., 2000) to examine more directly the neural substrates identified in our model and in attentional biases toward threatening information. The value of fMRI for this paradigm is that it allows us to identify the specific brain regions involved more precisely than do the behavioral and EEG paradigms we have used previously. For example, the data collected so far (replicated in two studies) suggest that the area of the posterior right hemisphere that is involved in responding to threat (presumably, the hypothesized arousal system) spans temporal, parietal, and occipital regions of the right hemisphere. Another boon of fMRI is that it facilitates our examination of the overlap between brain systems involved in emotion and attention, which has great promise to illuminate further the relationship between the two with regard to cognitive function.

Recent results from our second fMRI study (Heller et al., 2000) replicate the previous findings that implicated posterior regions of the right hemisphere in response to threat stimuli. These findings extend the previous data, however, in showing that the activation differs between participants who are unable to suppress the affective content of the words, as evidenced by a Stroop effect (i.e., they are slower to name the color of the word when it is a threatening rather than a neutral word), and those who are facilitated by the emotional words.

In this study, there was considerable individual variability in the effect of the emotional words on performance. Some individuals were faster to identify the color of the emotional words than the neutral words, whereas others were slower to identify the color of the emotional words than the neutral words. For the purposes of examining brain activity associated with these patterns of performance, we divided people in two different ways, one as a function of reaction time for appetitive words and one as a function of reaction time for threat words. These two groupings allow us to distinguish brain regions specifically involved in appetitive versus threat processing. We compared brain activity for the group that showed facilitation with that of the group that showed interference for threat words. We also compared brain activity for the group that showed facilitation with that of the group that showed interference for appetitive words.

A subset of 18 participants completed a variety of questionnaires to examine clinical and personality constructs relevant to anxiety. Despite the small sample size, patterns of reaction time were related to a number of these constructs, as well as to brain activity. Participants who showed facilitation to threat words exhibited a pattern of left dorsolateral prefrontal, left anterior temporal, and bilateral precuneus activation. Furthermore, this pattern was associated with higher scores on positive affect. These results suggest that individuals biased toward positive affect, and hence approach behavior, activate brain circuits involved in approach (e.g., left prefrontal and temporal regions). These regions overlap with regions engaged by selective attention tasks (left hemisphere frontal and parietal regions)——hence their better performance.

In contrast, people who showed interference to threat words demonstrated a pattern of right medial frontal, posterior left superior temporal, bilateral activation of occipital cortex, and bilateral deactivation of parietal cortex. This pattern was associated with higher scores on anxious arousal. These results suggest that for individuals prone to anxious arousal, threat words activate brain circuits associated with withdrawal and negative valence (including right frontal and parietal regions) and panic (occipital). Right medial frontal and posterior parietal regions on both sides have been implicated in both animal and human models of sustained attention and vigilance. This pattern of activation appears to have interfered with the selective attention required by the task. Bilateral deactivation of the parietal cortex may reflect an active attempt to suppress the attentional orientation or shift toward the threatening but task-irrelevant information.

Participants who showed facilitation to appetitive words had left prefrontal, left temporal, and bilateral parietal activation. These findings suggest that the brain circuits that are involved in appetitive facilitation are similar to those involved in facilitation to threat words, suggesting that facilitation involves a common dispositional bias toward approach.

In contrast, those with interference to appetitive words had right superior frontal, right middle temporal, and retrosplenial cortex activation, and this pattern was associated with higher scores on anhedonic depression, anxious apprehension, alexithymia, and negative affect. These results suggest that people who reacted aversively to the appetitive (all sex-related) stimuli engaged brain circuits involved in withdrawal and negative valence. Activation in retrosplenial cortex is consistent with other findings that this region is involved in emotionally arousing information processing, as well as in episodic memory.

These findings extend our previous research on anxiety and depressed mood by addressing brain regions involved in a task that required the regulation of emotional responses to threat and appetitive stimuli. The data suggest that individual differences on personality and symptom measures are associated with different patterns of reaction time, as well as with different patterns of activity in specific brain regions. Activity in these brain regions will affect patterns of cognition, attention, and emotion regulation.

A disposition toward positive affect was associated with activity in the neural circuits thought to be involved in approach behavior, as well as in promoting selective attention. On the other hand, anxious arousal seems to be linked to the activity of a right hemisphere system that plays an executive role in modulating attention and vigilance in response to threat. This right hemisphere system promotes sympathetic nervous system activity, spatial attention, visual scanning of the environment, and sensitivity to meaningful nonverbal cues. These characteristics are very adaptive in the context of a threatening situation. However, when threat is not present, or when an individual is prone to falsely perceive threat to be present (as is the case in many anxiety disorders), the activity of this emotional surveillance system interferes with accurate and quick responses to a task that requires selective attention.

Finally, interference in response to appetitive words was associated with self-reported anxious apprehension, anhedonic depression, alexithymia, and negative affect in this study, as well as with neural circuits that are associated with withdrawal and negative valence. We hypothesize that this pattern was characteristic of people who found the appetitive words (which were mostly sex-related) aversive or uncomfortable.

These findings take us a step further toward our goal of identifying more of the multiple brain regions involved in the many processes active in emotion. They suggest that states, traits, and symptoms are seamlessly intertwined with cognitive and attentional functions. Furthermore, these functions are supported by processing in specific brain regions that implement both emotional and cognitive processes.

REFERENCES

Almagor, M., Tellegen, A., & Waller, N. G. (1995). The Big Seven model: A cross-cultural replication and further exploration of the basic dimensions of natural language trait descriptors. *Journal of Personality and Social Psychology, 69,* 300–307.

American Psychiatric Association. (1994). *Diagnostic and statistical manual of mental disorders* (4th ed.). Washington, DC: Author.

Banich, M. T., Stolar, N., Heller, W., & Goldman, R. B. (1992). A deficit in right-hemisphere performance after induction of a depressed mood. *Neuropsychiatry, Neuropsychology and Behavioral Neurology, 5,* 20–27.

Beck, A. T., Rush, A. J., Shaw, B. F., & Emery, G. (1979). *Cognitive therapy of depression.* New York: Guilford Press.

Bruder, G. E. (1995). Cerebral laterality and psychopathology: Perceptual and event-related asymmetries in affective and schizophrenic disorder. In R. J. Davidson & K. Hugdahl (Eds.) *Brain asymmetry* (pp. 661–691). Cambridge, MA: MIT Press.

Compton, R. J., Banich, M. T., Mohanty, A., Milham, M. P., Miller, G. A., Scalf, P. E., & Heller, W. (2001). *Paying attention to emotion: An fMRI investigation of cognitive and emotional Stroop tasks.* Manuscript submitted for publication.

Compton, R. J., Heller, W., Banich, M. T., Palmieri, P. A., & Miller, G. A. (2000). Responding to threat: Hemispheric asymmetries and interhemispheric division of input. *Neuropsychology, 14,* 254–264.

Costa, P. T., & McCrae, R. R. (1980). Influence of extraversion and neuroticism on subjective well-being: Happy and unhappy people. *Journal of Personality and Social Psychology, 38,* 668–678.

Costa, P. T., Jr., & McCrae, R. R. (1992). *Revised NEO Personality Inventory (NEO-PI-R) and NEO Five-Factor Inventory (NEO-FFI) Professional Manual.* Odessa, FL: Psychological Assessment Resources.

Deldin, P. J., Keller, J., Gergen, J. A., & Miller, G. A. (2000). Right-posterior face processing anomaly in depression. *Journal of Abnormal Psychology, 109,* 116–121.

Diener, E., & Emmons, R. A. (1984). The independence of positive and negative affect. *Journal of Personality and Social Psychology, 47,* 1105–1117.

Diener, E., Larsen, R. J., Levine, S., & Emmons, R. A. (1985). Intensity and frequency: Dimensions underlying positive and negative affect. *Journal of Personality and Social Psychology, 48,* 1253–1265.

Digman, J. M., & Inouye, J. (1986). Further specification of the five robust factors of personality. *Journal of Personality and Social Psychology, 50,* 116–123.

Digman, J. M., & Takemoto-Chock, N. K. (1981). Factors in the natural language of personality: Re-analysis, comparison, and interpretation of six major studies. *Multivariate Behavioral Research, 16,* 149–170.

Ehlers, A., Margraf, J., Davies, S., & Roth, W. T. (1988). Selective processing of threat cues in subjects with panic attacks. *Cognition and Emotion, 2,* 201–219.

Eysenck, H. J. (1987). Comments on "The orthogonality of Extraversion and Neuroticism scales." *Psychological Reports, 61,* 50.

Foa, E. B., Ilai, D., McCarthy, P. R., Shoyer, B., & Murdock, T. (1993). Information processing in obsessive–compulsive disorder. *Cognitive Therapy and Research, 17,* 173–189.

Fujita, F., Diener, E., & Sandvik, E. (1991). Gender differences in negative affect and well-being: The case for emotional intensity. *Journal of Personality and Social Psychology, 61,* 427–434.

Gray, J. A. (1987). The neuropsychology of emotion and personality. In S. M. Stahl, S. D. Iversen, & E. C. Goodman (Eds.), *Cognitive neurochemistry* (pp. 171–190). Oxford, UK: Oxford University Press.

Heller, W. (1990). The neuropsychology of emotion: Developmental patterns and implications for psychopathology. In N. Stein, B. L. Leventhal, & T. Trabasso (Eds.), *Psychological and biological approaches to emotion* (pp. 167–211). Hillsdale, NJ: Erlbaum.

Heller, W. (1993). Neuropsychological mechanisms of individual differences in emotion, personality, and arousal. *Neuropsychology, 7,* 476–489.

Heller, W., Banich, M. T., Herrington, J. D., Mohanty, A., Fisher, J. E., Jacobson, B. L., Scalf, P., Erickson, K. I., Koven, N. S., Compton, R. J., & Miller, G. A. (2000, November). *Differential brain activation in response to positive and threat stimuli in an emotional Stroop paradigm.* Paper presented at the annual meeting of the Society for Research in Psychopathology, Boulder, CO.

Heller, W., Etienne, M., & Miller, G. A. (1995). Patterns of perceptual asymmetry in depression and anxiety: Implications for neuropsychological models of emotion and psychopathology. *Journal of Abnormal Psychology, 104,* 327–333.

Heller, W., & Nitschke, J. B. (1997). Regional brain activity in emotion: A framework for understanding cognition in depression. *Cognition and Emotion, 11,* 637–661.

Heller, W., & Nitschke, J. B. (1998). The puzzle of regional brain activity in depression and anxiety: The importance of subtypes and comorbidity. *Cognition and Emotion, 12*, 421–447.

Heller, W., Nitschke, J. B., Etienne, M. A., & Miller, G. A. (1997). Patterns of regional brain activity differentiate types of anxiety. *Journal of Abnormal Psychology, 106*, 376–385.

Heller, W., Nitschke, J. B., & Lindsay, D. L. (1997). Neuropsychological correlates of arousal in self-reported emotion. *Cognition and Emotion, 11*, 383–402.

Hope, D. A., Rapee, R. M., Heimberg, R. G., & Dombeck, M. J. (1990). Representations of the self in social phobia: Vulnerability to social threat. *Cognitive Therapy and Research, 14*, 177–189.

Hotard, S. R., McFatter, R. M., McWhirter, R. M., & Stegall, M. E. (1989). Interactive effects of extraversion, neuroticism, and social relationships on subjective well-being. *Journal of Personality and Social Psychology, 57*, 321–331.

Keller, J., Nitschke, J. B., Bhargava, T., Deldin, P. J., Gergen, J. A., Miller, G. A., & Heller, W. (2000). Neuropsychological differentiation of depression and anxiety. *Journal of Abnormal Psychology, 109*, 3–10.

Kendell, R. E., MacKenzie, W. E., West, C., McGuire, R. J., & Cox, J. L. (1984). Day-to-day mood changes after childbirth: Further data. *British Journal of Psychiatry, 145*, 620–625.

Keogh, E., French, C. C., & Reidy, J. (1998). Predictors of worry. *Anxiety, Stress, and Coping, 11*, 67–80.

Kirkcaldy, B. D. (1984). The interrelationship between state and trait variables. *Personality and Individual Differences, 5*, 141–149.

Ladavas, E., Nicoletti, R., Umilta, C., & Rizzolatti, G. (1984). Right hemisphere interference during negative affect: A reaction time study. *Neuropsychologia, 22*, 479–485.

Larsen, R. J. (1989). Personality as an affect dispositional system. In L. A. Clark & D. Watson (Chairs), *Emotional bases of personality*. Symposium conducted at the meeting of the American Psychological Association, New Orleans, LA.

Larsen, R. J., & Diener, E. (1985). A multitrait-multimethod examination of affect structure: Hedonic level and emotional intensity. *Personality and Individual Differences, 6*, 631–636.

Larsen, R. J., & Diener, E. (1992). Promises and problems with the circumplex model of affect. In M. S. Clark (Ed.), *Emotion* (pp. 25–59). Newbury Park: Sage.

Larsen, R. J., & Ketelaar, T. (1989). Extraversion, neuroticism and susceptibility to positive and negative mood induction procedures. *Personality and Individual Differences, 10*, 1221–1228.

Larsen, R. J., & Ketelaar, T. (1991). Personality and susceptibility to positive and negative emotional states. *Journal of Personality and Social Psychology, 61*, 132–140.

Levy, J., Heller, W., Banich, M. T., & Burton, L. A. (1983). Asymmetry of perception in free viewing of chimeric faces. *Brain and Cognition, 2*, 404–419.

Liotti, M., & Tucker, D. M. (1992). Right hemisphere sensitivity to arousal and depression. *Brain and Cognition, 18*, 138–151.

Mathews, A., & MacLeod, C. (1985). Selective processing of threat cues in anxiety states. *Behaviour Research and Therapy, 23*, 563–569.

McCrae, R. R., & Costa, P. T. (1987). Validation of the five-factor model of personality across instruments and observers. *Journal of Personality and Social Psychology, 52*, 81–90.

McCrae, R. R., & Costa, P. T. (1989). More reasons to adopt the five-factor model. *American Psychologist, 44*, 451–452.

McCrae, R. R., Costa, P. T., & Busch, C. M. (1986). Evaluating comprehensiveness in personality systems: The California Q-Set and the five-factor model. *Journal of Personality, 54*, 430–446.

McNally, R. J. (1998). Cognitive aspects of posttraumatic stress disorder. In E. Sanavio (Ed.), *Behavior and cognitive therapy today: Essays in honor of Hans J. Eysenck* (pp. 181–187). Oxford, UK: Elsevier Science.

McNally, R. J., Kaspi, S. P., Riemann, B. C., & Zeitlin, S. B. (1990). Selective processing of threat cues in posttraumatic stress disorder. *Journal of Abnormal Psychology, 99*, 398–402.

Meyer, G. J., & Shack, J. R. (1989). Structural convergence of mood and personality: Evidence for old and new directions. *Journal of Personality and Social Psychology, 57*, 691–706.

Nitschke, J. B., Heller, W., Imig, J., McDonald, R. P., & Miller, G. A. (2001). Distinguishing dimensions of anxiety and depression. *Cognitive Therapy and Research, 25*, 1–22.

Nitschke, J. B., Heller, W., & Miller, G. A. (2000). Anxiety, stress, and cortical brain function. In J. C. Borod (Ed.), *The neuropsychology of emotion* (pp. 298–319). New York: Oxford University Press.

Nitschke, J. B., Heller, W., Palmieri, P. A., & Miller, G. A. (1999). Contrasting patterns of brain activity in anxious apprehension and anxious arousal. *Psychophysiology, 36*, 628–637.

O'Malley, M. N., & Gillette, C. S. (1984). Exploring the relations between traits and emotions. *Journal of Personality, 52*, 274–284.

Otto, M. W., Yeo, R. A., & Dougher, M. J. (1987). Right hemisphere involvement in depression: Toward a neuropsychological theory of negative affective experiences. *Biological Psychiatry, 22*, 1201–1215.

Palmieri, P. A., Heller, W., & Miller, G. A. (2001). *Posttrauma anxiety and depression: Implications for conceptualization and assessment of PTSD*. Manuscript in preparation.

Peabody, D. (1984). Personality dimensions through trait inferences. *Journal of Personality and Social Psychology, 46*, 384–403.

Peabody, D., & Goldberg, L. R. (1989). Some determinants of factor structures from personality trait descriptors. *Journal of Personality and Social Psychology, 57*, 552–567.

Russell, J. A. (1980). A circumplex model of affect. *Journal of Personality and Social Psychology, 39*, 1161–1178.

Schmidtke, J. I., & Heller, W. (2001). *Personality, affect, and EEG: Predicting patterns of regional brain activity related to extroversion and neuroticism.* Manuscript submitted for publication.

Spielberger, C. D., Gorsuch, R. L., Lushene, R. E., Vagg, P. R., & Jacobs, G. A. (1983). *Manual for the state-trait anxiety inventory.* Palo Alto, CA: Consulting Psychologists Press.

Tellegen, A. (1985). Structures of mood and personality and their relevance to assessing anxiety, with an emphasis on self-report. In A. H. Tuma & J. D. Maser (Eds.), *Anxiety and the anxiety disorders* (pp. 681–706). Hillsdale, NJ: Erlbaum.

Thayer, R. E., Takahashi, P. J., & Pauli, J. A. (1988). Multidimensional arousal states, diurnal rhythms, cognitive and social processes, and extraversion. *Personality and Individual Differences, 9,* 15–24.

Warr, P. B., Barter, J., & Brownbridge, G. (1983). On the independence of positive and negative affect. *Journal of Personality and Social Psychology, 44,* 644–651.

Watson, D. (1988). Intraindividual and interindividual analyses of positive and negative affect: Their relation to health complaints, perceived stress, and daily activities. *Journal of Personality and Social Psychology, 54,* 1020–1030.

Watson, D., Clark, L. A., & Tellegen, A. (1988). Development and validation of brief measures of positive and negative affect: The PANAS scales. *Journal of Personality and Social Psychology, 54,* 1063–1070.

Watson, D., & Tellegen, A. (1985). Toward a consensual structure of mood. *Psychological Bulletin, 98,* 219–235.

Watts, F. N., McKenna, F. P., Sharrock, R., & Trezise, L. (1986). Colour naming of phobia-related words. *British Journal of Psychology, 77,* 97–108.

Williams, D. G. (1981). Personality and mood: State-trait relationships. *Personality and Individual Differences, 2,* 303–309.

CHAPTER 5

Incentive and Threat Reactivity
Relations with Anterior Cortical Activity

STEVEN K. SUTTON

Personality science has the exciting charge of investigating the intrapersonal processes that are common to all humans, along with exploring the components of those processes that lead to individual differences. One potentially fruitful area of investigation is basic motivational processes that drive and direct our behavior. An initial, possibly overly simplistic, division of motivation can be made by distinguishing motivational processes associated with incentives from those associated with threats. Any organism with the potential to selectively move about its environment must be able to organize mental, physiological, and environmental resources in order to turn incentives into rewards and keep threats from becoming punishments. Such systems have been proposed and described by numerous biobehavioral researchers (e.g., Clark & Watson, 1999; Depue & Collins, 1999; Gray, 1981; Kagan, Reznick, & Snidman, 1988; Konorski, 1967; Lang, 1995; Rothbart, Derryberry, & Posner, 1994; Tucker & Williamson, 1984). This chapter first presents some ideas associated with these concepts, then a sampling of research findings linking anterior cortical brain activity with incentive and threat motivational states and traits. By investigating relations between neurobiological functioning and motivation, we can take a step toward further understanding potential neurobiological substrates of personality.

INCENTIVE AND THREAT MOTIVATION SYSTEMS

As is implied by the nature of the stimuli used to label these two systems, the functions and supporting behaviors, cognitions, and feelings associated with each system are expected to differ in significant ways. For the *incentive* system, we would highlight (1) approach and goal pursuit behaviors; (2) cognition that supports the detection of and orientation toward positively valenced stimuli, along with the evaluation of the sequential movements required and adopted in order to make the incentive a reward; and (3) feelings that would best be described as eager, enthusiastic, and excited during the pre–goal-attainment period. For the *threat* system, we would highlight (1) an initial behavioral inhibition of ongoing activity at the time of threat detection, along with preparation for withdrawal and avoidance behaviors; (2) cognition that supports the detection of, vigilant attention toward, and evaluation of negatively valenced stimuli; and (3) feelings that would best be described as anxious, nervous, and tense. These two sets of terms describing the feelings for incentive and threat motivation easily map onto the constructs and self-report measures of positive and negative affect/activation (e.g., Watson, Clark, & Tellegen, 1988) and energetic and tense arousal (e.g., Thayer, 1989). They map only indirectly onto common discrete emotion constructs such as amusement, anger, disgust, embarrassment, happiness, sadness, and surprise. For example, happiness is associated with post–goal-attainment conditions, rather than the pre–goal-attainment pursuit of an incentive (eagerness).

Whereas the incentive and threat systems are considered independent in terms of their eliciting stimuli, it is important to consider the issue of coactivation. One reason for this is the predominant anticipatory and preparatory, rather than consummatory (Konorski, 1967), nature of these systems. They are repeatedly activated by stimuli to prepare one for appropriate action, irrespective of whether or not that action is engaged. Furthermore, our externally and internally generated environments continually present both incentives and threats. For example, as I drive my car to and from work, I repeatedly encounter opportunities to approach my endpoint goal. I also come across other incentives, such as a fast-food restaurant or coffee house. Furthermore, as I maneuver through this maze, I am repeatedly presented with threats to my physical and mental well-being. Similarly, coactivation stems from the fact that single entities within our environment may present both incentive and threat qualities. For example, the bear that you or your early evolutionary ancestor may be hunting can be dinner for you, or you dinner for it. Your boss has the potential to give you a raise or a promotion or to fire you.

Another important issue is the interaction of the incentive and threat systems. This interaction is likely to be mutually inhibitory in nature. This derives from the convergence of three facts: (1) our environment is often composed of a collection of incentives and threats; (2) the available resources called on by these systems are limited; and (3) at any given moment, one cannot both physically approach and withdraw from the same location. This proposal of mutual inhibition will most likely express itself at the behavioral level. However, this is also likely to occur at the cognitive level when information processing resources such as attention and working memory are limited. The feeling level may be least influenced by this mutual inhibition, although there is evidence that such inhibition occurs when one system is highly active (e.g., Thayer, 1989). This mutual inhibitory quality makes relative activation of either system an important consideration when studying motivational states.

Individual Differences in Motivation System Reactivity

Temperament has been defined as "constitutionally based individual differences in reactivity and self-regulation, influenced over time by heredity, maturation, and experience" (Rothbart & Ahadi, 1994, p. 55). Individual differences in the reactivity of the incentive and threat systems nicely fit this definition of temperament, be it in children or adults. The reactivity (or sensitivity or strength) of a motivation system reflects how rapidly and dominantly the system organizes resources in response to a pertinent stimulus. This general operating characteristic of the motivation system emphasizes *reactivity* rather than general level of activity. In other words, the "trait" is not the level at which your engine idles, but rather the increase in engine activity when you hit the gas pedal. The stable, enduring characteristic of each motivation system is not its activity level (which constantly fluctuates), but rather its reactivity (or sensitivity or strength)—the rapidity and efficiency of the motivation system to prepare the organism for action in response to a broad class of eliciting stimuli.

It is reasonable to presume that the sensitivity of these systems are unimodal and symmetric in distribution. Therefore, one expects that most people will be about average in system sensitivity and that these motivational systems are unlikely to account for much variance in most single situations in which numerous constructs are influential. The sensitivities of these systems also are proposed to be orthogonal, even though the systems themselves are proposed to mutually inhibit each other. Therefore, any combination of incentive and threat sensitivity is possible. Furthermore, given the idea of mutual inhibition, *relative* sensitivity of each system is an important consideration when studying the influence of motivational traits on current behavior, thoughts, and feelings. In other words, it is less an issue of how sensitive the incentive or threat system is but rather of which system is more sensitive, given that each system is continually being activated.

The proposal of individual differences in *reactivity* has implications for the measurement of motivational states and traits. First, reactions are transient and dynamic. Any identifiable reaction has multiple components. Some of the most prominent are onset, peak amplitude, and decay or recovery. Given this dynamic, it becomes important to make observations that allow one to accurately measure the component of interest. This is difficult when one is trying to observe a reaction to a single stimulus with the measurement tools that personality scientists use regularly, especially self-report measures. One alternative is to infer individual differences in reactivity by observing levels of activity over time and across situations. In essence, asking an individual to report his or her general level of affect can *approximate* the sensitivity of one's motivation system, which is directly related to one's reaction to stimuli rather than general level of activation.

A related implication is the importance of tracking the environment in which the person maneuvers. Not all environments are equal in terms of incentives and threats. And not all individuals in the same environment are equally positioned to approach the desired and avoid the undesired. Thus individual differences in incentive and threat sensitivity will not express themselves everywhere and anywhere. For example, an individual who is highly sensitive to incentives and lives in an environment that presents itself with few signals for reward will not express many approach behaviors nor feel generally eager or enthusiastic. With that said, it is also possible that an individual highly sensitive to incentives will more likely perceive more or less neutral, ambiguous, and novel stimuli as incentives. This, in turn, would generate feelings of eagerness and approach behaviors.

From these proposals about incentive and threat sensitivities, one can derive the following predictions. Individuals who are relatively high in incentive system sensitivity (1) will execute approach behaviors more readily and more forcefully in response to *known* incentives (conditioned stimuli), as well as to novel, potential incentives; (2) will more rapidly detect incentives in complex environments and will more likely attend to incentives than threats; (3) will develop stronger associations among incentives and positively valenced stimuli and constructs and, in turn, will more likely evaluate ambiguous stimuli as positively valenced; and (4) will experience higher momentary and general levels of eagerness and enthusiasm. Individuals who are relatively high in threat system strength or sensitivity (1) will more likely inhibit ongoing goal pursuit and vigilantly attend to threat, (2) will execute avoidant or withdrawal behaviors more readily and more forcefully, (3) will more rapidly detect and attend to threats in complex environments, (4) will develop stronger associations among threats and other negatively valenced stimuli and constructs, and (5) will experience higher momentary and general levels of anxiety and nervousness.

Neurobiological Substrates

Proposals concerning links between personality constructs and neurobiological structures and functioning (including neurotransmitter systems) have been around for a long time (e.g., Eysenck, 1967; Pavlov, 1955). Given the fundamental conceptual nature of the incentive and threat systems, we expect an associated fundamental neurobiology in humans and other animals, with some areas of overlap and some areas of specialization in terms of brain structures and neurotransmitter systems. For example, Depue and others (e.g., Depue & Collins, 1999) have argued that the mesolimbic dopamine neurotransmitter system and associated subcortical structures appear to be core neurobiological substrates of the incentive system, whereas the ceruleocortical noradrenergic neurotransmitter system and associated subcortical structures appear to be core neurobiological substrates of the threat system. The view proposed by Davidson (e.g., 1995) emphasizes approach and withdrawal as organizing dimensions of behavior and argues that one likely area of motivation system separation in primates is anterior cerebral lateralization. More specifically, for individuals who are strongly right-handed, it is proposed that left anterior cortical regions provide substrates for components of the incentive system and right anterior cortical regions provide substrates for components of the threat system.

It is not surprising that these systems have frontal lobe components, given the potential complexity of responding to incentives and threats and the general link between the frontal lobes and planful behavior. But why the asymmetry? One general reason is for more efficient, rapid, and accurate processing for each system (Kosslyn, 1987). Another general reason is to separate those processes that lead to behavioral inhibition and preparation for withdrawal or avoidance from those that move toward an incentive. Approaching threats and avoiding incentives is not conducive to mental health or survival. Furthermore, these can be thought of as competing systems that will, on occasion, need to acquire control over available resources in order to make the incentive a reward or to keep the threat from becoming a punishment. Asymmetry may aid this mutually inhibitory aspect of system functioning.

Other aspects of incentive and threat motivation suggest the importance of frontal lobe processes. For example, Davidson (1995) proposed that left anterior cortical regions help maintain images of goal states, which is critical for much of our goal-oriented behavior, given that many rewards are not present in our immediate environment. Furthermore, there is a sequential "take-a-step, evaluate progress, take-a-step" nature of moving toward a desired object, especially when the desired object is animate. This merges well with the sequential nature of language, especially the generation of speech, which is lateralized toward left anterior cortical regions. For the threat system, the idea of lateralization nicely merges with the cognitive process of vigilant attention that has been linked to right anterior cortical regions (for a review, see Posner, 1995). This also fits with the traditional notion that the right side of the cortex tends to support integrative processing of multiple sensory stimuli, the kind of processing one needs when evaluating the what, where, and how of a threat.

There also appears to be sufficient evidence from research in neurobiology to conclude that there are asymmetric projections from subcortical neurotransmitter systems to anterior cortical regions (see Robbins & Everitt, 1995; Tucker & Williamson, 1984). More specifically, the mesolimbic dopaminergic system, which ascends from subcortical structures associated with incentive motivational processes, appears to asymmetrically project to left anterior cortical regions. The ceruleocortical noradrenergic system, which ascends from subcortical structures associated with threat motivational processes, appears to asymmetrically project to right anterior cortical regions.

Technological and methodological limitations have made it difficult to study the long-purported links between neurobiological activity, motivation, and personality. However, recent advances in neuroimaging technology, as well as methodological advances in cognitive neuroscience and affective neuroscience, make it easier to test questions concerning these links. Not only has the technology become more powerful and precise, it has also become more affordable and accessible. As with any aspect of technology and research methodology, each has its strengths and weaknesses. Scalp electroencephalography (EEG) is one of the oldest, least invasive, and most accessible and affordable technology for assessing regional cortical activity. In the following studies, Fourier transform of EEG was used to compute power density values in the alpha band (8–13 Hz), which is a commonly used (inverse) index of cortical activity (see Pivik et al., 1993).

The measurement of brain electrical activity using scalp electrodes presents several problems that are common to personality research (e.g., acquiring reliable measures) and several problems that are unique to EEG (e.g., reducing nonneurogenic sources of electrical activity recorded by a scalp electrode). With sufficient training of personnel and attention to detail, these challenges are easily overcome. However, these issues must be addressed and appropriate analytic techniques applied. For excellent presentations of these issues, see Davidson, Jackson, & Larson (2000) and Duffy (1994).

SAMPLES OF RECENT RESEARCH

The following sections present several studies that highlight relations between anterior brain activity, threat, and incentive motivation. Some of these studies created motivationally relevant laboratory environments and assessed changes in anterior brain activity in response to these conditions. In other words, these studies investigated one aspect of the intrapersonal processes associated with incentive and threat motivational states. Other studies measured resting brain activity and assessed relations with trait-oriented aspects of motivation (e.g., sensitivity). Still other studies used initial measures of resting cortical activity to predict individual differences in reactions to motivationally relevant stimuli in an experiment.

Anterior Brain Activation and Motivational States

One relatively early study highlights the link between anterior brain activity, incentives, and threats. Sobotka, Davidson, and Senulis (1992) had unselected participants perform a simple reaction time task in which trials differed in terms of the nature of the motivational manipulation. On some trials, the incentive was a 25-cent reward for responding faster than an individually set criterion. On other trials, the threat was a 25-cent loss for not responding fast enough. The motivational nature of each trial was signaled for a 4-second period immediately prior to the presentation of the reaction stimulus. EEG was used to measure brain activity during the 4-second windows. Sobotka et al. (1992) found relatively greater left-sided midfrontal brain activity during incentive trials relative to threat trials.

In a study using positron emission tomography (PET) of glucose metabolism rather than EEG to record brain activity, eight female volunteers viewed an extended series of pictures to elicit incentive and threat motivation (Sutton et al., 1996). In the first of three sessions over a 15-day period, participants viewed neutral pictures drawn from the International Affective Picture System (Center for the Study of Emotion and Attention, 1995). In the second and third sessions, participants viewed either a set of threat-oriented or a set of incentive-oriented pictures, respectively (counterbalanced across participants). Not surprisingly, self-report and facial EMG showed that the neutral condition, with the initial experience with the PET procedures (e.g., being injected with a radioisotope for the first time), generated relatively high levels of anxiety. Therefore, the initial and threat conditions were combined and compared with the incentive condition. Consistent with the pattern of results from the self-report and facial EMG measures, participants exhibited significantly greater metabolic activity in *right* prefrontal cortical regions during the initial and threat sessions.

Other EEG studies used targeted populations in order to present a more powerful incentive or threat stimulus in the laboratory. For example, Davidson, Marshall, Tomarken, and Henriques (2000) had social phobics and nonphobic control participants prepare to make a public speech. During this 3-minute preparation period, EEG and cardiovascular measures were made. Social phobics reported higher levels of anxiety during this period. They also had higher heart rate and showed a greater increase in brain activity in right anterior temporal and lateral prefrontal regions. In other words, an anxiety-provoking situation (the anticipation of the public speech) generated greater right-sided anterior cortical brain activity in individuals who particularly find such situations threatening. Focusing more on incentive motivation, Zinser, Fiore, Davidson, and Baker (1999) presented chronic cigarette smokers who had abstained from smoking for 24 hours with a lit cigarette for 60 seconds prior to permitting inhalation. These individuals showed a strong increase in left midfrontal brain activity during this preconsummatory period.

Another study highlights the incentive and approach nature of left frontal activity. Harmon-Jones and Sigelman (2001) found that participants experiencing anger (which occurs in goal-striving contexts and promotes the displacement of goal-striving obstacles) showed greater left frontal activity. This finding also demonstrates the importance of conceptualizing discrete emotional states in terms of motivational dimensions, moving beyond the widely used dimensions of valence and arousal. That is, there is no simple mapping of valence on the incentive and threat motivation systems. Negative valence does not necessarily go with threat motivation, as is highlighted by these results. And incentive motivation may be associated with negatively valenced emotion when goal striving fails (e.g., sadness) or fails to proceed at an acceptable pace (e.g., frustration; Carver & Scheier, 1998).

Resting Anterior Brain Activity and Motivational Traits

Since the mid-1980s, several studies have assessed relations between resting anterior brain activity and various measures of individual differences in incentive and threat motivation. Many studies have found relations between resting left-sided anterior brain activity and greater sensitivity to incentives and between resting right-sided anterior brain activity and greater sensitivity to threats. To highlight this pattern of results and related issues, the following are three studies I performed in collaboration with Richard Davidson, along with shorter summaries of related research findings from other laboratories.

From 1991 through 1994, five cohorts of University of Wisconsin undergraduates provided resting EEG data in Richard Davidson's laboratory. A subset of participants from the latter three cohorts provided data for the following set of studies. Participants in each cohort initially volunteered for two sessions, for which each received course credit for participation. Of these unselected volunteers, only those who were strongly right-handed and had no history of psychiatric disorder, neurological disorder, or brain trauma remained in the study. Ninety-one of these persons subsequently agreed to participate in two non-EEG sessions for money. These two sessions were completed between 4 and 30 months following participation in the two resting EEG sessions.

EEG was recorded during eight 1-minute periods within each of two sessions, which were separated by 6 weeks. The participant is instructed to sit quietly with eyes opened or closed on four of the eight periods within each session. EEG data collection required about 15 minutes following 30–50 minutes of electrode placement by a pair of trained research assistants. As mentioned previously, many important issues must be addressed when recording brain activity using scalp electrodes. Some of these issues are presented here. For more information about general issues, see Davidson et al. (2000) and Duffy (1994). For more detailed information concerning the recording of resting EEG for this study, see Sutton and Davidson (1997).

EEG was recorded from 29 standard sites—13 homologous left–right pairs and 3 midline sites—following the 10/20 system (Jasper, 1958). Two electrode pairs also were placed around the eyes for the recording of eye movements and eyeblinks, which are primary sources of nonneurogenic electrical activity at EEG sites. This array of EEG electrodes covered cortical regions from the frontal pole (Fp) through the frontal lobe (F), the central sulcus (C), temporal lobe (T), and parietal lobe (P), with the most posterior sites over the parietal/occipital lobe border (PO). The three midline sites were Fz, Cz, and Pz (z referring to the zero line). For each electrode location on the left side of the head, there is a homologous electrode on the right side of the head. Each electrode site is referenced by the cortical region and a number. For example, the left and right midfrontal sites are F3 and F4, and the left and right lateral frontal sites are F7 and F8. The larger numbers refer to the greater distance from the midline.

There are numerous potential metrics for assessment of brain activity using EEG. In this case, Fourier transform was used to estimate power density values ($\mu V^2/Hz$) for the standard alpha band (8–13 Hz). Values in this band are generally accepted as an inverse index of cortical activity (see Pivik et al., 1993). Due to interindividual differences in the distribution of these values, they were normalized via log transformation. Furthermore, an asymmetry score was computed for each of the 13 left–right electrode pairs by subtracting the value for the left site from that of the right site. Positive (negative) asymmetry scores reflect relatively greater left-sided (right-sided) activation.

One reason for this computation is to control for nonneurogenic sources of individual differences in the computation of power density values. One nonneurogenic source is skull thickness, in which there is more interindividual variability than intraindividual variability. It is most important to attempt to control for this source of variability in an individual differences study that does not group participants and has a relatively small sample size. Computing an asymmetry score also has *conceptual* value in that the relative level of left-sided versus right-sided activity may better predict behavior given the purported mutually inhibitory relation between the incentive and threat systems. If both systems are continually activated and coactivated across situations and over time, then the relative sensitivity of the incentive versus threat system may account for more variance than either system on its own.

One important question concerning these measures of resting cortical brain activity is whether or not they have the psychometric characteristics one desires of a "trait." Cronbach's (1951) alpha can be used to estimate internal consistency reliability by treating individual 1-minute baselines as comparable to items on a questionnaire. And by acquiring resting EEG from two sessions separated by 6 weeks, intraclass correlations can be computed to estimate test–retest reliability. Asymmetry scores have been shown to have good internal consistency reliability and adequate test–retest reliability (e.g., Sutton & Davidson, 1997; Tomarken, Davidson, Wheeler, & Kinney, 1992). These estimates of reliability tend to be lower for anterior relative to central and posterior homologous pairs. This tendency highlights the need to aggregate both within and across sessions to get the best estimates of true scores. To further investigate this issue, Tomarken, Keener, and Neubauer (1994) assessed test–retest reliability across various combinations of resting EEG sessions; three initial sessions were completed within a few months, and another two sessions were completed about 1 year later. The intraclass correlation of the aggregate midfrontal asymmetry score across the three initial sessions and the aggregate across the two latter sessions was .82. This was considerably higher than the values computed within the initial or latter sessions, which were much more proximal in time.

Resting EEG Asymmetry and Self-Reported Motivational Strength

One question addressed with data from the last of these three cohorts asked whether or not resting anterior brain activity was related to self-report measures that would index the sensitivity of incentive and threat motivation (Sutton & Davidson, 1997). Forty-six participants (23 females) provided two reliable sessions of resting EEG data and completed two self-report measures twice. These were the dispositional/general version of the Positive and Negative Affect Schedule (PANAS-General; Watson, Clark, & Tellegen, 1988) and the BIS/BAS Scales (Carver & White, 1994). The PANAS-General was completed during each resting EEG session following EEG data collection (6 weeks later). The BIS/BAS Scales were completed once at the end of the second EEG session and once during a non-EEG session (4–6 months later).

These two self-report inventories were selected because they both have conceptual links to incentive and threat motivation, yet they index motivation system sensitivity in different ways. The PANAS-General presents two sets of 10 terms targeting positive affect/activation (PA) and negative affect/activation (NA). As stated previously, these scales map onto the feelings associated with incentive and threat motivation, respectively. The prediction is that someone with a more sensitive incentive threat system would both have greater left (right) anterior cortical activity while at rest and report higher general levels of PA (NA). The BIS/BAS Scales were created to measure individual differences in the strength of Gray's (e.g., 1981) Behavior Inhibition System (BIS) and Behavioral Activation (or Approach) System (BAS). Items for both scales inquire about *reactions* to pertinent stimuli rather than general levels of activity or preferences for certain conditions. Again, greater left (right) anterior activity is predicted to be related to higher BAS (BIS) scores. Given the procedures for computing EEG asymmetry scores, BAS/BIS and PA/NA difference scores also were calculated for each assessment, then averaged across the two assessments.

Consistent with predictions, the correlation between the BAS/BIS difference score and midfrontal (F3/F4) EEG asymmetry was .53 ($p < .005$), with significant correlations at other anterior sites. The correlations between the BAS/BIS difference score and EEG asymmetry at central and more posterior scalp sites were not significant (e.g., C3/C4 = .26, $p > .07$), and P3/P4 = .03). Moreover, the difference between the BAS/BIS with midfrontal correlation versus the BAS/BIS with parietal correlation was significant ($t(43) = 2.79, p < .01$). This underscores the specificity of these relations to the anterior cortical regions.

The correlation between the PA/NA difference score and midfrontal EEG asymmetry was also positive, but not significant at .16. Furthermore, the BAS/BIS difference score and midfrontal EEG asymmetry correlation was significantly greater than this PA/NA correlation ($t(43) = 2.87, p < .01$). This pattern of results emphasizes the link between anterior brain activity and the *sensitivity* of the incentive and threat motivation systems such that the BIS/BAS Scales more directly assess *reactions* to incentive and threat situations, whereas the PANAS-General addresses general levels of PA and NA. General levels of PA and NA clearly are linked to one's characteristic ways of reacting to incentives and threats but are also influenced more by environmental conditions that do not directly map onto the sensitivities of the motivation systems.

It is also valuable to contrast these correlations with correlations between resting EEG asymmetry and other personality measures that can conceptually be linked to left anterior activity and right anterior activity. For example, is anterior EEG asymmetry correlated with self-reported motivational state at the time of the EEG data acquisition? Immediately following the completion of EEG data acquisition, participants completed the PANAS with instructions to consider their *current* feelings (Watson et al., 1988). No association with anterior EEG asymmetry was observed. Furthermore, participants in some cohorts completed the Eysenck Personality Inventory (Extraversion, Neuroticism, and Psychoticism; Eysenck & Eysenck, 1964), the Affect Intensity Measure (Larsen, 1984), and the Life Orientation Test (Optimism & Pessimism; Scheier & Carver, 1985). In each case, the inventory was completed once, either during the first or second resting EEG session. None of the scales from these inventories was found to be significantly correlated with EEG asymmetry.

Other researchers have reported findings that link resting anterior brain activity with self-report measures. For example, Harmon-Jones and Allen (1997) reported positive correlations between EEG asymmetry and BAS scores. Tomarken and Davidson (1994) found that females who expressed a repressive-defensive coping style (minimizing negative events and affect and accentuating positive events and affect) exhibited greater resting left-sided anterior asymmetry than controls. Schmidt (1999) reported that left and right anterior brain activity is differentially associated with sociability and shyness, respectively. From an incentive–threat perspective, sociability reflects an incentive-oriented view of other individuals (often major sources of reward), whereas shyness reflects a threat-oriented view of others (often, also, major sources of punishment). Extending these ideas to other populations, Henriques and Davidson (1990, 1991) have shown that currently or previously depressed individuals (i.e., those who present a significant lack of incentive motivation) exhibit relatively less resting left frontal activity. In summary, there is a substantial set of studies demonstrating links between left- and right-sided anterior cortical activity with incentive and threat motivation sensitivity, respectively.

Resting EEG Asymmetry and Biased Information Processing

Given that one component of motivation is the detection, selection, and orientation toward incentives and threats, it appears likely that individual differences in the strength of these two systems would influence information processing in a way that is consistent with the stronger of the two systems under circumstances in which other factors are controlled for. To test this idea, relations between resting anterior brain activity and the processing of affect-laden information in a forced-choice judgment of association task were assessed (Sutton & Davidson, 2000a). The prediction was that individuals exhibiting relatively greater resting left-sided (right-sided) anterior brain activity would be more likely to judge the more positively (negatively) valenced of the word pairs as going together better.

Participants were 83 (38 males) volunteers who provided reliable resting EEG data and completed a repeated, simple choice task in which two word pairs were presented simultaneously on the left and right side of a 14-inch computer monitor. Each word pair was presented with one word above the other. The participant was instructed to choose the word pair that "went together best" by pressing the "z" (left) or "/" (right) key on a standard computer keyboard. In each case, the presented word pairs were easily associated. Therefore, it was unlikely that word pair selection was based on the semantic associability of the word pair. However, word pairs were selected to have either an unpleasant (e.g., hurt–cry, war–gun, starving–hunger, pain–ache), neutral (e.g., mail–box, wheel–cart, accordion–instrument, kitchen–stove), or pleasant (e.g., happy–glad, ocean–beach, art–beauty, doctor–help) affective tone. Each choice was between word pairs from different affective categories: unpleasant versus neutral, unpleasant versus pleasant, and pleasant versus neutral.

Overall selection of word pairs was converted to a performance measure called the *positivity index* for assessing relations with resting EEG asymmetry. The positivity index is the total number of times the participant selected the more pleasant, or positive, of the two word pairs presented. This is the sum of (1) the number of pleasant pairs selected in pleasant–neutral comparisons, (2) the number of pleasant pairs selected in pleasant–unpleasant comparisons, and (3) the number of neutral pairs selected in neutral–unpleasant comparisons. Therefore, this positivity index is a measure of cognitive bias that is conceptually and psychometrically most similar to the EEG asymmetry metric.

Consistent with predictions, those with relatively greater left-sided resting anterior brain activity selected the more positively valenced word pair more often. More specifically, there was a significant correlation between the positivity index and anterior frontal (AF3/AF4) resting EEG asymmetry of .29 ($p < .01$). The correlations were marginally significant between the positivity index and resting EEG asymmetry at the midfrontal (F3/F4; $r = .20$) and lateral frontal (F7/F8; $r = .21$) sites. These positive relations were specific to anterior brain regions in that the correlation between the positivity index and anterior frontal asymmetry was significantly greater than was the correlation with parieto-occipital (PO3/PO4) asymmetry.

Another intriguing finding was prompted by analyses of valence ratings by an independent set of raters. This showed that females, relative to males, rated word pairs in the unpleasant category as more unpleasant and word pairs in the pleasant category as more pleasant. Such differences suggest that males and females process the pleasant and unpleasant word pairs differently. This may extend to the paired comparison task. Females, who on average appear to treat valence as a more salient dimension of the word pairs than males, may be more likely to use this dimension when evaluating the word pairs. This, in turn, may mediate the relation between anterior asymmetry and the positivity index. Consistent with this idea, the correlation between anterior frontal asymmetry and the positivity index was significant for females ($r = .39$), but not for males ($r = .12$). However, these correlations were not significantly different from each other. It is worth noting that both males and females, on average, selected the more positive word pair more often than one would expect based on chance, and the two groups did not differ in this tendency.

In summary, resting anterior brain activity predicted judgments of associative strength when contrasting stimuli that systematically differed in affective tone. Individuals with relatively greater resting left anterior frontal activity more often selected the more pleasant of the two word pairs. This highlights the trait-like nature of incentive and threat motivation sensitivity, given the extended time between the resting EEG sessions and the performance of the word-pairs task. Clearly, relations among resting EEG asymmetry and biased information processing of affective stimuli require further study with different cognitive tasks that target more specific cognitive processes. However, it is possible that the influence of the incentive and threat systems on these processes may be complex and that the links may be best observed with more complex cognitive tasks and contrasting stimuli, as is the case with the word-pairs task.

Resting EEG Asymmetry and (Self-)Motivated Performance

A third question addressed in this study was whether or not resting anterior brain activity would predict behavior on laboratory tasks when incentives (or threats) were presented (Sutton & Davidson, 2000b). There are many ways to present incentives and threats in laboratory tasks. One common path (especially with college students) is to create incentive and/ or threat conditions through the presentation of success and/or failure feedback. The general prediction is that those with a relatively more sensitive incentive (threat) system would show better task performance when performance feedback is set at a high rate of success (failure). More specifically, those with relatively greater left-sided anterior EEG asymmetry are expected to show a greater responsiveness to task feedback when that feedback is predominantly positive.

To test this prediction, 76 participants (42 females) who had provided reliable resting EEG data from two sessions performed a simple, "go-oriented" button-press task between 4 and 28 months following completion of the EEG sessions. The button-press device had one central button and five peripheral buttons. Each button had an adjacent pair of lights. Following an initial introduction and demonstration of an individual trial, the participant completed 10 trials to become familiar with the task. Each trial began with the participant pressing the central button, which started the clock that timed the length of the trial. The lights at one of the five peripheral buttons would then come on (amber in color), which signaled the participant to press that peripheral button (which would turn the lights off). Then the lights at the central button would turn amber, going off when the participant pressed the central button. This sequence of "central button–peripheral button" was repeated five times within a single trial. The sequence of peripheral buttons was quasi-random. The end of each trial was signaled by a flashing of all peripheral lights. The participant could start the next trial as soon as he or she desired, with the exception that the next trial would automatically begin in 5 seconds.

The participant was instructed to perform each trial as quickly as possible without making any mistakes. The time required to complete each trial was recorded. The task was performed for 2-minute periods under one of two conditions. During the *practice* condition, in which no trial-by-trial performance feedback was provided, the end of a trial was always signaled with amber lights flashing at all peripheral buttons. During the *feedback* condition, success trials were signaled with flashing green lights and failure trials were signaled with flashing red lights. Success was computed using a moving time criterion that was individually titrated and adjusted on a trial-by-trial basis. The target success rate was 90% for each 2-minute period. Actual success rates ranged from 87% to 92%.

Given the high rate of success feedback, the total number of trials performed during the 2-minute period was used as a measure of motivated performance in this rather straightforward "go-task." Change (increase) in performance was computed by subtracting the number of trials completed in the practice condition from the number completed in the feedback condition. It was predicted that this metric would be positively correlated with left anterior EEG asymmetry. That is, those who exhibit relatively greater incentive motivation as indexed by resting EEG would show a greater increase in the number of trials completed when performance feedback was provided. This result may occur in addition to predicting individual differences in the number of trials completed for the two conditions. In fact, anterior EEG asymmetry was not correlated with the number of trials completed during either the practice or feedback condition.

In general, both males and females exhibited an increase in the number of trials completed during the feedback condition. For males, performance increased from the practice to the feedback condition by an average of 2.61 (SD = 1.79) trials completed, $t(33)$ = 8.51, p < .001. For females, performance increased by an average of 1.69 (SD = 2.26) trials completed, $t(41)$ = 4.85, p < .001. The difference between means was marginally significant, $t(74)$ = 1.94, p > .05.

Unlike in the word-pairs task, the correlation between anterior EEG asymmetry and the increase in performance was not significant when both males and females were included in the analysis. However, as shown in Figure 5.1, male participants with greater left midfrontal (F3/F4) resting EEG asymmetry exhibited a greater increase in task performance during the feedback condition. Figure 5.2 shows that females exhibited a nonsignificant negative correlation between midfrontal asymmetry measure and the increase in task performance. These correlations were significantly different for males and females (z = 2.18, p < .05).

In summary, resting activity in midfrontal brain regions predicted task performance improvements when success feedback was introduced. However, this relation was specific to male participants, who showed a medium-sized correlation between resting asymmetry and performance increases. The correlation for females was not significant. It is noteworthy that males, on average, exhibited an increase in trials completed that was marginally significantly greater than the average increase exhibited by females, suggesting that the performance feedback may be more motivationally relevant for men than for women.

These findings from the button-press task and word-pairs task provide additional support for the proposal that left and right anterior brain regions are components of the incentive and threat motivation systems and that measurement of anterior brain activity while one sits quietly can be used as an index of the sensitivity of each system. Furthermore, the results of these two studies suggest that the nature of the task is an important determinant of the expression of motivation system sensitivity. Future research will attempt to further expand on the critical characteris-

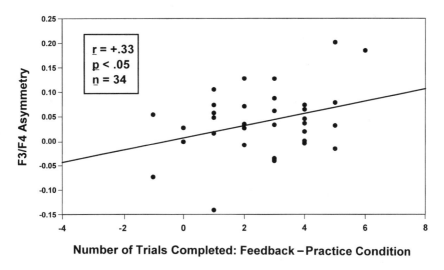

FIGURE 5.1. Resting anterior brain activity asymmetry and button-press task performance change in males.

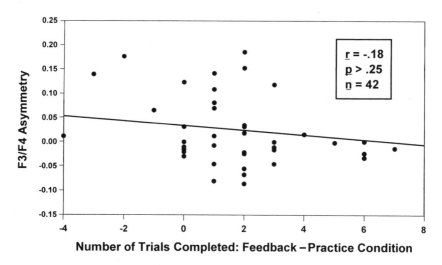

FIGURE 5.2. Resting anterior brain activity asymmetry and button-press task performance change in females.

tics of such tasks to better understand how system sensitivities express themselves. This emphasizes the importance of attending to other personality constructs that may influence the expression of individual differences in incentive and threat motivation.

Self-Reported Motivation Sensitivity

As described previously, Sutton and Davidson (1997) showed a strong correlation between midfrontal EEG asymmetry and the BAS/BIS difference scores for 46 individuals (23 females) who provided reliable EEG data across two sessions and reliable self-report from two administrations of the BIS/BAS Scales (Carver & White, 1994). Are these self-report measures of motivation sensitivity related to word-pairs or button-press task performance or both? More specifically, the BAS-Drive subscale (versus Reward Sensitivity and Fun Seeking subscales) was hypothesized to be related to the increase in button-press task performance when feedback was introduced. As with resting anterior EEG asymmetry, the correlation between the BAS-Drive subscale and the change in number of trials completed was moderately positive, $r(44) = .30$, $p < .05$. However, the correlation with the BAS/BIS difference score was not significant. Furthermore, neither the BAS/BIS difference score nor the individual (sub-)scale scores were significantly correlated with the positivity index on the word-pairs task. These results highlight the nonoverlapping nature of these various measures of incentive and threat system sensitivity. Obviously, concluding that the EEG measures are more sensitive than the self-report measures would be premature.

SUMMARY

One aim of this chapter was to present a sense of how neurobiological concepts and measures can contribute to personality science. As many can attest, researchers cannot ignore the potential for neurobiological substrates of intrapersonal processes and individual differences. It is suggested that incentive and threat motivation systems present tractable conceptual and methodological starting points for such research. Other personality processes certainly require incorporation in order for us to better understand the expression of incentive and threat sensitivities either inside or outside of the laboratory.

There are many advantages to using neurobiological and psychophysiological measures to address questions of interest to personality scientists. There are also several limitations. To some extent, the concepts of spatial and temporal resolution incorporate all of these limitations.

More specifically, even with the advent of high-density arrays that permit recording from 128 sites, scalp EEG measures will never provide the spatial resolution needed to strongly link specific cortical regions with particular behaviors and feelings. Other technologies, such as fMRI, might move us closer to that goal. However, a related concern is whether or not that is a valuable goal for personality science. In other words, the incremental validity acquired versus the cost of acquiring such data may not present an economical cost–benefit ratio.

With this said, the recent advances in technology make this an exciting domain for research. Whereas the technology has improved dramatically, it does not overcome poor conceptualization of processes and poor experimental design. It is critically important to use theory and findings from behavioral research to derive appropriate studies measuring neurobiological and psychophysiological activity. Furthermore, neuroimaging and psychophysiology research also will be limited by the "artificiality" of the environments and manipulations used to collect quality data. Therefore, it is critically important to link such research with research that can be argued to have more ecological validity.

There are numerous current and future directions for research on incentive and threat motivation systems as intrapersonal processes with individual differences in sensitivity of each system. First and foremost, the studies presented in detail herein require replication and extension. Current extensions should target more specific components of cognition associated with the processing of incentives and threats (e.g., attention, working memory) and should attempt to track motivational and emotional reactions with better temporal resolution. One example of this latter idea is the use of the acoustic startle probe eyeblink reflex methodology (for a review, see Lang, 1995) to assess reactions during the perception of incentives and threats, as well as the anticipation of pleasant and aversive stimuli.

Recent research using this tool targeted a population of individuals who purportedly have deficient reactions to threats—psychopaths. Patrick and his colleagues have presented a mix of incentive- and threat-oriented pictures to males with psychopathy. Relative to controls, psychopaths exhibited a weaker reaction to threatening pictures (e.g., Patrick, Bradley, & Lang, 1993). More recently, Sutton and Newman (2001) observed a similar diminished response to threatening pictures in females with psychopathy. Highlighting the importance of tracking the time course of the reaction, this diminished response was observed at 2 seconds, but not at 4.5 seconds, following picture onset. At 4.5 seconds, females with psychopathy exhibited the normative response to the threatening pictures.

Other areas of related research are linking measures of incentive and threat sensitivity with various aspects of neurobiological functioning. For example, Davidson, Coe, Dolski, and Donzella (1999) found that greater resting *right* frontal brain activity was associated with poorer immune functioning. This is consistent with the extensive set of research findings linking chronic stress with poorer immune functioning. Some of the most exciting research in this area has been conducted by Depue and his colleagues using neurochemical challenges to manipulate brain activity in the assessment of relations between motivation-oriented traits and neurotransmitter systems (e.g., White & Depue, 1999; Zald & Depue, 2001).

Another set of future directions emphasizes related psychological concepts and constructs. One highly related broad construct is emotion regulation, what one might describe as the dance partner of emotional reactivity. Within this broad domain, one can investigate neurobiological mechanisms that appear to be associated with other self-descriptive dimensions of temperament, such as impulsivity and disinhibition at one extreme and constraint at the other (e.g., Clark & Watson, 1999). This concept and related dimensions have been repeatedly associated with serotonergic activity. Also within this broad domain, there is the more conscious aspect of emotion regulation, by which one voluntarily develops and chooses behavioral and cognitive techniques to enhance or reduce emotional reactions (e.g., Gross, 1999; Jackson, Malmstadt, Larson, & Davidson, 2000). Another related broad concept within personality science is self-regulation. In fact, the extensive overlap of concepts from these two domains with different developmental histories provides an excellent base for generating new research questions (Carver, Sutton, & Scheier, 2000).

In summary, this chapter presents two broad biobehavioral systems as tractable research constructs when considering the biologically based components of personality. The incentive and threat motivation systems respond to pertinent stimuli, organizing available resources in preparation for and execution of action in the pursuit of rewards and the avoidance of punishments. Personality researchers are encouraged to consider these two systems as viable research complements (or alternatives) to traditional descriptive dimensions of personality that purportedly have a biological basis. One highlighted component is that the personality trait (i.e., the stable, enduring characteristic of the individual) is found in an operating characteristic of the system—reactivity or sensitivity. Another highlighted component is the importance of relative activity levels (states) and relative sensitivities (traits). These features have implications for conceptualizing, as well as testing, the influence of these systems on motivated behavior.

It is an exciting time in personality science, as well as in cognitive science, affect science, and the neurosciences. There are many opportunities for significant advances in understanding intrapersonal processes and individual differences, especially through the use of ideas, methods, and findings from related domains to address questions of particular interest to personality scientists. There also are many opportunities to intertwine, if not merge, various perspectives within personality science. The value of a multimethod, multitrait approach to personality has long been acknowledged. At present, there is a nice confluence of conceptual, methodological, and technological advances that makes this an excellent time for applying this approach, especially to questions concerning relations between personality and neurobiology.

ACKNOWLEDGMENTS

The following individuals provided invaluable assistance in the data collection and data processing for the three studies presented in detail in this chapter: Terry Ward, Darren Dottl, Bonny Donzella, Isa Dolski, Bridget Cavanaugh, Andrea Norris, Amy Parsons, Jennifer Passehl, and Aimee Reid. Furthermore, those studies were partly supported by a postdoctoral fellowship to S. K. Sutton from the NIMH Postdoctoral Training Program in Emotion Research (T32-MH18931; R. J. Davidson, Director), and a Young Investigator Award from the National Alliance for Research on Schizophrenia and Depression to S. K. Sutton.

I am indebted to Richie Davidson for the opportunity to develop my research ideas and gain experience with various methodologies and technologies during my years of postdoctoral training at the University of Wisconsin. I also thank my colleagues at the University of Miami, Chuck Carver, Sheri Johnson, and Ray Winters, for valuable intellectual exchanges and for comments on a previous version of this chapter.

REFERENCES

Carver, C. S., & Scheier, M. F. (1998). *On the self-regulation of behavior*. Cambridge, UK: Cambridge University Press.

Carver, C. S., Sutton, S. K., & Scheier, M. F. (2000). Action, emotion, and personality: Emerging conceptual integration. *Personality and Social Psychology Bulletin, 26*, 741–751.

Carver, C. S., & White, T. L. (1994). Behavioral inhibition, behavioral activation, and affective responses to impending reward and punishment: The BIS/BAS scales. *Journal of Personality and Social Psychology, 67*, 319–333.

Center for the Study of Emotion and Attention. (1995). *The International Affective Picture System: Photographic slides*. Gainesville, FL: Center of Research in Psychophysiology, University of Florida.

Cronbach, L. J. (1951). Coefficient alpha and the internal structure of tests. *Psychometrika, 16*, 297–334.

Clark, L. A., & Watson, D. (1999). Temperament: A new paradigm for trait psychology. In L. A. Pervin & O. P. John (Eds.), *Handbook of personality: Theory and research* (2nd ed., pp. 399–423). New York: Guilford Press.

Davidson, R. J. (1995). Cerebral asymmetry, emotion, and affective style. In R. J. Davidson & K. Hugdahl (Eds.), *Brain asymmetry* (pp. 361–387). Cambridge, MA: MIT Press.

Davidson, R. J., Coe, C. L., Dolski, I., & Donzella, B. (1999). Individual differences in prefrontal activation asymmetry predict natural killer cell activity at rest and in response to challenge. *Brain, Behavior, and Immunity, 13,* 93–108.

Davidson, R. J., Jackson, D. C., & Larson, C. L. (2000). Human electroencephalography. In J. T. Cacioppo, L. G. Tassinary, & G. G. Berntson (Eds.), *Handbook of psychophysiology* (pp. 27–52). New York: Cambridge University Press.

Davidson, R. J., Marshall, J. R., Tomarken, A. J., & Henriques, J. B. (2000). While a phobic waits: Regional brain electrical and autonomic activity in social phobics during anticipation of public speaking. *Biological Psychiatry, 47,* 85–95.

Depue, R. A., & Collins, P. F. (1999). Neurobiology of the structure of personality: Dopamine, facilitation of incentive motivation, and extraversion. *Behavioral and Brain Sciences, 22,* 491–569.

Duffy, F. H. (1994). The role of quantified electroencephalography in psychological research. In G. Dawson & K. W. Fischer (Eds.), *Human behavior and the developing brain* (pp. 93–133). New York: Guilford Press.

Eysenck, H. P. (1967). *The biological basis of personality.* Springfield, IL: Thomas.

Eysenck, H. P., & Eysenck, S. G. B. (1964). *Eysenck Personality Inventory.* San Diego: Educational and Industrial Testing Service.

Gray, J. A. (1981). A critique of Eysenck's theory of personality. In H. J. Eysenck (Ed.), *A model for personality* (pp. 246–276). Berlin, Germany: Springer-Verlag.

Gross, J. J. (1999). Emotion and emotion regulation. In L. A. Pervin & O. P. John (Eds.), *Handbook of personality: Theory and research* (2nd ed., pp. 525–552). New York: Guilford Press.

Harmon-Jones, E., & Allen, J. J. (1997). Behavioral activation sensitivity and resting frontal EEG asymmetry: Covariation of putative indicators related to risk for mood disorders. *Journal of Abnormal Psychology, 106,* 159–163.

Harmon-Jones, E., & Sigelman, J. (2001). State anger and prefrontal brain activity: Evidence that insult-related relative left-prefrontal activation is associated with experienced anger and aggression. *Journal of Personality and Social Psychology, 80,* 797–803.

Henriques, J. B., & Davidson, R. J. (1990). Asymmetrical brain electrical activity discriminates between previously depressed subjects and health controls. *Journal of Abnormal Psychology, 99,* 22–31.

Henriques, J. B., & Davidson, R. J. (1991). Left frontal hypoactivation in depression. *Journal of Abnormal Psychology, 100,* 535–545.

Jackson, D. C., Malmstadt, J. R., Larson, C. L., & Davidson, R. J. (2000). Suppression and enhancement of emotional responses to unpleasant pictures. *Psychophysiology, 37,* 515–522.

Jasper, H. H. (1958). The ten-twenty electrode system of the International Federation. *Electroencephalography and Clinical Neuropsychology, 10,* 371–375.

Kagan, J., Reznick, J. S., & Snidman, N. (1988). Biological bases of childhood shyness. *Science, 240*, 167–171.

Konorski, J. (1967). *Integrative activity of the brain: An interdisciplinary approach.* Chicago: University of Chicago Press.

Kosslyn, S. (1987). Seeing and imagining in the cerebral hemispheres: A computational approach. *Psychological Review, 94*, 148–175.

Lang, P. J. (1995). The emotion probe: Studies of motivation and attention. *American Psychologist, 50*, 372–385.

Larsen, R. J. (1984). Theory and measurement of affect intensity as an individual difference characteristic. *Dissertation Abstracts International, 5*, 2297B. (University Microfilms No. 84-22112)

Patrick, C. J., Bradley, M. M., & Lang, P. J. (1993). Emotion in the criminal psychopath: Startle reflex modulation. *Journal of Abnormal Psychology, 102*, 82–92.

Pavlov, I. P. (1955). *Selected works* (S. Belsky, Trans.). Moscow: Foreign Languages.

Pivik, R. T., Broughton, R. J., Coppola, R., Davidson, R. J., Fox, N., & Numer, M. R. (1993). Guidelines for the recording and quantitative analysis of electroencephalographic activity in research contexts. *Psychophysiology, 30*, 547–558.

Posner, M. I. (1995). Attention in cognitive neuroscience: An overview. In M. S. Gazzaniga (Ed.), *The cognitive neurosciences* (pp. 615–624). Cambridge, MA: MIT Press.

Robbins, T. W., & Everitt, B. J. (1995). Arousal systems and attention. In M. Gazzaniga (Ed.), *The cognitive neurosciences* (pp. 703–720). Cambridge, MA: MIT Press.

Rothbart, M. K., & Ahadi, S. A. (1994). Temperament and the development of personality. *Journal of Abnormal Psychology, 103*, 55–66.

Rothbart, M. K., Derryberry, D., & Posner, M. I. (1994). A psychobiological approach to the development of temperament. In J. E. Bates & T. D. Wachs (Eds.), *Temperament: Individual differences at the interface of biology and behavior* (pp. 219–255). Hillsdale, NJ: Erlbaum.

Scheier, M. F., & Carver, C. S. (1985). Optimism, coping, and health: Assessment and implications of generalized outcome expectancies. *Health Psychology, 4*, 219–247.

Schmidt, L. A. (1999). Frontal brain activity in shyness and sociability. *Psychological Science, 10*, 316–320.

Sobotka, S. S., Davidson, R. J., & Senulis, J. A. (1992). Anterior brain electrical asymmetries in response to reward and punishment. *Electroencephalography and Clinical Neurophysiology, 83*, 236–247.

Sutton, S. K., & Davidson, R. J. (1997). Prefrontal brain asymmetry: A biological substrate of the behavioral approach and inhibition systems. *Psychological Science, 8*, 204–210.

Sutton, S. K., & Davidson, R. J. (2000a). Resting anterior brain activity predicts the evaluation of affective stimuli. *Neuropsychologia, 38*, 1723–1733.

Sutton, S. K., & Davidson, R. J. (2000b). Resting midfrontal brain activity predicts motivated behavior. *Psychophysiology, 37*(Suppl.), S96.

Sutton, S. K., Larson, C. L., Ward, R. T., Holden, J. E., Perlman, S. E., & Davidson,

R. J. (1996). The functional neuroanatomy of the appetitive and aversive motivation systems: Results from an FDG-PET study. *Neuroimage, 3,* S240.

Sutton, S. K., & Newman, J. P. (2001). Affective reactions to unpleasant pictures in female psychopaths. *Psychophysiology, 38*(Suppl.), S93.

Thayer, R. E. (1989). *The biopsychology of mood and arousal.* New York: Oxford University Press.

Tomarken, A. J., & Davidson, R. J. (1994). Frontal brain activation in repressors and non-repressors. *Journal of Abnormal Psychology, 103,* 339–349.

Tomarken, A. J., Davidson, R. J., Wheeler, R. E., & Kinney, L. (1992). Psychometric properties of resting anterior EEG asymmetry: Temporal stability and internal consistency. *Psychophysiology, 29,* 576–592.

Tomarken, A. J., Keener, A., & Neubauer, D. L. (1994). Long-term stability of frontal brain asymmetry: It helps to aggregate. *Psychophysiology, 31*(Suppl.), S97.

Tucker, D. M., & Williamson, P. A. (1984). Asymmetric neural control systems in human self-regulation. *Psychological Review, 91,* 185–215.

Watson, D., Clark, L. A., & Tellegen, A. (1988). Development and validation of brief measures of positive and negative affect: The PANAS scales. *Journal of Personality and Social Psychology, 54,* 1063–1070.

White, T. L., & Depue, R. A. (1999). Differential association of traits of fear and anxiety with norepinephrine- and dark-induced pupil reactivity. *Journal of Personality and Social Psychology, 77,* 863–877.

Zald, D. H., & Depue, R. A. (2001). Serotonergic functioning correlates with positive and negative affect in psychiatrically healthy males. *Personality and Individual Differences, 30,* 71–86.

Zinser, M. C., Fiore, M. C., Davidson, R. J., & Baker, T. B. (1999). Manipulating smoking motivation: Impact on an electrophysiological index of approach motivation. *Journal of Abnormal Psychology, 108,* 240–254.

PART II

PERSONALITY DEVELOPMENT IN ITS SOCIAL CONTEXT

CHAPTER 6

Models of Development

MICHAEL LEWIS

Models of development represent worldviews about human nature and environments that create a human life course (Lewis, 1997; Reese & Overton, 1970; Riegel, 1976). Models of personality development also reflect these views, and the data from normal and abnormal lives need inform our theories of personality development. The trait notion of personality (Block & Block, 1980) and the idea of the invulnerable child (Anthony, 1970; Garmezy, 1974; Rutter, 1981), for example, both share the view that some fixed patterns of behavior are usually unaffected by environmental factors. Likewise, information about regression to old behavior patterns requires that we reconsider the notion that all developmental processes are transformations; that is, the belief that old behavior patterns are transformed into new ones, so that the old ones disappear. Clearly, models of development are applicable to studying personality development. In fact, I would argue that personality and development represent different foci of the same question: Are there enduring—over time and place—features of individuals that remain consistent?

Models of development have been considered by many writers, and the interested reader is referred to Reese and Overton (1970) and, more recently, Lewis (1997). I particularly like Riegel's (1978) scheme for considering models that involve the child and the environment. In his scheme, each of these two elements can be an active or a passive agent. The passive child–passive environment model is of relatively less interest because it arose from the views of John Locke and David Hume but now receives little attention. In such a model, the environment does not try to affect behavior, and the child is a passive "blank tablet" on which is received information from the world around it. Such models originally had some use, for example, in our understanding of short-term memory. These memories were likened to a small box that was sequentially filled. When a new memory was entered and there was no more room, the first (or oldest) memory dropped out. Although such a view of memory is no longer held, other views, especially in perception, share many of the features of this model. Gibson's (1969) notion of affordance, for example, suggests such a model because innate characteristics of the child extract the given features of the environment. Such models are by their nature often mechanistic.

The passive child–active environment model is an environmental control view, because in it the environment actively controls, by reward and punishment, the child's behavior. The characteristics of this environment may differ, as may the nature of the reinforcers, but the child's behavior is determined by its environment. We are most familiar with this model in operant conditioning (Skinner, 1953). It is a model much favored by many therapists and is used in diverse areas, such as behavior modification treatment to alter maladaptive behavior, as well as in theories that explain normal sex-role learning by parental or peer reinforcement (Bem, 1987; Fagot & Patterson, 1969).

A third model is that of an active person and a passive environment. These models have in common an active child extracting and constructing its world from the material of the environment. Piaget's theory fits well within this framework (Piaget, 1952), although some have argued that Piaget may be a preformationalist (passive child–passive environment) in that in his theory all the structures children create are identical (Bellin, 1971). Given the active organismic view of Piaget, it is easy to see that, although the child needs the environment to construct knowledge, the environment itself plays little role (Lewis, 1983). Linguistic theorists, such as Chomsky (1957, 1965) and Lennenberg (1967), believe that biological linguistic structures are available for children to use in their construction of language in particular environments. Whether such views are better placed in the passive child–passive environment model is questionable, although the critical feature of this model should not be lost. In the therapeutic situation, we often employ such a model when we attempt to help patients alter their behavior (active person); we discount the role of the environment.

The last model is most familiar to developmentalists because of its interactive nature. An active person and an active environment are postulated as creating, modifying, and changing behavior. These interactive models take many forms, varying from the interactional approach of Lewis (Lewis, 1972; Lewis & Feiring, 1991) to the transactional models of Sameroff and Chandler (1975). They also include Chess and Thomas's (1984) and Lerner's (1984) goodness-of-fit model and, from a developmental psychopathology point of view, the notion of vulnerability and risk status (Garmezy, Masten, & Tellegen, 1984; Rutter, 1979). In his attempt to understand cognitive development, Luria (1976) argued that cognitive structures themselves are the consequence of an interaction between the nature of the environment and an active child. Such a view of interaction is often found in research on cultural differences (Cole, 1996).

Even though Riegel's (1978) approach is useful, other systems of classification are available. For example, both passive child and passive and active environment models are mechanistic in that either *biological givens* within the organism or *environmental structures* outside the organism act on the child. On the other hand, both active child models must be interactive because organisms almost always interact in some way with their environment, which, given its structure (whether active or passive), affects the ongoing interaction. In the models of development as they are related to personality, we use a combination of approaches.

Here I consider three models of the development of personality: a *trait or status model*, a *contextual or environmental model*, and an *interactional model*. Although each of these models has variations, the interactional model is the most variable. Because attachment theory remains central to normal and maladaptive development, I use it often as an exemplar in the discussion. These three models, which are prototypes of the various views of the development of personality, make clear how such models diverge and how they can be used to understand the etiology of personality.

TRAIT OR STATUS MODEL

The trait or status model is characterized by its simplicity. It holds to the view that a trait, or the status of the child at one point in time, is likely to predict a trait or status at a later point in time. A trait model is not interactive and does not provide for the effects of the environment. In fact, in the most extreme form, the environment is thought to play no role either in effecting its display or in transforming its characteristics. A particular trait may interact with the environment, but the trait is not changed by that interaction.

Traits are not easily open to transformation and can be processes, coping skills, attributes, or tendencies to respond in certain ways; the candidate most often considered in the developmental literature is temperament. Within personality research, traits are similarly defined, but today we are more likely to refer to the Big Five traits (see Goldberg, 1990). Traits are often thought to be innate. However, traits also can be acquired through learning or through more interactive processes; that is, they are the result of early experiences. Once a trait is acquired, it remains relatively unaffected by subsequent interactions. The trait model is most useful in many instances, for example, when considering potential genetic or biological causes of subsequent personality characteristics. A child who is born with a certain gene or a set of genes is likely to display specific behavioral patterns at some later time. This model characterizes some of the research in the genetics of personality. The early work of Kallman (1946), for example, on heritability of schizophrenia supports the use of such a model, as does the lack or presence of certain chemicals on depression (e.g., Puig-Antich, 1982). In each of these cases, the presence of particular features is hypothesized as likely to affect behavior and personality. Although a trait model is appealing in its simplicity, there are any number of problems with it; for example, considering psychopathology, not all people who possess a trait or have a particular status at one point in time are likely to show subsequent psychopathology or the same type of psychopathology (Saudino, 1997). The fact that all children of schizophrenic parents do not themselves become schizophrenic, or that not all monozygotic twins show concordance vis-à-vis schizophrenia suggests that other variables need to be considered (Gottesman & Shields, 1982; Kringlon, 1968). We return to this point again; however, it is important to note that the failure to find a high incidence of schizophrenic children of schizophrenic parents led to the postulation of such notions as resistance to stress, coping styles, and invulnerability. Each of these terms has a traitlike feature to it.

From a developmental perspective, the trait model also is useful when considering traits that are not genetically or biologically based. For example, the attachment model, as proposed by Bowlby (1969) and Ainsworth (1973), holds that the child's early relationship with its mother, in the 1st year of life, is likely to determine the child's adjustment throughout life. The security of attachment that the child shows at the end of the 1st year of life is the result of the early interaction between the mother and the child. Once the attachment is established, it acts as a trait affecting the child's subsequent behavior. That is, once established, it acts like any other trait; that is, it may interact with the environment but is not altered by it (see Ainsworth, 1989; Ainsworth & Marvin, 1995).

Figure 6.1 presents the trait model using the traditional attachment construct. Notice that the interaction of the mother and child at T_1 produces the intraorganism trait, C_{t1}, in this case, a secure or an insecure attachment. Although attachment is the consequence of an interaction, once established, it is the trait (C_{t1}) residing in the child that leads to C_{t2}. There is no need to posit a role of the environment except as it initially produces the attachment. The problems with a trait view of the attachment model have been addressed by many (Lamb, Thompson, Gardner, & Charnov, 1985; Lewis, Feiring, & Rosenthal, 2000); nevertheless, it is a widely held view that the mother–child relationship in the 1st year of

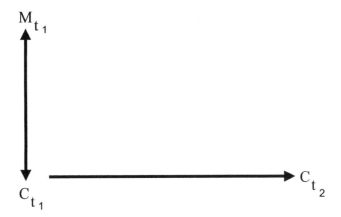

FIGURE 6.1. Trait model using the attachment construct.

life can affect the child's subsequent personality through affecting his or her social–emotional life, as well as his or her mental health.

Moreover, there is the belief that a trait can act as a protective factor in the face of environmental stress. Secure attachment is seen as an invulnerability factor. In developmental theory, the concept of invulnerability is similar to a trait model; that is, there are attributes of children that appear to protect them from subsequent environmental stress. These attributes (or traits) serve to make the child stress-resistant. Such a mechanism is used to explain why not all at-risk children develop psychopathology (Garmezy et al., 1984; Rutter, 1979).

Figure 6.2 presents the invulnerability model from the point of view of an acquired trait. Notice that at t_1, the environment is positive, so the child acquires a positive attribute. At t_2, the environment becomes negative; however, the attribute acquired at t_1 protects the child (the child remains positive). At each additional point in time (t_3, $t_4...t_n$), the environment may change; however, this change has little effect on the child because the intraorganism trait is maintained. It is increasingly clear that secure attachment is not a protective factor in terms of the child's reaction to subsequent stress (Lewis et al., 2000).

Trait models in personality theory are not new, although their popularity has changed over time (Allport & Allport, 1921; Goldberg, 1990). The problems identified in personality research apply here as well, namely, the recognition that individual traits are likely to be situation specific (Mischel, 1965). As such, they can only partially characterize the organism. For example, a child may be securely attached to his or her mother but insecurely attached to his or her father or older sibling. It would there-

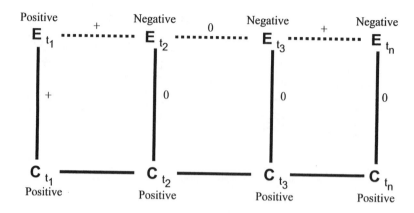

FIGURE 6.2. Invulnerability model from point of view of an acquired trait.

fore be hard to characterize the child as insecurely attached simply because he or she is insecurely attached to one family member but not to the others (Fox, Kimmerly, & Schafer, 1991). Prediction from an insecure attachment trait to subsequent behavior would be difficult without knowing the child's total attachment pattern. For example, a girl who is securely attached to mother but insecurely attached to father may be likely to be able to form good peer relationships with women but not with men. Likewise, a girl who is securely attached to father but insecurely attached to mother may be likely to be able to form good peer relationships with men but not with women. Thus attachment is situationally based rather than trait based. This would dilute attachment from a trait located within the individual to a set of specific relationships, depending on the different attachments formed. Thus to characterize the child in a simple way, such as secure or insecure, may miss the complex nature of traits, especially those likely to be related to personality factors or even to psychopathology. Equally problematic, in the trait notion such models leave little room for the impact of environment on subsequent developmental growth or dysfunction. Environments play a role in children's development in the opening year of life and continue to do so throughout the lifespan (Lewis, 1997, 1999a).

CONTEXTUAL OR ENVIRONMENTAL MODEL

The prototypic environmental model holds that exogenous factors influence development. Two of the many problems in using this model are (1) our difficulty in defining what environments are and (2) the failure to consider the impact of environments throughout the lifespan. In fact, the strongest form of the developmental environmental or contextual model argues for the proposition that adaptation to current environment throughout the life course has a major influence on our behavior and on our personalities. Moreover, such a model is familiar to students of personality because it represents the idea that context, to a large degree, determines behavior. As environments change, so too does the individual (Lewis, 1997). This dynamic and changing view of environments and adaptation is in strong contrast to the earlier models of environments as forces that act on the individual and that act on the individual *only in the early years of life.*

Because other people make up the important aspect of our environment, work on the structures of the social environment is particularly relevant, and an attempt has been made to expand the numbers of potentially important people in the child's environment (Lewis, 1984), as well as to create an analysis of the structure of the social environment itself (Lewis, 1987b). Although considerable effort has been focused on the importance of the mother on the child's development, other persons, including fathers, siblings, grandparents, and peers, clearly have importance in shaping the child's life (Bronfenbrenner & Crouter, 1983; Dunn, 1993; Fox et al., 1991; Lewis, 1984).

The role of environments in the developmental process has been underplayed because most investigators seek to find the structure and change within the organism itself. Likewise, in the study of personality development, even though we recognize that environments can cause both normal and abnormal behavior, we prefer to treat the person—to increase coping skills or to alter specific behaviors—rather than to change the environment (Lewis, 1997). Yet we can imagine the difficulties that are raised when we attempt to alter specific maladaptive behaviors in environments in which such behaviors are adaptive—a point well taken by Szasz (1961).

For example, our belief that the thrust of development resides in the organism rather than in the environment, in large part, raises many problems. At cultural levels, we assume that violence (and its cure) must be met in the individual—a trait model—rather than in the structure of the environment. The rate of murders committed with handguns in the United States is many times higher than in any other Western society. We seek responsibility in the nature of the individual (e.g., XYY males, or the genetics of antisocial behavior) when the alternative of environmental structure is available. In this case, murders may be due more to the availability of handguns. The solution to the high murder rate in the United States might be the elimination, through punishment, of the possession of weapons. Thus we conclude either that Americans are by their genetic nature more violent than Europeans or that other Western societies do not allow handguns and therefore have lower murder rates (see Cairns & Cairns, 2000).

The general environmental model that I have suggested (Lewis, 1997) holds that children's behavior always is a function of the environment in which the behavior occurs, because the task of the individual is to adapt to its current environment.[1] As long as the environment appears consistent, the child's behavior will be consistent; if the environment changes, so, too, will the child's behavior. It is the case that maladaptive environments produce both normal and abnormal behavior. From a developmental point of view, I would hold that maladaptive behavior is caused by maladaptive environments; if we change those environments, we may be able to alter the behavior.

Figure 6.3 presents this model. The environment (E) at t_1, t_2, and t_3 all influence the child's behavior at each point in time. The child's behavior at C_{t1}, C_{t2}, and C_{t3} appears consistent, and it is, as long as E remains consistent. In other words, the continuity in C is an epiphenomenon of the continuity of E across time. Likewise, lack of consistency in C reflects the lack of consistency in the environment. The child's behavior changes over t_1 to t_3 as the environment produces change. Even though it appears that C is consistent, it is so because E is consistent. Consistency and change in C are supported by exogenous rather than by endogenous factors.

Such a model of change as a function of the environment can be readily tested, but rarely is it done. This failure reflects the bias of the trait model in developmental theory. Consider the attachment model (Figure 6.1). Although it is recognized that the environment affects attachment at t_1, the child's status or trait at t_1 (C_{t1}) is hypothesized to determine the child's other outcomes, C_{t2}, C_{t3}, and so forth. Rarely is the envi-

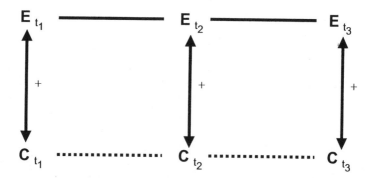

FIGURE 6.3. Model of change as a function of the environment.

ronment, and the consistency of the environment, factored into the model as a possible cause of subsequent child behavior. Consider that poor parenting produces an insecure child at C_{t1}, and this parenting remains poor at t_2, t_3. Without considering the continuing effects of poor parenting, it is not possible to make such a conclusion. That most developmental research in this area fails in this regard constitutes evidence for the lack of interest in the environmental model.

This problem is found throughout the study of personality development. Depressed women are assumed to cause concurrent, as well as subsequent, depression in children (Zahn-Waxler, Cummings, McKnew, & Radke-Yarrow, 1984). What is not considered is the fact that depressed mothers at t_1 are also likely to be depressed at t_2 or t_3. What role does the mother's depression at these points play in the child's subsequent behavior? We can only infer the answer, given the limited data available. The question that needs to be asked is: What would happen to the child if the mother was depressed at t_1 but not at t_2 or t_3? This type of question suggests that one way to observe the effect of the environment on the child's subsequent behavior is to observe those situations in which the environment changes.

Although the environmental model can be made more complex, this model suggests, in all cases, that the child's concurrent health status is determined by the environment. Should the environment change, then the child's status will change. The degree to which the environment remains consistent is the degree to which the same behavior will be consistently found within the child. Therefore, the environmental model is characterized by the view that holds that the constraints, changes, and consistencies in children's personality rest not so much with intrinsic structures located in the child as in the nature, structure, and environment of the child (Lewis, 1997).

INTERACTIONAL MODEL

Although the trait model is most often used in research, the interactional model is usually held to be the one which, from a theoretical point of view, is most likely to account for the development and change in personality. This mismatch between theory and research has serious implications for the growth of our knowledge about human development. Interactional models vary; some researchers prefer to call them "interactional" and others "transactional" (Lewis, 1972; Sameroff & Chandler, 1975). All these models have in common the role of both child and environment in determining the course of development. In these models, the nature of the environment and the characteristics or traits of the child are needed to explain concurrent, as well as subsequent, behavior and adjustment. Such models usually require an active child and an active environment; however, they need not do so. What they do require is the notion that behavior is shaped by its adaptive ability and that this ability is related to environments. Maladaptive behavior may be misnamed because the behavior may be adaptive to a maladaptive environment. The stability and change in children's personality need to be viewed as a function of both factors, and, as such, the task of any interactive model is to draw us to the study of both features. In our attachment example, the infant who is securely attached as a function of the responsive environment in the 1st year will show competence at a later age as a function of the earlier characteristic, as well as of the nature of the environment at that later age (see Lewis, 1999b).

One of the central issues in developmental theories that are interactive in nature is the question of transformation. Many models can be drawn of how concurrent behavior is a function of traits and environment. In one, both trait and environment interact and produce a new set of behaviors. However, neither the traits nor the environment are transformed, that is, altered, by the interaction. An example of this is the goodness-of-fit model. In another model, traits and environments interact such that a trait remains (is not transformed) but is not visible in one environment, although it is visible in another. The vulnerable child is an example of this. In still another model, both trait and environment interact, producing a new set of behaviors that transform both the trait and the environment. From a developmental perspective, this is the most transformational model because the old behaviors give rise to new behaviors, and the environment itself is altered by the exchange. The number and nature of the various interactional models is considerable. We focus on three of them in order to demonstrate their importance for our theories about the development of personality.

Goodness-of-Fit Model

According to the goodness-of-fit model, discord arises when the child's characteristics do not match the environmental demand, or, stated another way, the environmental demand does not match the child's characteristics (Lerner, 1984; Thomas & Chess, 1977). Notice that maladjustment is the consequence of the mismatch. It is not located in either the nature of the child's characteristics or in the environmental demand. Because of this, such a model can be accused of "relativism." Some researchers would argue that certain environmental demands, by their nature, will cause pathology in the same way that certain child characteristics, by their nature, will cause them. Although this may be the case in extremes, the goodness-of-fit model suggests that psychopathology is the consequence of the mismatch between trait and environment, and that, as such, it is an interactive model.

In terms of transformation, such a model is relatively silent. Even so, it would seem reasonable to imagine that new behaviors arise due either to the match or mismatch, but these new behaviors do not require the old behaviors to be transformed or eliminated. The active child in an inactive environment may learn to move more slowly, but the trait of activity is not lost or transferred. The environment, too, may change, because less is required of the child, but the values or goals underlying the requirement remain and are not changed.

In exploring early sex-role behavior in children and maternal attitudes about sex role on subsequent adjustment, a goodness-of-fit model appeared to best explain the data. Lewis (1987a) observed the sex-role behavior of 2-year-olds in terms of how much the children played with "male" and "female" toys. There were large individual differences; some boys played more with boys' toys than girls' toys, and some boys played more with girls' toys than boys' toys. The same was true for the girls. Mothers were given the Bem Sex Role Inventory (1987), and we were able to determine their sex-role orientation. Some mothers were traditional, whereas others were more androgynous in their sex-role beliefs. We found that school adjustment, as rated by the teacher, was neither dependent on the mother's belief nor the child's sex-role play. Rather, adjustment was dependent on the goodness-of-fit between the child's play and the mother's belief. For example, boys showed subsequently better adjustment if their mothers were androgynous in belief and if they played equally with boy and girl toys, as well as if mothers were traditional and the boys played more with boy than girl toys. Adjustment at 6 years was worse if there was no fit—for example, if the mothers were traditional and the boys were androgynous or if the mothers were androgynous and the boys were more male-toy oriented. The same was true for girls. The goodness-of-fit between the individual and his or her environment, rather than the nature of the child's behavior itself, may be more important for the development of maladaptive behavior. One therapeutic solution, then, is to alter the maladaptive behavior of the individual; the other is to alter the nature of the fit. Matching children by their characteristics to teachers' traits reduces educational mismatch and increases academic achievement.

Vulnerability Model

The vulnerable child is an important example of the usefulness of a nontransformational interactive model. A vulnerable child possesses some traits that place him or her at risk. If the environment is positive, the at-risk features are not expressed, and the child appears to be adjusted. Over repeated exposures to the positive environment, the child appears adjusted; however, if given an instant or two of a negative environment, the child will show abnormal behavior. It is obvious from this example that the positive environmental experiences were unable to transform traits that remained independent of their interaction with the environment and were expressed only under particular circumstances. Although there are few data on the topic, it is possible that the traits are influenced by the environment such that repeated positive exposures make the response to a negative environment less severe. Under such conditions, we approach a more complete transformational model.

Transformational Model

These types of developmental models, which require that all features that make up an interaction are themselves composed of all features and are transformed by their interaction, are called transactional models (Sameroff, 1975). For example, if the child's characteristics at C_{t1} interact with the environment E_{t1} to produce a transformed C_{t2} and E_{t2}, then it is likely that C_{t1} and E_{t1} also were transformed from some earlier time $t_{(n-1)}$ and that, therefore, each feature is never independent of the other. Such models reject the idea that child traits or environmental characteristics are ever independent or exist as "pure" forms; here there is an ultimate regression of effects. Moreover, these features interact and transform themselves at each point in development. The linear functions that characterize the other models are inadequate for the transformational view. The parent's behavior affects the child's behavior; however, the parent's behavior was affected by the child's earlier behavior.

Lewis and Feiring (1989), for example, have found that intrusive mothers of 3-month-olds are likely to have insecurely attached children at 1 year. However, the mothers' overstimulation appears to be related to their children's behavior. Many of these 3-month-olds are asocial; that is, they prefer to play with and look at toys rather than people, and this leads to overstimulation as their mothers try to get the children to interact with them. Is it the overstimulation or intrusiveness of the mother or the asocial trait of the child or both that lead to the insecurely attached child at 1 year? Insecure attachment at 1 year can be transformed given the proper environment, and an insecure attachment can transform a positive environment into a negative one. Consider the irritable child who interacts with a positive environment and produces a negative environment that subsequently produces a negative, irritable child. The causal chain does not simply pass in a continuous fashion either through the environment or through the irritable child, as the trait or environmental models would have it. In fact, it is a circular pattern of child cause affecting the environment and the environment cause affecting the child. Such models have intrinsic appeal but are by their nature difficult to test. Recent theories of dynamic systems are now becoming more available that may allow us to explore this in more detail (Thelen & Ulrich, 1991; Thom, 1975; Zeeman, 1976). Even so, it is difficult not to treat a child or an environmental characteristic as a "pure" quantity, though we might know better. As such, we tend to test the interactive models that require less transformation.

LONGITUDINAL STUDIES

Although the literature reflects a strong belief in an interactional model of personality development, the actual research conducted follows more of a trait model. In one of the largest and best longitudinal studies, children's temperament at 3 years was related to personality characteristics at 18 years. Caspi and Silva (1995) claim to demonstrate high consistency over age levels that preserves individual differences from childhood to young adulthood. Such studies as these argue for a trait model in which earlier differences can be seen at later ages. No attempt is made to look at the environment at both ages and relate it to this consistency. But how consistent are the findings? In one study, Caspi, Henry, McGee, Moffitt, and Silva (1995) found only a modest relation between temperament ratings at 3 and 5 years and behavioral problems between 9 and 15 years. Most correlations are not significant, and the ones that are account for less than 12% of the variance (Caspi et al., 1995, Tables 3 and 4). Not much better results were found when looking at 3- to 21-year outcomes (Newman, Caspi, Moffitt, & Silva, 1997). We, too, have been looking at a longitudinal study following children from birth until 18 years (see Lewis et al., 2000; Rosenthal, Feiring, & Lewis, 1998).

In the Rosenthal et al. (1998) study, we examined volunteering behavior of young adults when they were 18–21 years old and related their prosocial behavior to their earlier cognitive, social adjustment, stress, and family data. No earlier participant characteristics, such as their early IQ, sociability, or attachment relationship to their mothers, were related to their volunteering behavior. In a regression analysis, these factors did not account for a significant percent of the variance. However, the concurrent factors, when the children were 18 years old, were related to their volunteering and included some individual characteristics but mostly environmental factors, such as more cohesive families, more families whose other members volunteered, and whether or not the 18-year-olds belonged to an organization that had volunteering as part of its mission.

These results suggest that early individual characteristics, as posited in the trait model, are not related to later social behavior such as volunteering. What was related to young adult volunteering was what the young adults were like at the time that volunteering behavior was observed. At this age, it was the social environment that was more related to volunteering than the particular characteristics of the 18-year-olds themselves. Such findings as these suggest that the trait model is not adequate for observing the developmental process; rather, it was the concurrent environment that was most related.

In another study, the three models proposed—trait, environment, and interaction models—were examined by looking at the relation between early attachment relationship and subsequent young adults' attachment and psychopathology (Lewis et al., 2000). In addition to the standard 1-year-old attachment procedure, adult attachment scores were obtained, along with teachers', mothers', and adolescents' ratings of psychopathology. In order to obtain measures of environment that might be related to the stability or change in children's attachment relationships, a family or environment variable was obtained—divorce status of the parents when the children were young adults. Divorce status was used as a measure of the caregiving environment because divorce has direct impact on parents and children, as it affects the emotional and social experiences of the family (Davies & Cummings, 1994). The results have been reported elsewhere (Lewis, 1999b; Lewis et al., 2000). Eighty-four children (48 girls) were seen and followed in this study. The results indicated that there was no continuity in attachment, such that security of attachment at 1 year bore no relation to young adult attachment. Moreover, security of attachment at 1 year was unrelated to the young adults' level of emotional disturbance or maladjustment. Again, the trait model did not hold.

What did seem to be the case is that young adults' attachment to their parents at 18 years is related to the young adults' social environments at 18. Divorce status of the family when the children are young adults also was related to their maladjustment whereas their 1-year attachment status was not. These data support the environmental model. Although general developmental theory would argue for an interactional approach, our data revealed no such effect. The early attachment of the child and the divorced family environment did not add any variance that was not explained by the environmental model itself. Although there is some evidence in the developmental literature for an interactional approach, the data are not that strong (Lewis, 1999c). Moreover, without a consideration of the environment over time, it is still relatively unproven whether any interactional model accounts for more of the variance than does an environmental model alone. As is discussed subsequently, without the proper environmental measurement, any serious test of the various developmental models is not possible.

Recently we have been exploring the precursors of body dissatisfaction, as by the time children become young adults they show large individual and group differences in how they view their bodies. As has been reported many times, young adult women have greater body dissatisfaction than men (Rosenblum & Lewis, 1999). Data from the periods of infancy (0–3 years), childhood (6–9 years), and early adolescence (13 years) that contained information on such variables as family relationships (attachment), IQ, peer friendships, self-consciousness, and maladjustment were available and related to body dissatisfaction when the children were young adults. Also available were data on the same variables taken at the same time the young adults reported on their body dissatisfaction.

The results paralleled those found in the other longitudinal studies. First, few earlier variables taken during infancy, childhood, or early adolescence predicted much of the variance in 18-year-old's body dissatisfaction. Second, the association between body dissatisfaction and concurrent variables accounts for more variance than the earlier variables. Finally, the social network, in particular the same-sex-peer network, is consistent over age. It is the one factor most related to body dissatisfaction, with children who have more same-sex peers having greater body dissatisfaction.

Such findings as these show that earlier traits or characteristics have little relation to later personality characteristics and that the concurrent environment is most predictive of these characteristics. These results, in general, hold across most longitudinal studies. It has been labeled a simplex pattern, as prediction grows weak as the two age points increase in time.

THE NEED FOR PREDICTION

Underlying each model of development and, therefore, underlying the development of personality is the hope that change is lawful and, therefore, predictable. As we all know, however, lawfulness is not necessarily synonymous with prediction. From the point of view of trait models, the prediction is predicated on the belief that either the learned or the biologically determined trait will continue to express itself throughout the life course. The problem with such a view is that, at least in the first third of the life cycle, it does not hold very well, with perhaps only 20–30% of the variance over time explained. It is possible that the measurement issue may be the problem. With better measures, consistency could be shown to be greater. Unfortunately, the findings, for the most part, are so pervasive across a wide domain of functioning that such an argument is difficult to defend.

From a developmental perspective, however, the trait model is a difficult one to properly test. The reason for this problem rests on how phenotype is related to genotype (see Kagan, 1980). Consider this problem: in the first 10 years of life, a child's behavioral repertoire expands rapidly, so that there are relatively few behaviors at the beginning of life and a multitude later. This being the case, the genotype must necessarily utilize different behaviors at different points in time in order to express itself. The ability of any theory to specify behaviors or sets of behaviors that remain in service of the same genotype does not exist. For example, crying in infancy is a measure both of asking for help, as the infant cannot speak, and of expressing an emotion. Once the child learns to communicate through speech, the cries that functioned as a communicatory vehicle start to drop out.

The trait model of development fits well with trait notions in terms of personality structure. Goldberg's (1990) and McCrae and Costa's (1990) view about the Big Five personality traits certainly fit into this model. Indeed, as we shall see shortly, this model has received considerable support. Surprisingly, though, McCrae and Costa (1990) do not look at consistency in these traits by examining the intercorrelational matrix created by comparing individual differences at one age with those at another. Rather, they use the mean data by age as a way of arguing consistency. Although such an argument may be acceptable in the personality literature, from a developmental perspective it does not make too much sense. Caspi and colleagues, however, had tried such a trait formulation using the more recognized attempts at looking at individual consistency across time (see Caspi & Roberts, 2001). Unfortunately, from a trait perspective, their findings show only a very modest consistency, often accounting for less than 12% of the variance. This problem of consistency, a necessary condition for a trait view, is discussed in the next section.

The trait model's problems with prediction create problems for the model, but similar problems exist for the environmental and for the interactional models as well. Even so, the problem is not as great, because it is well recognized that environments can and do change and that the changes can be random (Bandura, 1982; Lewis, 1997) and not necessarily predictable. The environmental models have fewer problems with prediction because, as has been repeatedly pointed out, environmental and interactional models do not require prediction for their verification (Featherman, 1983; Lewis, 1999a).

THE CASE FOR CONTEXT

Although the data in support of a trait model of personality are weak, it should be clear that a trait model may be more reasonable for certain personal characteristics than others. No developmental model alone can explain change over time. For example, our idea about ourselves, that this is "me," that I have feelings, cognitions, and beliefs, may be a function of one model, whereas how sociable one is may require another.

Although I have argued against a notion of strong continuity, the idea of "me" as existing as "me" over long periods of time and the tendency I have to explain my current life by events that I imagined occurred in the past are very strong. Arguing against continuity and a trait model is always difficult, and one is often abused for having such a notion, because it questions a fundamental sense of ourselves. For the past 50 years, this has been the fate of those who challenge the idea of an enduring personality over time and context. Although I have argued against continuity of personality (Lewis, 2001), I have done so because of the need to focus our attention on the often neglected and important role of context. It is a misunderstanding to think that the contextual or environmental argument proposed speaks against continuity of personality or of traits. None of us yet knows the answer to this. What is important is the need to strongly consider context and to remove its effects from our analysis of continuity (or consistency) of individual characteristics over time.

Without knowing about context, whether it is consistent and stable over time, we cannot disassociate consistency as a personality trait from consistency of the context. Although there are small across-age consistency correlations that are significant and would support, in part, the idea that continuity in personality traits appears to exist, we do not know if such correlations reflect context consistency rather than the consistency of the trait. For example, if a 1-year-old child raised by a depressed mom is observed at 5 years, it is important to know if at 5 years the child's mother is still depressed. If she is, then the characteristics of the child and their consistency may be the consequence of the consistency of the mother's depression. A depressed mother affects her child at 1 year and affects her child at 5 years in the same fashion. The child's consistency may be epiphenomenal to the environmental consistency. In order to observe whether the consistency in the child characteristic is due to the consistency in the environment, we must look at cases in which the environment changes over time, as well as those in which it remains the same. If the characteristic of the child were to be consistent over time when the environment is not consistent, we would have strong support for the idea that personality characteristics, once formed, tend to be consistent over time. Unfortunately, the literature about development usually does not obtain measures of environmental consistency or change. Without environmental measures, the idea that we are measuring consistency of a personality trait independent of context is unwarranted.

Environments can be considered in many different ways. The trait theorists for the most part have chosen to deal with environment by making environment a part of the characteristic of the individual. So, for example, people with certain types of personality characteristics are likely to choose certain environments. This being the case, it is easy to conclude that the consistency of the environment reflects only the consistency of the person's characteristic. Although this assumption may be true, it is certainly not a test of the proposition that personality characteristics or traits exist independent of context. Indeed, by following such an argument, the trait theorists have made it impossible to answer the legitimate question about contextual influences. It is interesting to note in this regard that both trait and gene theorists reduce environmental effects to characteristics of the individual. In this way, the argument for contextual influences is eliminated. The possibility of or the need for contextual factors in these cases is eliminated by definition but not by fact.

In this chapter, I have approached the topic of continuity and discontinuity of personality characteristics by looking at the data in the early period of the lifespan. How do the data for the earlier part of the lifespan, the first two dozen years, agree with the data obtained across the whole lifespan? There appears to be general agreement that the correlations (or stability) of personality characteristics are quite low for the first 30–40 years of life but become stronger at later ages (Caspi & Roberts, 2001). This is explained in such terms as *crystallization* (Caspi & Roberts, 2001), *consolidation, increased stability* (McCrae, 2001), and *fixed*. It is not at all clear what these phrases really mean. There are several possibilities; one is that the personalities of people continue to develop and change until about 30 or even 50 years of age. But what does this mean? If it is changing, why is it? Is this a random change, a change in a direction, or a change brought about by changes in the environment? It is not enough to say *crystallization* or *consolidation*—we have to see what those terms signify. A second possibility, and the one that I offer and elaborate on later, is that for the first 30 years of life the environment is changing rapidly, and thereafter it becomes more regular. The cause of low correlations (.30 or so) over time in the first 30 years of life and the higher correlations over time later (.70) is due to the change in the stability of the environment. In a word, when the context settles down, so does personality. A third possibility has to do with the meaning of questionnaires. Past a certain age a person's answers to questionnaires may become stable and have consistent meaning. Thus Kagan (2001), like Frege, argues that a woman's answers to questions about her sociability represent her sense of meaning of extroversion or introversion but not the referential meaning. What we may be observing is not the consistency in personality characteristics but that the meaning of a question may undergo a change; thus the greater stability later reflects the stability of meaning.

If we were willing to consider and to study environments, we might have some good basis with which to study personality development. Even a single measure of environment would surely show that children and young adults go through a large number of contextual changes in the first 30 years: going from home to public school, from family to peers, different places to live, new jobs, getting married, and having children. Are not each of these powerful contextual variables? However, after 30 years, people begin to "settle down," to have a job or career, to live in a home, to be married, and so forth. Thus the 30–plus-year period is marked by relatively few powerful contextual changes. When context becomes simplified and does not change very rapidly, then across-age correlations are higher. The existing correlations from early childhood, childhood, adulthood, and old age, as reported, support the idea of personality consistency changes over the lifespan, provided that we take environments seriously. That there are but a few measures of environments besides socioeconomic status (an economic, not psychological, variable) suggests that the field at large is more interested in measures of the person rather than measures of the contexts.

As a field, we have argued for a very powerful hypothesis. We have argued that personality characteristics of individuals are enduring across time and context. In this chapter, I have raised the question of whether or not the data from the past 75 years of development and study supports this powerful hypothesis. It is not supported in the first third of life, and the correlations are, overall, rather weak for the rest of the lifespan. Even so, I suspect that we cannot resolve these differences because they speak to basic worldviews. Nevertheless, we do need to ask if the data obtained show strong or weak effects. Given the very strong form of the hypothesis on personality that has been suggested, the data show only a weak effect. Whether we should be satisfied with weak effects given the strong hypothesis is something that needs to be answered. More important, to what use can we put such data? I suspect that in order for us to progress in our common study of personality and its development, we need to consider many different tasks. The measurement of environments by far is one of our greatest challenges. Without the study of measurement of environments, we do not yet have the means to answer the questions nor test the models proposed. I certainly do not mean to claim that we do, only that in the early part of life, when environments and traits are considered, the role of environment shows powerful effects. This should be considered as we strive to address the problem of personality development across the lifespan.

NOTE

1. Here I refer to the objective environment, if it could be measured. This environment is not the subjective environment as seen by the child, although the difference between objective and subjective measures of the environment remains a problem that needs careful study.

REFERENCES

Ainsworth, M. D. S. (1973). The development of infant–mother attachment. In B. M. Caldwell & H. N. Ricciuti (Eds.), *Review of child development research* (Vol. 3, pp. 1–95). Chicago: University of Chicago Press.

Ainsworth, M. D. S. (1989). Attachment beyond infancy. *American Psychologist, 44,* 709–716.

Ainsworth, M. D. S., & Marvin, R. S. (1995). On the shaping of attachment theory and research: An interview with Mary D. S. Ainsworth. *Monographs of the Society for Research in Child Development, 62*(2–3, Serial No. 244).

Allport, F. H., & Allport, G. W. (1921). Personality traits: Their classification and measurement. *Journal of Abnormal and Social Psychology, 16,* 1–40.

Anthony, E. J. (1970). The behavior disorders of children. In P. H. Mussen (Ed.), *Carmichael's manual of child psychology* (pp. 667–764). New York: Wiley.

Bandura, A. (1982). The psychology of chance encounters and life paths. *American Psychologist, 37,* 747–755.

Bellin, H. (1971). The development of physical concepts. In T. Michel (Ed.), *Cognitive development and epistemology* (pp. 85–119). New York: Academic Press.

Bem, S. L. (1987). Masculinity and femininity exist only in the mind of the perceiver. In J. M. Reinish, L. A. Rosenblum, & S. A. Sanders (Eds.), *Masculinity/femininity: Basic perspectives* (pp. 304–314). New York: Oxford University Press.

Block, J., & Block, T. H. (1980). The role of ego control and ego resiliency in the organization of behavior. In W. Collins (Ed.), *Minnesota Symposium on Child Psychology* (Vol. 13, pp. 325–377). Hillsdale, NJ: Erlbaum.

Bowlby, J. (1969). *Attachment and loss: Vol. 1. Attachment.* New York: Basic Books.

Bronfenbrenner, U., & Crouter, A. C. (1983). The evolution of environmental models in developmental research. In W. Kessen & P. H. Mussen (Eds.), *Handbook of child psychology: Vol. 1. History, theory, and methods* (pp. 357–414). New York: Wiley.

Cairns, R. B., & Cairns, B. D. (2000). The natural history and developmental functions of aggression. In A. J. Sameroff, M. Lewis, & S. M. Miller (Eds.),

Handbook of developmental psychopathology (2nd ed., pp. 403–430). New York: Kluwer Academic/Plenum Press.

Caspi, A., Henry, B., McGee, R. O., Moffitt, T. E., & Silva, P.A. (1995). Temperamental origins of child and adolescent behavior problems: From age three to age fifteen. *Child Development, 66*, 55–68.

Caspi, A., & Roberts, B. W. (2001). Personality development across the life course: The argument for change and continuity. *Psychological Inquiry, 12*(2), 49–66.

Caspi, A., & Silva, P. A. (1995). Temperamental qualities at age 3 predict personality traits in young adulthood: Longitudinal evidence from a birth cohort. *Child Development, 66*, 489–498.

Chess, S., & Thomas. A. (1984). *Origins and evolution of behavior disorders.* New York: Brunner/Mazel.

Chomsky, N. (Ed.). (1957). *Syntactic structures.* The Hague, Netherlands: Mouton.

Chomsky, N. (Ed.). (1965). *Aspects of the theory of syntax.* Cambridge, MA: MIT Press.

Cole, M. (1996). *Cultural psychology: A once and future discipline.* Cambridge, MA: Harvard University, Belknap Press.

Davies, P. T., & Cummings, E. M. (1994). Marital conflict and child adjustment: An emotional security hypothesis. *Psychological Bulletin, 116*, 387–411.

Dunn, J. (1993). *Young children's close relationships: Beyond attachment.* Newbury Park, CA: Sage.

Fagot, B. I., & Patterson, G. R. (1969). An in vivo analysis of reinforcing contingencies for sex role behaviors in the preschool child. *Developmental Psychology, 1*, 566–568.

Featherman, D. L. (1983). *Biography society and history: Individual development as a population process.* (CDE Working Paper), University of Wisconsin, Madison, WI.

Fox, N. A., Kimmerly, N. L., & Schafer, W. D. (1991). Attachment to mother/attachment to father: A meta-analysis. *Child Development, 62*(1), 210–225.

Garmezy, N. (1974). The study of competence in children at risk for severe psychopathology. In E. Anthony & C. Koupernik (Eds.), *The child in his family* (Vol. 3, pp. 77–98). New York: Wiley.

Garmezy, N., Masten, A. S., & Tellegen, A. (1984). The study of stress and competence in children: A building block for developmental psychopathology. *Child Development, 55*, 987–1111.

Gibson, J. J. (1969). *Principles of perceptual learning and development.* New York: Appleton-Century-Crofts.

Goldberg, L. R. (1990). An alternative "description of personality": The Big Five factor structure. *Journal of Personality and Social Psychology, 59*, 1216–1229.

Gottesman, I., & Shields, J. (Eds.). (1982). *Schizophrenia: The epigenetic puzzle.* New York: Cambridge University Press.

Kagan, J. (1980). Perspectives on continuity. In O. G. Brim & J. Kagan (Eds.), *Constancy and change in human development* (pp. 26–74). Cambridge, MA: Harvard University Press.

Kagan, J. (2001). The need for new constructs. *Psychological Inquiry, 12*(2), 84.

Kallman, F. J. (1946). The genetic theory of schizophrenia: An analysis of 691 schizophrenic twin index families. *American Journal of Psychiatry, 103,* 309–322.

Kringlon, E. (1968). An epidemiological twin study of schizophrenia. In D. Rosenthal & S. Kety (Eds.), *The transmission of schizophrenia* (pp. 49–63). New York: Pergamon Press.

Lamb, M. E., Thompson, R., Gardner, W., & Charnov, E. (1985). *Infant–mother attachment: The origins and developmental significance of individual differences in strange situation behavior.* Hillsdale, NJ: Erlbaum.

Lennenberg, E. H. (1967). *Biological foundations of language.* New York: Wiley.

Lerner, R. H. (1984). *On the nature of human plasticity.* New York: Cambridge University Press.

Lewis, M. (1972). State as an infant–environment interaction: An analysis of mother–infant interaction as a function of sex. *Merrill–Palmer Quarterly, 18,* 95–121.

Lewis, M. (1983). Newton, Einstein, Piaget, and the concept of self. In L. S. Liben (Ed.), *Piaget and the foundations of knowledge* (pp. 141–177). Hillsdale, NJ: Erlbaum.

Lewis, M. (1984). Social influences on development: An overview. In M. Lewis (Ed.), *Beyond the dyad* (pp. 1–12). New York: Plenum Press.

Lewis, M. (1987a). Early sex role behavior and school age adjustment. In J. M. Reinish, L. A. Rosenblum, & S. A. Sanders (Eds.), *Masculinity/femininity: Basic perspectives* (pp. 202–226). New York: Oxford University Press.

Lewis, M. (1987b). The social development of infants and young children. In J. Osofsky (Ed.), *Infant development* (2nd ed., pp. 419–493). New York: Wiley.

Lewis, M. (1997). *Altering fate: Why the past does not predict the future.* New York: Guilford Press.

Lewis, M. (1999a, Summer). Do environments matter at all? [Review of the book, *The nurture assumption: Why children turn out the way they do*]. *Social Policy,* 34–43.

Lewis, M. (1999b). Contextualism and the issue of continuity. *Does infancy matter?: Infant behavior and development, 22*(4), 413–444.

Lewis, M. (1999c). On the development of personality. In L. Pervin & O. John (Eds.), *Handbook of personality* (2nd ed., pp. 327–346). New York: Guilford Press.

Lewis, M. (2001). Continuity and change: A reply. *Psychological Inquiry, 12*(2), 110–112.

Lewis, M., & Feiring, C. (1989). Infant, mother, and mother–infant interaction behavior and subsequent attachment. *Child Development, 60,* 831–837.

Lewis, M., & Feiring, C. (1991). Attachment as personal characteristic or a measure of the environment. In J. L. Gewirtz & W. M. Kurtines (Eds.), *Intersections with attachment* (pp. 1–21). Hillsdale, NJ: Erlbaum.

Lewis, M., Feiring, C., & Rosenthal, S. (2000). Attachment over time. *Child Development, 71*(3), 707–720.

Luria, A. R. (1976). *Cognitive development: Its cultural and social foundations.* Cambridge, MA: Harvard University Press.

McCrae, R. R. (2001). Traits through time. *Psychological Inquiry, 12*(2), 85–87.

McCrae, R. R., & Costa, P. T., Jr. (1990). *Personality in adulthood.* New York: Guilford Press.

Mischel, W. (1965). *Personality assessment.* New York: Wiley.

Newman, D. L., Caspi, A., Moffitt, T. E., & Silva, P. A. (1997). Antecedents of adult interpersonal functioning: Effects of individual differences in age 3 temperament. *Developmental Psychology, 33*(2), 206–217.

Piaget, J. (1952). *The origins of intelligence in children.* New York: International Universities Press.

Puig-Antich, J. (1982). Psychobiological correlates of major depressive disorder in children and adolescents. In L. Greenspan (Ed.), *Psychiatry 1982: Annual review* (pp. 41–64). Washington, DC: American Psychological Association.

Reese, H. W., & Overton, W. F. (1970). Models of development and theories of development. In L. R. Goulet & P. B. Baltes (Eds.), *Life-span developmental psychology: Research and theory* (pp. 115–145). New York: Academic Press.

Riegel, K. R (1976). *Psychology of development and history.* New York: Plenum Press.

Riegel, K. R. (1978). *Psychology, mon amour: A countertext.* Boston: Houghton Mifflin.

Rosenblum, G., & Lewis, M. (1999). The relations among body-image, physical attractiveness, and body mass in adolescence. *Child Development, 70*(1), 50–64.

Rosenthal, S., Feiring, C., & Lewis, M. (1998). Political volunteering from late adolescence to young adulthood: Patterns and predictors. *Journal of Social Issues, 54*(3), 477–493.

Rutter, M. (1979). Protective factors in children's responses to stress and disadvantage. In M. W. Kent & J. G. Rolf (Eds.), *Primary prevention of psychopathology: Vol. 3. Social competence in children* (pp. 150–162). Hanover, NH: University Press of New England.

Rutter, M. (1981). Stress, coping and development: Some issues and some questions. *Journal of Child Psychology and Psychiatry, 22*, 323–356.

Sameroff, A. (1975). Transactional models in early social relations. *Human Development, 18*, 65–79.

Sameroff, A., & Chandler, M. J. (1975). Reproductive risk and the continuum of caretaking causality. In F. D. Horowitz (Ed.), *Review of child development research* (Vol. 4, pp. 187–244). Chicago: University of Chicago Press.

Saudino, K. J. (1997). Moving beyond the heritability question: New directions in behavioral genetic studies of personality. *Current Directions in Psychological Science, 6*(4), 86–90.

Skinner, B. F (1953). *Science and human behavior.* New York: Macmillan.

Szasz, T. S. (1961). *The myth of mental illness.* New York: Harper & Row.

Thelen, E., & Ulrich, B. D. (1991). Hidden skills: A dynamic systems analysis of treadmill stepping during the first year. *Monographs of the Society for Research in Child Development, 56*(1, Serial No. 223).

Thom, R. (1975). *Structural stability and morphogenesis*. Reading, MA: Benjamin.

Thomas, A., & Chess, S. (1977). *Temperament and development*. New York: Brunner/Mazel.

Zahn-Waxler, C., Cummings, E. M., McKnew, D. H., & Radke-Yarrow, N. (1984). Altruism, aggression, and social interactions in young children with a manic-depressive parent. *Child Development, 55*, 112–122.

Zeeman, E. C. (1976). Catastrophe theory. *Scientific American, 234*, 65–83.

CHAPTER 7

Evolutionary and Developmental Perspectives on the Agentic Self

PATRICIA H. HAWLEY
TODD D. LITTLE

The concept of agency in human behavior is quite widespread but possesses many faces (Bandura, 1997; Blatt & Blass, 1986; Chapman, 1984; Little, Hawley, Henrich, & Marsland, in press). The central goal of this chapter is to examine two different, yet complementary, levels of meaning associated with the development of agency. The first level relates to the evolutionary basis of personal agency. Contrary to common perceptions that evolutionary perspectives address only human universals, our perspective emphasizes individual-by-context interactions in a way that gives rise to meaningful predictions about individual differences in agency and the circumstances in which these differences are expected to emerge. The second level relates to the individual's ontogenetic sense of personal agency. As described in more detail later, one's sense of personal agency stems from goal-driven actions. It functions as a personal resource for facing the challenges that emerge throughout development (Little, 1998). In other words, how individuals meet and overcome such life-course challenges is the proximal, or surface, level of personal agency.

The evolutionary and developmental perspectives that we espouse share a common origin; namely, an organismic metatheory (Little, in press; Little et al., in press)—that is, a perspective that considers the organism or individual to be an active agent in his or her own development. Our organismic perspective is not teleological in that it does not espouse an ideal end state toward which all organisms aspire. Instead, it is agnostic in regard to direction and probabilistic in terms of potential outcomes. From this vantage point, most of human behavior is defined as actions.

Actions are those behaviors that are both volitional and goal directed in nature. Individuals are inherently active and self-regulating in their choice and execution of actions, and their actions are thus purposeful and self-initiated. That is, actions result from selective choices that emanate primarily from the individual and yet derive from sources that are common to all individuals.

An organismic perspective also suggests that the actions emanating from the individual are motivated to service basic needs of the individual. Resource control theory (Hawley, 1999), our focal instantiation of the evolutionary perspective, posits that acquiring and utilizing material and social resources is a driving force in behavior because these resources are necessary for the survival and reproduction of the individual. Action control theory (e.g., Little, 1998; Little, in press), our focal instantiation of the developmental perspective, posits that actions also service basic psychological needs for competence and relatedness. Although these needs are not new to the study of human behavior (Bakan, 1966; Deci & Ryan, in press; Hogan & Hogan, 1991; White, 1959), we attempt to integrate both ontogenetic and phylogenetic perspectives.

AN EVOLUTIONARY PERSPECTIVE

Personal agency varies among individuals; that is, individuals are more or less agentic in their actions, varying from helpless to empowered. To some, however, employing evolutionary approaches to the study of individual differences may seem in some sense oxymoronic. Evolutionary biology and evolutionary psychology, for example, typically have focused on species-typical adaptations and mechanisms. From biological perspectives, phenotypic (and thereby genotypic) variability is the raw material on which natural selection operates. Selection in general is seen as a homogenizing force that culls less optimal variants in favor of those that foster survival and reproduction (Willams, 1966). Members of any population differ from one another in what is seen as largely inconsequential ways; individual differences are noise in the evolutionary process that results from nonselective mechanisms such as mutation, recombination, and drift. Studies in evolutionary psychology accordingly focus on topics such as mate selection, with little consideration for individual-difference variables (e.g., Cosmides & Tooby, 1995), with the exception perhaps of demographics such as gender, age, and socioeconomic status (e.g., Buss, 1994).

This species-general approach to evolutionary psychology confronts long-held beliefs in other fields of psychology that individual differences are anything but inconsequential. Personality theorists, for example, have long shown how individual differences are related to adaptation across the lifespan. Only more recently has it been suggested that these differences are themselves related to reproductive success (Buss, 1999; Hawley, 1999).

Work in behavioral genetics has shown that a good portion of this variation in personal characteristics is heritable (e.g., Plomin & Caspi, 1999). Heritability is often considered to support evolutionary arguments, as "adaptations" must have a genetic component. Paradoxically, however, the more the variability in a population on a certain trait is due to genetic differences (i.e., heritability), the less likely it is that the trait is an "adaptation." Naturally selected adaptations tend to have by definition very low heritabilities because there is little variation across individuals (e.g., a four-chambered heart). In other words, "heritable diversity is inversely proportional to adaptive importance" (Tooby & Cosmides, 1990, p. 49). One may legitimately wonder, then, what role evolution may play on traits across which we so obviously differ (e.g., agency).

Part of the reluctance to incorporate individual-difference variables into evolutionary perspectives may stem in part from misunderstandings concerning the relative contributions of the gene and the environment to phenotypic characteristics. Evolution by natural selection is—and always has been—a highly contextual theory. Biological considerations of environment include the microenvironment of the gene (including other components of the genome and somatic environment), as well as the ecological environment (Williams, 1966). Many of the effects of the ecological environment on phenotypic adaptation are well known and well accepted (e.g., climate, resources, predators). Less understood and less well studied, however, are the effects of demographics and social environments such as the family constellation (Belsky, Steinberg, & Draper, 1991; Sulloway, 1996) or the peer group (Hawley & Little, 1999). Draper and colleagues, for example, have proposed that adolescent sexual behavior may be "calibrated" by early environmental conditions (e.g., father absence for girls; Belsky et al., 1991; Draper & Harpending, 1982). Psychologists may be skeptical at least partially because "adaptation" in the evolutionary sense is closely tied to genetic inheritance. Yet, at the same time, we more readily accept the "internal representations" formed by the mother–infant attachment relationship as an early calibration that presumably affects later reproductive behavior (Bowlby, 1969; Belsky, 1997; Sroufe, 1992).

These environmental effects or calibrations can serve to maintain meaningful variance in phenotypic traits (e.g., strategic specialization; Maynard Smith, 1974). For example, strategies employed by individuals may be influenced by the strategies adopted by others. An individual may enjoy a higher average payoff by choosing a suboptimal strategy or niche occupied by fewer competitors (e.g., Buss, 1999; Mealey, 1995; Sulloway,

1996). Some authors have proposed that the brain's function is to generate behavior relevant for adaptive issues appropriate to environmental circumstances (Cosmides & Tooby, 1995; Pinker, 1997). Some behaviors, for good reason, are not under personal control (e.g., breathing) whereas others are (e.g., mate selection). As such, the brain is keenly attuned to these environmental circumstances, such as the level of available oxygen, the characteristics of available mates (Buss, 1994), or the properties of the self (*reactive heritability*; Tooby & Cosmides, 1990).

Grand theories of personality have always sought to identify the core of human nature (a goal shared by evolutionary psychologists). A brief survey suggests that theoretical biologists and personality theorists have entertained common notions about what is important for human adaptation, ontogenetic or phylogenetic. One sees, for example, themes of balancing sex and aggression (Freud), affection and competition (Adler), intimacy and status (McClelland), superiority striving (Adler), and dominance feelings (Maslow). Given that these fundamental motives are universal, common across many species (e.g., de Waal, 1982), moderately heritable and ecologically modifiable, and, theoretically if not actually, related to differential reproductive success, then they are appropriate for incorporation into evolutionary models. Indeed, evolutionary models may foster a deeper understanding and give rise to interesting and testable predictions that have yet to be entertained.

RESOURCE CONTROL THEORY AND HUMAN AGENCY: CREATING WINNERS AND LOSERS

Similar to several personality theories, theories of motivation (e.g., Ryan, 1993), and models of social competence (e.g., Rubin & Rose-Krasnor, 1992), resource control theory has the balancing of self and other goals at its core. This theoretical perspective is based on the assumption that humans, like other social species, should optimally behave in ways that facilitate personal resource acquisition while at the same time maintaining friendly bonds with other group members. The necessity of meeting one's needs and simultaneously being a good group member underlies the evolution of much of human behavior and psychological organization: It implies that individuals must balance being egoistic and other-oriented (Alexander, 1979; Charlesworth, 1996; Trivers, 1971). Competition for resources in the presence of others is the mechanism underlying natural selection (an idea Darwin derived from reading Thomas Malthus; but see Williams, 1966, for important exceptions). Modern theoreticians have speculated about why we live in groups, and resource acquisition is one of these pulls (e.g., Alexander, 1979). Together these two premises lead directly to a quandary that Darwin himself recognized—that the presence of others intensifies intragroup competition for the very resources that the group acquires. In other words, "cooperative" relationships are inevitably contaminated by competition.

Because resources in any social group are essentially limited, there will be group members who are better able to acquire and defend resources through various means than other group members. That is, outside of a perfect world, there will be winners and losers. Resource control theory refers to such winners as "social dominants" (Hawley, 1999). In contrast to familiar traditional ethological approaches that define social dominance in terms of aggression (e.g., Bernstein, 1981; Strayer & Strayer, 1976), resource control theory defines social dominance in terms of relative success at resource competition. Within-group (i.e., between-person) competition is the source of the dominance hierarchy, which from this point of view is merely an ordering of individuals according to their relative competitive abilities (cf. Bernstein, 1981; Strayer & Strayer, 1976). Accordingly, socially dominant individuals by definition experience the lion's share of wins, whereas social subordinates experience a disproportionate quantity of losses.

This updated view is consistent with key findings in the ethological literature. "Alphas," for example, have long been known to be preferred social partners, to be socially central, to be looked up to, to be considered attractive mates, and to exude confidence. Resource control theory maintains that the reason is not that they can physically dominate others, but rather that these dominant individuals—who may not, in fact, be overly aggressive—are superior competitors for resources that all group members are predisposed to covet. They are socially central because they demonstrate the skills that would make other individuals also better off.

Two consequences of this reasoning confront accepted theories but, oddly, are consistent with common sense. First, dominant individuals, even if they use aggressive strategies, demonstrate competency. Although aggression is most commonly viewed as the hallmark of social incompetence (e.g., Coie, 1996; Erdley & Asher, 1998), highly respected powerful individuals often have a "dark side" (e.g., politicians, CEOs, etc; see, e.g., Hogan, Raskin, & Fazzini, 1990). In fact, moderate aggression makes for good leadership (Hogan, Curphy, & Hogan, 1994).

Second, prosociality is not entirely other serving. Trivers (1971, 1985) brilliantly described the nature of cooperative human relationships, the emotional–cognitive mechanisms for their maintenance, and conditions of their dissolution. His theory of reciprocal altruism suggests that affiliative relationships are essentially founded on a series of exchanges by which each attempts to maximize benefits and minimize costs while appearing to be a benevolent alliance partner. The best candidates for friendships exude helpfulness, trustworthiness, and honesty. If one is convincing, one will likely be rewarded with many loyal (resource-yielding) partnerships. Charlesworth also picked up this theme in his theoretical treatment of cooperation as a competitive strategy (e.g., Charlesworth, 1996).

In line with these two consequences to evolutionary reasoning, we propose that at least two strategies for resource control should emerge: direct strategies (i.e., coercion, aggression) and indirect strategies (i.e., prosociality, cooperativeness). In principle, both strategies in various combinations should emerge in social groups perhaps in accordance with forces consistent with strategic specialization and reactive heritability (Tooby & Cosmides, 1990). That is, coercion may pay off in a group of passive others, in which resistance and risk of escalation is low, and may be best carried off by one with a larger or stronger physique.

Strategies need not be adopted because there is a "gene" for them (this is exceedingly unlikely), but rather because the "competition module" of the brain is ideally suited to estimate whether one has a chance to prevail and which strategy has a higher chance of leading to success. Males of many species display and size each other up before one has second thoughts or, less frequently, they actually fight (Lorenz, 1966). Humans also rely on physical cues such as posture and voice to make quick assessments about the status of others (e.g., Gregory & Webster, 1996). Strategies are maladaptive if they are suited to past conditions but not to present ones (e.g., agonistic behavior may be reasonable in a contentious sibling circle but not among more peaceful peers). The entire competitive atmosphere should also push some individuals to choose alliance formation over aggression. If alliances cannot be won easily, ingratiation may be the best one can do. We return to the discussion of strategies later.

THE SEEDS OF AGENCY

Resource-related interactions are by no means limited to the cutthroat world of monkeys or corporate America. They begin the day when one lets out a cry that is quieted only by access to the breast (e.g., Bowlby, 1969). Attachment researchers have long argued that the manner in which the primary caregiver attends and responds to infant signals is an important foundation of personality development. These early resource-related interactions form the basis of the child's beliefs in his or her own effectiveness and lovability (e.g., Ainsworth, 1969; Sroufe, 1992).

No one considers these early mother–infant interactions to be indicators of social dominance. We would not conclude that the infant is socially dominant to his or her mother simply because he or she is efficacious at extracting resources from her. Not long after, however, the child encounters interactions that are related to social dominance, namely, in the peer group.

We believe that these early (e.g., toddlerhood; Hawley & Little, 1999) win–loss experiences set the stage for the development of personal agency. Indeed, these early experiences may further sow the seeds of agency that may be planted by the mother–infant bond. As mentioned, and as any day care worker can attest, in any nursery group there are winners and, therefore, also losers. Winners presumably are learning that their goals can be met, that they can control their environment, that their efforts pay off, and that future efforts are likely to pay off as well. Early win experiences may calibrate one to behave agentically across situations in ways that make agency appear to be a stable trait. Similarly, children who experience losses early on (in what are often viewed as trivial disputes over toys) may be at risk for learning that they cannot achieve their goals or control their environment in the presence of peers, that their efforts will not pay off, and that future efforts are futile.

Social dominance is a context-dependent quality. One must be in the presence of others to be dominant (i.e., to be superior in competitive ability). The "henpecked" child in one context may come to suddenly "rule the roost" when the context changes. Nonetheless, social dominance should be related to personal traits associated with ability and motivational factors. In preschoolers, for example, we found persistence to be an important predictor of winning, along with contextual variables such as time spent at the day care (as a proxy for experience with peers) and relative developmental age (Hawley & Little, 1999; Hawley, in press). In contrast to ethological studies that equate social dominance with aggression, we did not find boys to be at an advantage over girls. Nor would we expect them to be in light of our theoretical position.

Not only should dominance be predictable, but it should also serve as an effective predictor of meaningful social outcomes outside of the context of competition. In other words, is the social dominance hierarchy simply something that we as adults notice, or does it carry meaning to the children involved? We addressed this question by employing Kenny and LaVoie's (1985) social relations model to uncover regularities in children's interaction patterns with their peers (Hawley & Little, 1999). By observing most of the possible child–child pairings, we were able to disentangle the relative contributions of the individuals involved in each interaction from relationship-level characteristics. Thus we were able to explore whether the relationship between individual-level characteristics and social behavior was moderated by social dominance outside of the context of competition.

Social dominance was indeed related to behavior outside of the context of competition. A child's social dominance predicted the degree to which he or she was willing to play with a toy in the presence of a peer and, conversely, the degree to which he or she deferred to his or her partner and imitated the partner. For example, when a child was paired with a subordinate peer, he or she actively used the toy. When the same child was with a dominant peer, he or she was more likely to defer, even in the absence of threat. In other words, win–loss experiences effectively metacommunicated appropriate social behavior, even to toddlers.

This pattern of results furthermore suggests to us that resource-directed interactions are indeed rich contexts in which personal agency can be expressed and solidified. Children appear to be sensitive to them from very early on, as would be expected of a construct that is central to human social structure. In these interactions, children at the extremes (very high rank and very low rank) are receiving a consistent story with very different home messages: "the world is my oyster" versus "I am the pawn of others' wishes." At the high end, we might expect a developing child with characteristics not unlike the silverback gorilla (confidence in appearance and action, socially central, surgent). At the other extreme, the child may be at risk to be submissive, socially peripheral (if not victimized), and withdrawn.

In any hierarchy, few individuals are at the extremes. Most children of middle rank experience both wins and losses depending on with whom they are interacting—those more dominant to themselves or less. Win experiences may foster a sense of personal agency in mid-ranking children that subordinates do not enjoy. It may be, however, that those occupying the highest ranks will be more likely to experience autonomy within the context of resource-directed behavior. Middle-ranking children may resort to strategies such as cooperation, alliance formation, and ingratiation toward high-ranking others. They may know how and be able to achieve their goals, but they may nonetheless sometimes experience control of their behavior as more external than internal to themselves.

BALANCING SELF AND OTHERS' GOALS AND THE EMERGENCE OF STRATEGIES

Prosocial strategies of resource control expertly capitalize on the social group's mediation of material access by fostering cooperative relationships and treating others in ways that encourage goodwill, reciprocity, and loyalty (e.g., helping, sharing, and appearing altruistic). Coercive strategies disregard these positive bonds to gain direct access to resources by, for example, taking, monopolizing, and thwarting others. Importantly, both strategies underlie winningness and therefore lead to (and are the result of) personal agency. Even though coercive strategies may bear a social cost such as loneliness, presumably as a result of alienating peers (Hawley, Little, & Pasupathi, in press), both prosocial and coercive strategies are superior to adopting no strategy: Subordinates neither orient toward resources in the environment nor capitalize on the mediating effect of others. Thus these individuals risk not meeting their material and social needs.

If this line of reasoning is correct, we should see the emergence of subgroups of individuals based on the degree to which they employ the two proposed strategies of resource control. Accordingly, these groups of individuals should differ on key personality characteristics that would (1) move them toward resources in the first place (e.g., surgency) and (2) move them toward one strategy or another (e.g., agreeableness, hostility). Additionally, differential resource acquisition should be associated with the employment of the strategies; that is, resource controllers should engage in more aggression, prosociality, or both than noncontrollers. Furthermore, as a consequence to relative effectiveness in resource control, the subgroups should differ in the degree to which they experience personal agency and, therefore, well-being.

In studying preadolescents and adolescents, we find patterns that are consistent with our expectations. First, these groups of children can be divided into five groups based on relative levels of the self-reported degree to which they utilize prosocial (e.g., "I get what I want by being helpful") and coercive (e.g., "I get what I want by making threats") strategies of resource control. Prosocial controllers report using only prosocial strategies, coercive controllers report using only coercive strategies, bistrategic controllers report using both, subordinates report using neither, and typical children report midrange on either one or both. Most children are typical.

Importantly, the groups differ in many characteristics, as would be expected, including ways that are not of central importance here (but see Hawley et al., in press; Hawley, 2001). It is useful, for example, to compare the most successful and the least successful groups—the bistrategics and the subordinates. Recall that resource control theory posits that others will gravitate toward successful controllers, prefer them, and compete among themselves to be with them. Because the successful controller's material and social needs are being met, they will feel good about their competitive abilities, good about their social abilities, and overall enjoy positive well-being and even health (Sapolsky, 1999). All of this goodness will come despite the fact that the successful controller may be aggressive; perhaps even because he or she is aggressive. In contrast, noncontrollers lose all the way around. Indeed, negative emotional responses such as ill-being may function as an effective signal to the individual indicating that his or her current behavior is not optimally adaptive and that another strategy should be explored or goals should be changed (Nesse & Lloyd, 1992).

We have found that children who endorse both strategies are by far the most successful resource controllers in their own opinions and in the opinions of others (i.e., peers). In addition, they are well liked, perceived as the most popular, and report themselves to be among the happiest, least lonely, and most socially agentic children of the schoolyard. They describe themselves as being hostile and aggressive, as well as prosocial and among the most socially skilled. In contrast, subordinate children are the least effective at resource control and are seen as such by others. They are the least liked, perceived as the least popular, rejected by other children, and report themselves to be among the least happy, most lonely, and least socially agentic children. Typical children are midway between the extremes on these characteristics. We know of no other theory that would predict this pattern of results. It should be noted, however, that our theoretical stance is essentially directional in terms of specifying causes and effects. Given that these data are cross-sectional, causal direction cannot be assured.

Our underlying orientation, however, is consistent with work on social dominance and sociopharmacology. McGuire and associates, for example, have demonstrated that hierarchy ascendance is associated with serum serotonin elevations (Brammer, Raleigh, & McGuire, 1994; McGuire, Raleigh, & Brammer, 1984). In the presence of others, top-ranked male vervets had higher than average serotonin levels. When removed from the group, they returned to normal levels (i.e., dominance requires the presence of others). In the absence of the reigning alpha, a new male rose in the hierarchy and, accordingly, enjoyed elevated serotonin until the reigning male returned. The authors concluded that elevated serotonin was both a cause and effect of successful ascendance. The effects of serotonin on mood and behavior are well known: Low levels of serotonin are associated with low self-esteem, anxiety, and depression. Pharmacologically enhanced serotonin (e.g., serotonin reuptake inhibition) decreases anxiety and increases sociability and assertiveness (Frank & Thase, 1999). That is, it increases qualities associated with winningness.

In a similar vein, social subordinance in nonhuman primates has been linked with hypercortisolism, an exaggerated stress response (Sapolsky, Alberts, & Altmann, 1997). Chronic stress response increases risk for certain diseases (Sapolsky, 1999). Similar associations have been found in human populations in terms of socioeconomic status, the supposed human analog to suboptimal resource control at a societal level. Thus low rank is evidently not only bad for well-being but also quite likely bad for health, once again underscoring the selective advantage of skilled and successful competition.

This evolutionary argument suggests that organismic adaptation requires basic motivational systems that move individuals to meet their material needs (i.e., competence needs) and to seek (resource-mediating) social relationships (i.e., relatedness needs). In other words, optimal adaptation implies drives that move the individual to seek both resources and social relationships simultaneously. This duality of motivation is especially true in infancy, when basic survival depends on both. In our view, this duality of motivation is a lifespan source of behavior and beliefs. Throughout the life course, the individual's choice of day-to-day actions and goals would reflect both the general resource orientation of the individual and the preferred strategy for acquisition. Moreover, the choices in actions would also be made in light of the context in which one is engaged.

A DEVELOPMENTAL PERSPECTIVE

Given the organismic penchant for motivated actions, development is predominantly self-guided and the individual gives form and meaning to his or her actions throughout development. These actions give rise to a sense of agency, and they are instigated by the agentic strivings of the individual. Agentic actions are autonomous actions in the sense that they originate from the individual and are self-chosen (see, e.g., Deci & Ryan, in press; Little, Lopez, & Wanner, 2001). In other words, the development of agency and the various functions of agency in development are clearly interwoven processes. Much of our ability to understand both changes in agency and the influences of agency depends on understanding the mechanisms by which actions come about and how actions (and their consequents) are evaluated.

Social learning theorists have outlined numerous mechanisms by which learning about oneself and one's actions can occur. Direct experiences of success and failure have well-documented effects on the likelihood of future behaviors occurring. Vicarious experiences, too, have been clearly implicated as a mechanism of learning. Related to these processes, direct instruction from knowledgeable others and performance feedback from evaluative others are both powerful influences affecting the development of one's sense of self. The emotional nature (e.g., shame vs. pride) and magnitude of one's reactions to these various sources of information further shape and solidify the impact of what has been learned. Adding to this list of features is the direction and quality of social comparisons that are available. Little, Oettingen, Baltes, and their colleagues (e.g., Little,

Oettingen, Stetsenko, & Baltes, 1995) have provided a set of cross-cultural studies that support the idea that some contexts offer more veridical social comparison opportunities than other contexts (see also Little, 1998, for a review).

In comparison to these well-documented mechanisms, relatively little attention has been directed at the functions of symbolic actions in shaping the agentic self. Symbolic actions refer to the internal mental representations of actions, their rehearsals, their interpretations and reinterpretations, and the manner in which actions are integrated into unifying schemas and representations of the self. In this regard, many of Piaget's ideas on the development of cognition are directly applicable to understanding the development of the self. Equilibration, assimilation, and accommodation are the processes by which symbolic actions shape the development of the self (Chapman, 1984). These mechanisms of change are also shaped by the time units that mark development.

A key question in the development of self-related characteristics and processes is the time unit that governs growth, change, or transformations across the life course. Clearly, time can be marked as a simple chronological progression (i.e., age in years, months, days). For various reasons, however, chronological age may be an imprecise index or proxy of development. For example, maturational time and its markers (e.g., mental age, pubertal onset) have routinely been employed to better gauge developmental levels of individuals. Another marker that is clearly relevant for the development of agency is episodic time. Many key events would qualify as potential markers, including an illness, a first kiss, a personal loss, retirement, getting a license to drive, and so on. To complicate the developmental importance of such events is the issue of calibration for these events. For instance, the event of receiving a driver's license can be calibrated as age at which it was received or it can be calibrated as relative time in relation to some meaningful criteria (e.g., early, on-time, or late acquisition). Still another index of developmental influence is experiential time. Grade in school, for example, is commonly used to mark academic learning experiences.

These learning mechanisms, together with the episodes, events, experiences, and maturations attendant to development of the agentic self, give rise to various beliefs and judgments about how things function and which forms function best. The profile of control judgments can be used as a mirror on the agentic self. Beliefs about what it takes to accomplish goals (e.g., causality beliefs, strategy beliefs) offer a glimpse of one's worldview (see Figure 7.1). Such beliefs about the utility of actions are both means specific and context specific. For example, in the school context, beliefs about the usefulness of effort versus ability have shown distinctive patterns across age and sociocultural context (Little & Lopez, 1997). Beliefs

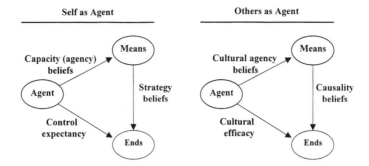

FIGURE 7.1. Relations among the three constituents of human action, both when the self is the agent and when others are the agents. Means can vary from personal attributes such as effort and ability to external aids such as friends and teachers.

about what one possesses in terms of capabilities (e.g., ability, perseverance, reliant relationships) offer a glimpse of the means one has available to pursue goals (see Figure 7.1). In the social domain, beliefs about the utility of effort and ability can be contrasted with other potential means such as aggressiveness and helpfulness. Such beliefs about the personal possession or usability of means are an integral part of the self-regulatory system because they reflect the orientation one would take in interactions with others. For example, a belief in the ability to effectively aggress versus a belief in the ability to be effectively helpful would differ by strategy orientation. The sets of beliefs illustrate the various forms and functions of personal agency.

The lifespan–life course perspectives on the functions and forms of agency can be exemplified by looking at the developmental trends and trajectories of control-related judgments. This literature has been characterized by a lack of congruence across studies; some show growth, some show decline, and still others indicate no changes. In their review of this literature, Grob, Little, and Wanner (1999) suggested that the lack of congruence depends on the various types of judgment one can make and the specific goal domain being examined. Grob et al. (1999) explored this hypothesis in a cross-sectional study of more than 600 Swiss adolescents and adults. They assessed four types of control judgments for each of three life domains (personal, social, and societal). The first type of judgment was the general control expectancy over the goal domain—feeling able to influence (1) personal goals such as health and intellectual growth, or (2) social goals such as establishing and maintaining close relationships, or (3) societal goals such as contributing to a cleaner environment or more tolerant social order. The other types of control judgments made of these goal domains were the personal importance of the goal, the degree to which one still strives to attain the goal, and the comparative control (i.e., relative to my peers do I have more or less control).

The findings strongly supported the "it depends" hypothesis. For example, striving to attain a social goal, such as a harmonious relationship with a significant other, was rated highest of the goal domains and did not change across the lifespan. Personal goal striving showed a steady decline with age. The comparative control of these two goal domains showed identical rainbow curves. In adolescence and again in old age, participants rated their control of social and personal goals as less than their peers' control. The arch of the curve, which indicated a sense of comparative control that exceeded that of one's peers, reached its apex at about age 45. The importance of societal goals was rated as high as social and personal goals in early adulthood and rose steadily across the lifespan; unfortunately, the perceptions that one can actually control societal events started low and steadily decreased across development (Grob et al., 1999).

The consequences of attaining goals can also vary as a function of the point along the life course at which a particular goal is attained and as a function of life-context moderators such as gender. For example, Shahar, Grob, and Little (2001) examined the relationship between depression and the reported attainment of the goal of achieving an intimate relationship. In young adulthood (ages 18–39), there were no differences on depression—males and females who either had or had not achieved intimate-relationship status were similar in their low levels of depressive symptomology. In mid-age, on the other hand, substantial gaps appeared to emerge; in fact, all four groups differed. Males who had not attained intimate-relationship status showed the highest levels of depression, followed by females who had not, then males who had, and then females who had. By old age, the gender differences disappeared, but the effect of either having attained or not having attained an intimate relationship was pronounced. Those persons who had not established an intimate relationship reported greater depressive symptoms than those who had achieved intimacy with another person.

Control perceptions can also vary in the type of event for which one perceives a sense of control. Clearly, desirable events would be preferred targets of goal pursuit. However, undesirable events can also be perceived as being within one's control. Kunzmann, Little, and Smith (2000) showed that control of desirable events was related to positive affect both cross-sectionally and longitudinally in a representative sample of very old persons (70 to 100+ years). The same sample of the longitudinal survivors revealed that perceived control of the undesirable events in one's life was also positively related to positive affect. As Kunzmann et al. (2000) note, this outcome is contrary to most theoretical positions and to much empirical work regarding the decidedly negative effects of perceived control over the undesirable events in one's life. The surviving sample differed significantly from the dropout subgroup on a number of important dimensions, including extroversion, emotional stability, and physical health. The authors suggested that such aspects of the self function as a personal resource that serves to aid an individual's continued fight to maintain an agentic self. Particularly in this age group, control of undesirable events connotes the potential for future changes that are desired and hence bolsters the motivational underpinnings of actions that support one's organismic pursuits. This counterintuitive finding highlights the need to examine both context- and self-related factors to understand the adaptive or maladaptive function of control-related perceptions across the lifespan.

The Kunzmann et al. (2000) study also highlights the downside of a loss of control. In both the cross-sectional and longitudinal samples, older individuals who felt that other people had control of their day-to-day affairs showed elevated levels of negative affect and reduced levels of positive affect. In old age, the perception that others are in control of one's personal activities becomes more realistic. The broader action control model of perceived control suggests that two types of control perceptions regarding others' influence may be relevant (Baltes, 1996). Although the participants in the Kunzmann et al. (2000) study experienced dependency and associated poor emotional outcomes, one can nonetheless maintain a sense of personal control by utilizing others for personal goal attainment. From this perspective, the onus of control of others is still held within the individual, and the sense of personal agency is still maintained. Having the skill to solicit and recruit the assistance of others has clear adaptive advantages. Problem-focused prosocial coping strategies (e.g., enlisting others to address a stressor) are strongly associated with positive outcomes (Little et al., 2001).

FINAL THOUGHTS

Human agency need not necessitate positive outcomes. Environmental feedback need not foster optimal functioning, especially when the environment is poor in material and social resources that would provide positive feedback. Agency can simply mean making the best of what may be a very bad situation. Indeed, this is the crux of adaptation in evolutionary models. Strategies arise that individuals use to get by. Adaptive behavior in one context may be extremely maladaptive behavior in another context. For example, in extreme circumstances, it is plausible that agentic behavior would warrant incarceration when viewed from the macro social level yet be adaptive in the micro context.

The evolutionary perspective outlined here suggests some continuity of goals over the lifespan (social vs. material) but is consistent with developmental perspectives calling for changes in specifics over time. These two levels of analysis are compatible. Each perspective takes into consideration a specific stratum of the structure of the self. Because both perspectives share a common metatheoretical basis (i.e., the organismic origin of actions), they provide complementary views that can be linked synergistically in cases in which the distal motivations of actions are tied directly to the proximal regulatory processes that guide them. In other words, by uniting an evolutionary perspective with an action control perspective, the two levels of analysis of human behavior can be applied to understand the development of the self more broadly. The driving force behind behavior (evolutionary basis) and the supporting action control profile of specific beliefs and behaviors (developmental basis) offer a unified set of theoretically derived constructs for understanding both the why and the how of behavior across the lifespan.

ACKNOWLEDGMENTS

Parts of this work were supported by a Guggenheim Foundation grant awarded to Patricia Hawley and a Yale College Social Sciences grant awarded to Todd D. Little.

REFERENCES

Ainsworth, M. D. (1969). Object relations, dependency, and attachment: A theoretical review of the infant–mother relationship. *Child Development, 40,* 969–1025.

Alexander, R. D. (1979). *Darwinism and human affairs.* Seattle, WA: University of Washington Press.

Bakan, D. (1966). *The duality of human existence.* Boston: Beacon Press.

Baltes, M. M. (1996). *The many faces of dependency in old age.* New York: Cambridge University Press.

Bandura, A. (1997). *Self-efficacy: The exercise of control.* New York: Freeman.

Belsky, J. (1997). Attachment, mating, and parenting: An evolutionary interpretation. *Human Nature, 8,* 361–381.

Belsky, J., Steinberg, L., & Draper, P. (1991). Childhood experience, interpersonal development, and reproductive strategy: An evolutionary theory of socialization. *Child Development, 62,* 647–670.

Bernstein, I. S. (1981). Dominance: The baby and the bathwater. *Behavioral and Brain Sciences, 4,* 419–457.

Blatt, S. J., & Blass, R. B. (1996). Relatedness and self-definition: A dialectic model of personality development. In G. Noam & K. W. Fischer (Eds.), *Development and vulnerability in close relationships* (pp. 309–338). Mahwah, NJ: Erlbaum.

Bowlby, J. (1969). *Attachment and loss: Vol 1. Attachment.* New York: Basic Books.

Brammer, G. L., Raleigh, M. J., & McGuire, M. T. (1994). Neurotransmitters and social status. In L. Ellis (Ed.), *Social stratification and socioeconomic inequality: Vol. 2. Reproductive and interpersonal aspects of dominance and status* (pp. 75–91). Westport, CT: Praeger/Greenwood.

Buss, D. M. (1994). The strategies of human mating. *American Scientist, 82,* 238–249.

Buss, D. M. (1999). *Evolutionary psychology: The new science of the mind.* Boston: Allyn & Bacon.

Chapman, M. (Ed.). (1984). Intentional action as a paradigm for developmental psychology: A symposium. *Human Development, 27,* 113–144.

Charlesworth, W. R. (1996). Co-operation and competition: Contributions to an evolutionary and developmental model. *International Journal of Behavioral Development, 19,* 25–39.

Coie, J. D. (1996). Prevention of violence and antisocial behavior. In R. D. Peters & R. J. McMahon (Eds.), *Banff International Behavioral Sciences Series: Vol. 13. Preventing childhood disorders, substance abuse, and delinquency* (pp. 11–18). Thousand Oaks, CA: Sage.

Cosmides, L., & Tooby, J. (1995). From evolution to adaptations to behavior: Toward an integrated evolutionary psychology. In R. Wong (Ed.), *Biological perspectives on motivated activities* (pp. 11–74). Norwood, NJ: Ablex.

De Waal, F. (1982). *Chimpanzee politics.* Baltimore, MD: Johns Hopkins University Press.

Deci, E. L., & Ryan, R. F. (Eds.). (in press). *Handbook of self-determination research.* Rochester, NY: University of Rochester Press.

Draper, P., & Harpending, H. (1982). Father absence and reproductive strategy: An evolutionary perspective. *Journal of Anthropological Research, 38,* 255–273.

Erdley, C. A., & Asher, S. R. (1998). Linkages between children's beliefs about the legitimacy of aggression and their behavior. *Social Development, 7,* 321–339.

Frank, E., & Thase, M. E. (1999). Natural history and preventative treatment of recurrent mood disorders. *Annual Review of Medicine, 50,* 453–468.

Gregory, S. W., & Webster, S. (1996). A nonverbal signal in voices of interview partners effectively predicts communication accommodation and social status perceptions. *Journal of Personality and Social Psychology, 70,* 1231–1240.

Grob, A., Little, T. D., & Wanner, B. (1999). Control judgments across the lifespan. *International Journal of Behavioral Development, 23,* 833–854.

Hawley, P. H. (1999). The ontogenesis of social dominance: A strategy-based evolutionary perspective. *Developmental Review, 19,* 91–132.

Hawley, P. H. (2001). *Prosocial and coercive configurations of resource control: A case for the well-adapted Machiavellian.* Manuscript submitted for publication.

Hawley, P. H. (in press). Social dominance and prosocial and coercive strategies of resource control in preschoolers. *International Journal of Behavioral Development.*

Hawley, P. H., & Little, T. D. (1999). On winning some and losing some: A social relations approach to social dominance in toddlers. *Merrill–Palmer Quarterly, 45,* 185–214.

Hawley, P. H., Little, T. D., & Pasupathi, M. (in press). Winning friends and influencing peers: Strategies of peer influence in late childhood. *International Journal of Behavioral Development.*

Hogan, R., Curphy, G. J., & Hogan, J. (1994). What we know about leadership: Effectiveness and personality. *American Psychologist. 49,* 493–504.

Hogan, R., & Hogan, J. (1991). Personality and status. In D. G. Gilbert & S. S. Connolly (Eds.), *Personality, social skills, and psychopathology* (pp. 137–154). New York: Plenum Press.

Hogan, R., Raskin, R., & Fazzini, D. (1990). The dark side of charisma. In E. K. Clark & M. B Clark (Eds.), *Measures of leadership* (pp. 343–354). West Orange, NJ: Leadership Library of America.

Kenny, D. A., & LaVoie, L. (1985). Separating individual and group effects. *Journal of Personality and Social Psychology, 48,* 339–348.

Kunzmann, U., Little, T. D., & Smith, J. (2000). Is age-related stability of subjective well-being a paradox?: Cross-sectional and longitudinal evidence from the Berlin Aging Study. *Psychology and Aging, 15,* 511–526.

Little, T. D. (1998). Sociocultural influences on the development of children's action-control beliefs. In J. Heckhausen & C. S. Dweck (Eds.), *Motivation and self-regulation across the life span* (pp. 281–315). New York: Cambridge University Press.

Little, T. D. (in press). Agency in development. In R. Silbereisen & W. H. Hartup (Eds.), *Expert views on human development.* East Sussex, England: Psychology Press.

Little, T. D., Hawley, P. H., Henrich, C. C., & Marsland, K. (in press). Three views of the agentic self: A developmental synthesis. In E. L Deci & R. M. Ryan (Eds.), *Handbook of self-determination research* (pp. 000–000). Rochester, NY: University of Rochester Press.

Little, T. D., & Lopez, D. F. (1997). Regularities in the development of children's causality beliefs about school performance across six sociocultural contexts. *Developmental Psychology, 33,* 165–175.

Little, T. D., Lopez, D. F., & Wanner, B. (2001). Children's action-control behaviors (coping): A longitudinal validation of the behavioral inventory of strategic control. *Anxiety, Stress, and Coping, 14,* 315–336.

Little, T. D., Oettingen, G., Stetsenko, A., & Baltes, P. B. (1995). Children's action-control beliefs and school performance: How do American children compare with German and Russian children? *Journal of Personality and Social Psychology, 69,* 686–700.

Lorenz, K. (1966). *On aggression.* New York: Harcourt, Brace, & World.

Maynard Smith, J. (1974). The theory of games and the evolution of animal conflict. *Journal of Theoretical Biology, 47,* 202–221.

McGuire, M. T., Raleigh, M. J., & Brammer, G. L. (1984). Adaptation, selection, and benefit–cost balances: Implications of behavioral–physiological studies of social dominance in male vervet monkeys. *Ethology and Sociobiology, 5,* 269–277.

Mealey, L. (1995). The sociobiology of sociopathy: An integrated evolutionary model. *Behavioral and Brain Sciences, 18,* 523–599.

Nesse, R. M., & Lloyd, A. T. (1992). The evolution of psychodynamic mechanisms. In J. Barkow, L. Cosmides, & J. Tooby (Eds.), *The adapted mind: Evolutionary psychology and the generation of culture* (pp. 601–624). New York: Oxford University Press.

Pinker, S. (1997). *How the mind works.* New York: Norton.

Plomin, R., & Caspi, A. (1999). Behavioral genetics and personality. In L.A. Pervin & O.P. John (Eds.), *Handbook of personality: Theory and research* (2nd ed., pp. 251–276). New York: Guilford Press.

Rubin, K. H., & Rose-Krasnor, L. (1992). Interpersonal problem solving. In V. B. V. Hassett & M. Hersen (Eds.), *Handbook of social development* (pp. 283–323). New York: Plenum Press.

Ryan, R. M. (1993). Agency and organization: Intrinsic motivation, autonomy, and the self in psychological development. In J. E. Jacobs (Ed.), *Nebraska symposium on motivation: Vol. 40. Developmental perspectives on motivation* (pp. 1–56). Lincoln: University of Nebraska Press.

Sapolsky, R. M. (1999). The physiology and pathophysiology of unhappiness. In D. Kahneman & E. Diener (Eds.), *Well-being: The foundations of hedonic psychology* (pp. 453–469). New York: Russell Sage Foundation.

Sapolsky, R. M., Alberts, S. C., & Altmann, J. (1997). Hypercortisolism associated with social subordinance or social isolation among wild baboons. *Archives of General Psychiatry, 54,* 1137–1143.

Shahar, G., Grob, A., & Little, T. D. (2001). *Control judgments and well-being across the life span.* Manuscript submitted for publication.

Sroufe, A. L. (1992). Relationships, self, and individual adaptation. In A. J. Sameroff & R.N. Emde (Eds.), *Relationship disturbances in early childhood: A developmental approach* (pp. 70–94). New York: Basic Books.

Strayer, F. F., & Strayer, J. (1976). An ethological analysis of social agonism and dominance relations among preschool children. *Child Development, 47,* 980–989.

Sulloway, F. (1996). *Born to rebel.* New York: Pantheon.

Tooby, J., & Cosmides, L. (1990). On the universality of human nature and the uniqueness of the individual: The role of genetics and adaptation. *Journal of Personality, 58,* 17–68.

Trivers, R. L. (1971). The evolution of reciprocal altruism. *Quarterly Review of Biology, 46,* 35–57.

Trivers, R. (1985). *Social evolution.* Menlo Park, CA: Cummings.

White, R. W. (1959). Motivation reconsidered: The concept of competence. *Psychological Review, 66,* 297–333.

Williams, G. C. (1966). *Adaptation and natural selection: A critique of some current evolutionary thought.* Princeton, NJ: Princeton University Press.

CHAPTER 8

Birth Cohort, Social Change, and Personality

The Interplay of Dysphoria and Individualism in the 20th Century

JEAN M. TWENGE

Every generation is a secret society and has incommunicable enthusiasms, tastes, and interests which are a mystery both to its predecessors and to posterity.

—JOHN JAY CHAPMAN

Men resemble the times more than they resemble their fathers.

—ARAB PROVERB

Imagine that you are a young person living in the United States in 1930. If you were suddenly transported to the year 2002, which things would be most strikingly different? You might notice that people lock their doors and are afraid that their children will be shot at school. Cities are filled with people who live alone and feel emotionally disconnected from other human beings. Individuals of every race and ethnicity work, eat, and converse together. Women, even mothers with small children, work outside the home. People define their identities individually, rather than as parts of families or workplaces, and Americans are unafraid to brag about themselves, pursue their own self-fulfillment, or divorce and remarry in search of happiness.

Put simply, a visitor from 1930s America would find that the year 2002 was essentially another culture. As a result, our visitor would notice that, on average, the residents of the year 2002 had different levels of personality traits compared with the average citizen of 1930. In other words, there were generational differences (or birth cohort differences) in personality. As a general rule, cultures can have considerable effects on personality, emotion, and cognitions (e.g., Choi, Nisbett, & Norenzayan, 1999; Heine & Lehman, 1997; Nisbett & Cohen, 1996; Suh, Diener, Oishi, & Triandis, 1998). With birth cohort differences, the cause is time period rather than region, but the principle is the same. These differences are not genetic, and they are (for the most part) not a result of variations in individual family environment. Instead, they stem from changes in the larger sociocultural environment: the social trends and *Zeitgeists* of particular times. The history of the 20th century is characterized by shifts in two primary areas: dysphoria and individualism. After exploring the theoretical and methodological background relevant to birth cohort differences, this chapter focuses on the empirical evidence for the personality changes produced by these two interlocking trends.

REASONS TO CONSIDER BIRTH COHORT CHANGE

Genetic and Environmental Influences on Personality

Most studies assume that genetics and individual family environment represent the only two influences on personality traits. In their study of identical twins reared apart, Bergeman, Plomin, McClearn, Pedersen, and Friberg (1988) state that "in the absence of selective placement, any similarity" between the twins "is due to genetic influences" (p. 400). Loehlin (1989) makes a similar statement. However, these authors seem to assume that the environment stops at the door of the family home. As many theorists and researchers have argued, the larger sociocultural environment can have a substantial effect on personality and development (e.g., Caspi, 1987; Elder, 1974, 1981a; Gergen, 1973; Nesselroade & Baltes, 1974; Ryder, 1965; Schaie, 1965; Stewart & Healy, 1989; Woodruff & Birren, 1972). Examining "nonshared" environment (Plomin & Daniels, 1987) does not solve this problem, because twins (identical or fraternal) are necessarily the same birth cohort; thus the larger sociocultural environment is still "shared" environment (but "shared" environment outside of the family). Thus birth cohort might be a nongenetic explanation for the similarity between identical twins raised apart.

Considering birth cohort might add to our understanding of shared environmental effects, especially as most studies have found that family environment is only a weak influence on personality traits that explains less than 10% of the variance (e.g., Bergeman et al.,1988; Langinvaionio, Kaprio, Koskenvuo, & Lonngvist, 1984; Loehlin, 1992; Rowe, 1990;

Shields, 1962). These results have led prominent authors to assert that personality traits are genetic, endogenous structures uninfluenced by the environment (e.g., McCrae et al., 2000). Research on birth cohort differences helps answer the challenge posed by Matthews and Deary (1998) who wrote: "with so much good evidence for broad heritability effects, the onus is on environmentalists to make clear hypotheses about the effects of specific environmental factors on personality and test them" (p. 120).

Overestimation of Heritability

The fact that twins share a birth cohort also means that these studies have likely overestimated the heritability estimates for personality traits. Almost all of the studies examining genetic and environmental effects on personality have included samples of only one birth cohort (or samples very close in birth cohort). If more cohorts were included, then the variance in personality would likely increase. If genetics explains a finite amount of personality, a study with more cohorts would shrink the percentage of the variance pie explained by genetics. For example, assume that genetics explains about 40% of a pie of variance with people from only one birth cohort. If more birth cohorts are included and the variance increases, the percentage of this larger pie that is explained by genetics will decrease below 40%.

Dickens and Flynn (2001) also address the possible exaggeration of heritability estimates, using the specific example of intelligence. Intelligence seems to be highly heritable, but IQ scores have increased substantially in recent birth cohorts (Flynn, 1987). Dickens and Flynn (2001) argue that genetics and environment may be correlated, producing a multiplier effect such that environmental influences are obscured. In addition, influences of the larger cultural environment may produce a social multiplier effect on IQ such that small environmental shifts may multiply into larger environmental changes that affect IQ. A similar argument could easily be made for personality traits. For example, a rise in the crime rate multiplies into numerous environmental influences as more people are victimized, the media covers the rise in crime, people talk about crime more, and individuals take steps to protect themselves. These shifts could lead to changes in anxiety, neuroticism, and possibly other personality traits.

A Contradiction: Cross-Sectional versus Longitudinal Studies of Personality Traits

Acknowledging birth cohort differences would also resolve a striking paradox in personality research: Longitudinal studies have often found remarkable consistency in personality traits as people age (e.g., Conley,

1984; Costa & McCrae, 1988; Costa, McCrae, & Arenberg, 1980; Finn, 1986; Kelly, 1955), whereas cross-sectional studies purporting to measure age differences have often found large effects (e.g., Bendig, 1960; Costa et al., 1986; S. B. G. Eysenck & Eysenck, 1969; H. J. Eysenck & Eysenck, 1975; Gutman, 1966). Birth cohort can explain this: In a cross-sectional study, the individuals of different ages also belong to different birth cohorts (Baltes & Nesselroade, 1972; Buss, 1974; Nesselroade & Baltes, 1974; Schaie, 1965; Woodruff & Birren, 1972; see also Table 8.1). On the other hand, longitudinal studies usually follow one birth cohort as they age. Thus at least some of the conflict between the results of longitudinal and cross-sectional studies may be explained by birth cohort differences in personality traits. This contradiction suggests that birth cohort differences in personality may be widespread.

HOW DOES THE LARGER ENVIRONMENT PRODUCE BIRTH COHORT CHANGE?

As one of the first generational theorists, Karl Mannheim (1928/1952) introduced the concept of a "generation unit," or a group of individuals who experience the same major historical events while young. Many other historical and social circumstances also shape a generation, with social circumstances often directly influencing personality (Elder, 1981a). This occurs not just by living through a certain historical era but by experiencing it at a certain age; the same event or environment means different things to individuals of different ages (Mannheim, 1928/1952; Ryder, 1965; Stewart & Healy, 1989). Glen Elder presented the classic example of this in his study of the Great Depression; he found that men and women who experienced the Depression as children showed different outcomes from those who lived through it as adolescents (Elder, 1979, 1981a, 1981b). Childhood and adolescent experiences may be especially important in the formation of cohort effects in personality, as the "critical periods" for much personality and attitude development most likely lies at these ages (e.g., Bengtson, Furlong, & Laufer, 1974; Elder, 1974, 1981a,

TABLE 8.1. Developmental Methods

Method	Source of variation	Held constant
Cross-sectional	Age and cohort	Period
Longitudinal	Age and period	Cohort
Time lag	Cohort and period	Age

1981b; Lambert, 1972; Ryder, 1965; Stewart & Healy, 1989). This shaping of individuals at young ages ultimately leads to cultural change, as one generation succeeds another in a society (Bengtson et. al., 1974; Lambert, 1972).

Until recently, however, birth cohort effects were rarely examined. When they were, they were often treated as a nuisance rather than as an interesting psychological and sociological effect. Caspi (1987) stressed the role of history and cohort in personality development and noted how psychologists have often ignored these elements:

> People are exposed to a slice of historical experience in the process of moving across age-graded roles, and throughout history the social meaning of these roles vary accordingly. Unfortunately, historical variation in life experience remains more of a problematic issue than a research option and line of advance in personality research. . . . Psychologists are more concerned with generalizing specific findings across historical epochs than with incorporating specific historical conditions in the assessment of lives. Indeed, personality research is often carried out without a sense of history, without recognition that phenotypic expressions represent a point of articulation between historical, social and ontogenetic processes. History must enter the picture in problem formulation and model development to ensure a satisfactory analysis of lives. (p. 1211)

Thus birth cohort can have significant effects on personality and the life course and should be examined with interest rather than be considered error variance.

METHODS FOR ADDRESSING BIRTH COHORT EFFECTS

The best method for examining birth cohort effects is the time-lag method, an underutilized method in psychology. Time lag examines samples of the same age at different points in historical time (see Table 8.1). Same-age samples collected over different years allow the inference that any differences must be due to birth cohort or time period effects. In some cases, researchers have these data themselves, gathered over the course of a long career (e.g., Dyer, 1987; Spence & Hahn, 1997). Performing a meta-analysis, however, is usually the best way to perform a time-lag analysis, because many samples of the same age group (e.g., college students) have been collected over the years from many sources. In my research, I have modified meta-analysis in this way, gathering reports of mean scores on various measures over time. I have often called this method "cross-temporal meta-analysis" due to its utility for studying change over time (see, e.g., Twenge, 2000; the method was first used in Twenge, 1997). In a cross-temporal meta-analysis, the main statistic is the correlation between the mean scores and the year in which the data were collected. A significant positive correlation means that a trait has increased over time, whereas a significant negative correlation means that a trait has decreased over time. The percentage of variance explained by birth cohort can be determined using the regression equation, calculating the difference between the scores at the earliest and latest year and using the average standard deviation reported for individual samples. (This is more accurate than estimating the variance from the correlation. Because the data points come from samples instead of individuals, the correlations are stronger than they would be if all individuals from the samples were included. Using the regression equation avoids committing this "ecological fallacy" for the variance estimate). Means on measures can also be matched with social indicators (e.g., the crime rate, the divorce rate) from the corresponding years to determine how the trait covaries with aspects of the social environment.

EMPIRICAL EVIDENCE FOR BIRTH COHORT EFFECTS

There is empirical evidence for birth cohort effects in many areas of personality, attitudes, behavior, and life choices. Here I review the evidence for two domains: dysphoria (including anxiety/neuroticism and depression) and individualism and views of the self (individualism, self-esteem, extraversion, and assertiveness). These two trends are most likely linked (e.g., Seligman, 1988, 1990). The empirical evidence for birth cohort effects in both areas is summarized in Table 8.2.

Changes in Dysphoria

Depression

The empirical evidence suggests that depression is on the rise (Klerman & Weissman, 1989; Lewinsohn, Rohde, Seeley, & Fischer, 1993; Robins, Helzer, & Weissman, 1984; for reviews, see Seligman, 1988, 1990). The change is so striking that some authors have referred to the 20th century as an "age of melancholy" (Hagnell, Lanke, Rorsman, & Ojesjo, 1982; Klerman, 1978). The Robins et al. (1984) study found that a cohort born during the 1940s was 5 to 10 times more likely to experience depression than a cohort born during the 1910s. Overall, about 9% of the 1940s cohort reported having an incident of major depression sometime in their lifetime. About 5% of a cohort born in the 1960s has reported a major

TABLE 8.2. Summary of Birth Cohort Differences in Personality Traits and Self-Conceptions

Trait	Population	Change	Reference(s)
Dysphoria			
Depression	General population, relatives of depressed individuals	Up since 1940s	Klerman & Weissman (1989); Lewinsohn, Rohde, Seeley, & Fischer (1993); Robins et al. (1984)
Neuroticism/anxiety	College students and schoolchildren	Up since early 1950s	Twenge (2000)
Individualism			
Individualism	Archival data, college students	Up since medieval times, but especially since late 1960s	Baumeister (1987); Gough (1991); Remley (1988)
Self-esteem	College students	Up since late 1960s	Twenge & Campbell (2001)
Extraversion	College students	Up since late 1960s	Twenge (2001a)
Assertiveness	College women and high school girls	Follows social status of women: Up 1930–1945, down 1946–1967, up 1968–1993	Twenge (2001b)

depressive incident to date. This statistic is especially alarming because the 1960s cohort was aged only 18 to 24 years at the time and thus had not yet passed through the riskiest times for depression. Lewinsohn et al. (1993) found that cohorts born in the 1970s also experienced high levels of depression. Although these studies were based on retrospective accounts, they all point in the direction of increasing dysphoria. Another study found that 26% of survey respondents in 1996 said they were headed for a nervous breakdown, compared with 19% in 1957 (Swindle, Heller, Pescosolido, & Kikuzawa, 2000).

Why is depression more common in recent birth cohorts? Klerman and Weissman (1989) suggest a number of possibilities, including decreases in social connections (as evidenced, for example, by increasing geographic mobility and the higher divorce rate). These might also be described as increasing "social anomie," a term coined by Durkheim (1897/1951) to describe social isolation and disconnection. As Seligman (1988, 1990) argues, the forces of modernization must explain much of the rise in depression, because more traditional cultures have not experienced the same cohort effect for depression. For example, the rate of depression for the old-order Amish in Pennsylvania is about one fifth to one tenth the rate of the general U. S. population (Egeland & Hostetter, 1983; Egeland, Hostetter, & Eshleman, 1983; Seligman, 1988, 1990). The Amish are a farming culture rooted in the customs of the 19th century; their communities are close-knit. As mainstream American culture has grown more urbanized and increased in social isolation and anomie, rates of depression have skyrocketed.

Anxiety

Just as higher depression rates have led to the label "the age of melancholy," other authors have labeled the 20th century "the age of anxiety" (e.g., Spielberger & Rickman, 1990, p. 69). Have people actually grown more anxious, or does hindsight bias lead us to believe that people were less anxious in the past? Depression and anxiety are linked (e.g., Tanaka-Matsumi & Kameoka, 1986), so it seems likely that anxiety would increase as well. However, the depression studies were based on retrospective accounts, which are necessarily somewhat unreliable (Lewinsohn et al., 1993), and some researchers argue that anxiety and depression arise from different sources (e.g., Barlow, 1988; Tellegen, 1985).

I conducted a meta-analysis of college students and schoolchildren who had responded to anxiety inventories between the 1950s and the 1990s (Twenge, 2000). This technique avoids the dangers inherent in retrospective accounts (such as those used in the depression studies) because respondents completed the anxiety measures in reference to their current state. The meta-analysis represented 170 samples of college students (40,192 individuals) and 99 samples of children aged 9 to 17 (12,056 individuals).

The results for both groups were the same: Mean scores on measures of anxiety increased a standard deviation from the 1950s to the 1990s. The increase was steady and linear. College students' scores increased on all four measures examined (the Taylor Manifest Anxiety Inventory, the Eysenck Personality Inventory Neuroticism scale, the Eysenck Personality Questionnaire Neuroticism scale, and the State–Trait Anxiety Inventory). Children's scores increased on the Children's Manifest Anxiety Scale. The increase was so large that the average score for children in the 1980s was higher than that reported for a sample of child psychiatric patients from the late 1950s (Levitt, 1959). For both samples, the change of one standard deviation means that the average respondent from the 1980s or 1990s would outscore all but 16% of respondents from the 1950s. It also means that birth cohort accounts for about 20% of the variance in anxiety/neuroticism as a personality trait (because this estimate was calculated using means and sample standard deviations instead of the correlation, it avoids committing the "ecological fallacy.") This is considerably more than the 5% to 10% usually explained by individual family environment.

If anxiety has increased, what are the causes? Why is modern life anxiety producing? First, dangers in the environment have increased. Crime rates are much higher than in the 1950s. During much of the period of the 1950s to the 1990s, children and adults worried that nuclear war might destroy the entire population at any time. AIDS also remains a threat to the health of adolescents and adults (as documented more thoroughly in Twenge, 2000, these environmental factors have been linked to anxiety on the individual level as well). In many ways, the world today seems to be a more dangerous place. Given that anxiety is basically a fear reaction, this may help explain the rise in this trait. When I matched anxiety scores with statistics on crime rates, worry about nuclear war, and AIDS cases, there was a consistent, positive relationship; anxiety scores were high when these environmental dangers were also high. As correlations, these analyses cannot prove causation, but they do show which environmental influences occur at the same time as higher or lower anxiety scores.

In addition, modern life is more individualistic and less socially connected than it once was; we experience more social anomie (Durkheim, 1897/1951). People marry later and get divorced more often. We have fewer siblings and fewer children of our own. Cross-country moves are common. Memberships in social and community groups are at historic lows, especially compared with the 1950s and 1960s (Putnam, 2000). People do not even visit friends as much as they once did. Increasingly, high school students disagree with the statement that "Most people can be trusted" and agree that "You can't be too careful with people" (Fukuyama, 1999; Smith, 1997). Social disconnection may be a crucial cause of anxiety and depression (Cohen & Wills, 1985; Baumeister & Leary, 1995; Baumeister & Tice, 1990). These statistics were also correlated with anxiety; anxiety was also high at times in which social connections were low (the divorce rate was high, more people lived alone, the birth rate was low, and people reported not trusting others). On the other hand, economic indicators (unemployment, the percentage of children in poverty) were not correlated with anxiety when matched historically.

Summary

Levels of dysphoria, including anxiety and depression, have increased in recent decades. These changes are linear and considerable. Evidence suggests that these changes are linked with historical trends toward increasing environmental threat and decreasing social connectedness. Birth cohort explains 20% of the variance in anxiety/neuroticism, and rates of depression have increased five- to tenfold between cohorts born early in the century and those born after 1945.

Changes in Views of the Self: Individualism, Self-Esteem, Extraversion, and Women's Assertiveness

Individualism

By all indications, Americans are becoming more individualistic. As Baumeister (1987) documented, the general trend in Western society has been toward a more self-focused conception of the individual. During medieval times, Western society was more collectivist; people defined themselves in terms of their connections to their families and communities. Everyone knew their place and stayed within it. Sons adopted the profession of their fathers (or the profession their fathers apprenticed them to). Marriages were arranged. Over the next few centuries, however, the Western self became more defined as an individual entity. Free choice and the preferences of the individual became more important.

This trend accelerated during the late 1960s and early 1970s. As Frum (2000) noted, the much reviled decade of the 1970s produced fundamental changes in American culture that are now embedded in our social ethos. Whereas duty to country and social norms once ruled American life, rampant individualism soon became the rule. "Doing your own thing" was increasingly fashionable. Seligman (1988) wrote: "the site of action shifted from outside the self to within the self" (p. 52). The emergence of this "California self" was accompanied by increasing distrust of larger social institutions and societal traditions in general. The result, Seligman argued, is an "individualism without commitment to the common good" (p. 55), not coincidentally also a formula for widespread depression.

Many of the breakdowns of social connections discussed in reference to anxiety have their root in this 1970s individualism: the higher divorce rate, the lower birth rate, and the decreasing popularity of formal social and community groups. The popular culture of the time promoted self-fulfillment, self-love, and "being your own best friend" (Ehrenreich & English, 1978). Pollsters noted that "the rage for self-fulfillment" had spread everywhere (Yankelovich, 1981, p. 3). It was no coincidence that the young people of the time were soon slapped with the label "the 'Me' Generation." Empirical evidence from psychology also suggests that the individualistic philosophy was growing in popularity. One study examined the characteristics valued by parents. Whereas American parents in the postwar era valued obedience in their children, by the 1970s and 1980s they placed more importance on independence and good judgment (Remley, 1988). Harrison Gough (1991, cited in Roberts & Helson, 1997) found that scores on an individualism measure (derived from the California Psychological Inventory) increased markedly between the 1950s and the 1980s.

Self-Esteem

This self-focus and individualism also had consequences for self-esteem: Increasingly, proclaiming that you loved, cherished, and valued yourself was no longer an immodest proposition (Jones, 1980; Rosen, 1998; Swann, 1996). Not only did the general societal ethos promote the self, but also a "self-esteem movement" (an offshoot of the "human potential" and "self-growth" movements) gained prevalence, arguing that "the basis for everything we do is self-esteem" (MacDonald, 1986, p. 27, as cited in Seligman, 1995). In general, self-esteem became an almost ubiquitous topic in the academic literature, as well as in the popular media (see Twenge & Campbell, 2001, for a discussion).

Working with my colleague Keith Campbell, I performed a metaanalysis on college students' scores on the Rosenberg Self-Esteem Scale (RSE) between 1968 and 1994. We found that college students' self-esteem scores increased about two thirds of a standard deviation over this 26-year period (Twenge & Campbell, 2001). Thus 1990s college undergraduates scored considerably higher in self-esteem than had their late-1960s counterparts. It is possible that today's undergraduates actually do feel better about themselves compared with the college students of the 1960s. It could also be that college students now speak the language of self-esteem and understand that one is supposed to possess copious amounts of this supposedly precious substance. Given the strong and documented shift toward individualism in the culture, however, it is likely that at least some of the change results from this increasing focus on the self. After all, if one is a functioning, happy human being, focusing on the self is more likely to lead to self-love than self-hate (e.g., Taylor & Brown, 1988).

Extraversion

Given this shift toward individualism, one might think that people also became more introverted. After all, the classic image of the introvert is someone who gets by alone and focuses inward. However, a plausible argument for increasing extraversion can also be made. The ethos of individualism did not change people's fundamental need to feel connected to each other (Baumeister & Leary, 1995). Thus in some ways increasing individualism led people to be more social and outgoing because, quite simply, they had to be. In earlier eras of close-knit families and small communities, people knew each other all of their lives. Even if they lived in a city, they knew their neighbors. They met the parents of their children's schoolmates in PTA or Kiwanis clubs. They often lived in one city and worked at one job all of their lives.

The cult of individualism began to change all of this. Families became more fractured. Neighborhood clubs and social groups dropped out of favor (Putnam, 2000). People moved more and changed jobs more often. Children interacted with their peers in day care centers and thus learned social skills at earlier ages. In general, the economy shifted from industry to service, and thus from jobs where you interacted only with your coworkers to jobs where you dealt with numerous, ever-changing customers every day. (It remains to be seen how recent trends in electronic communication, in which no face-to-face interaction occurs, will affect this environment). In sum, the societal trend has been toward meeting new people more often and toward more fluid and changeable relationships. In this world, being extraverted is no longer a quirk of genetics; it is a virtual requirement (e.g., Whyte, 1956). When you are expected to leave your birth family at a young age and create an entirely new support system of your own, being outgoing becomes essential. Extraversion, in its classic form, is not simply about liking to be with people; it is about liking to be with many people (such as at a party) and being comfortable meeting new people. In modern society, both family and career depend, at least in part, on being extraverted.

The available evidence suggests that extraversion began to increase in American college students beginning in the late 1960s. In a recent paper (Twenge, 2001a), I found that American undergraduates scored 0.79 to 0.97 standard deviations higher on extraversion scales in 1993 than in 1966 (the measures were the Extraversion scales of the Eysenck Personality Inventory and the Eysenck Personality Questionnaire). I trace these changes to several sources, including the move toward a service economy, day care, and the encouragement of free expression. Apparently the modern person needs a higher level of extraversion to successfully relate to a growing and impersonal collection of other individuals in the modern urban landscape.

Assertiveness

One trait closely linked with individualism is assertiveness, which is often defined as standing up for one's personal rights (Wilson & Gallois, 1993).

Assertiveness is closely linked with status and male gender roles (Eagly, 1983; Miller, 1986; Slater, 1970). For example, several studies have demonstrated that employed women have higher assertiveness levels than those not in the paid labor force (e.g., Clarey & Sanford, 1982; Wertheim, Widom, & Wortzel, 1978). The striking changes in women's status and roles over the century suggest that women's assertiveness levels might show substantial birth cohort differences. According to Eagly's (1987) social role theory, sex differences in personality traits arise because men and women are trained for different roles in life and then move on to perform those roles. Thus, when women's roles change, so should their personalities. This appears to be an entrenched folk belief as well (Diekman & Eagly, 2000).

The changes in women's status over the 20th century have been curvilinear rather than linear. The basic pattern shows an increase in women's status prior to and including World War II, a decrease in status postwar, and an increase in status after the late 1960s. For example, women's age at first marriage was actually higher in 1940 (21.5) than in 1960 (20.3); it rose slowly after the early 1960s. The median did not reach 21.5 again until 1979 (thus women married younger in 1978 than in 1940). College degrees also followed this pattern: in 1920, 34% of college degrees went to women; 40% in 1930; 41% in 1940; 32% in 1952; and 35% in 1960. The percentage of college degrees awarded to women did not reach the 1940 statistic of 41% again until 1965. Thus a smaller percentage of college degrees were awarded to women during the 1950s and early 1960s than during the 1930s. By the early 1990s, women earned the majority of college degrees (56% in 1997). This pattern also appears in the percentage of doctorates granted to women, which was 15% in 1930 but dropped to 9% by 1955. It did not reach the 1930 figure of 15% again until 1972 (thus women earned a higher percentage of doctorates in 1930 than they did in 1970). In 1993, women earned about 37% of doctorates (41% in 1997), demonstrating the rapid pace of change over 20 years.

Using the cross-temporal meta-analysis method, I found that college women's assertiveness followed the same pattern as their status and roles: It increased between the 1930s and World War II, decreased postwar, and increased again after the late 1960s (Twenge, 2001b). Within each era, the shifts in assertiveness averaged 0.44 standard deviations; overall, birth cohort explained about 14% of the variance in women's assertiveness. Women's assertiveness scores were correlated with historical statistics matched for each year, including median age at first marriage, labor force participation, and educational attainment. In contrast, college men's scores on assertiveness did not show significant birth cohort changes. During the most recent time period included in the study, sex differences in assertiveness decreased from a male advantage of 0.40 standard deviations in 1968 to no difference ($d = -.07$) in 1993. Thus assertiveness, once a solid sex difference favoring men, is now a personality trait with no discernible differences between men and women. Thus, as women's roles have changed, their personalities have reflected the traits needed for these new roles (Eagly, 1987).

Summary

There has been a strong trend toward individualism in American culture, particularly since the 1970s. Perhaps as a result, college students reported increasing levels of self-esteem from the late 1960s to the early 1990s. Levels of extraversion also rose, as being outgoing became increasingly necessary in the workplace and in social life. The substantial changes in women's roles from one era to the next produced changes in women's assertiveness.

IMPLICATIONS FOR PERSONALITY RESEARCH AND THEORY

Influences on Personality Traits

What do these results mean for personality psychology as a field? First, they demonstrate that the environment can have a substantial effect on personality traits, including those in the Big Five. These results are directly contrary to theories that assert that "personality traits are endogenous dispositions, influenced not at all by the environment" (McCrae et al., 2000, p. 175). These authors specifically exclude environmental influences from the figure that illustrates their model of personality traits and go on to say that "personality traits are more or less immune to environmental influences" (p. 175; see also McCrae & Costa, 1996, 1999). The strong effects of the sociocultural environment, as outlined in this chapter, suggest that such statements are untrue.

In general, birth cohort (as a proxy for the larger social environment) should be considered as an influence on personality. The larger social environment should be included among environmental influences (for twin studies, it is a shared environmental influence beyond the family). This seems especially important considering the small amount of variance explained by individual family environment in most studies (e.g., Bergeman et al.,1988; Langinvaionio et al., 1984; Loehlin, 1992; Rowe, 1990; Shields, 1962).

Of course, some changes in the larger social environment lead to changes in the individual family environment. The high divorce rate, for example, is a social trend that affects individual families. Thus at least some birth cohort changes are mediated through the individual family. The larger environment enters people's worlds in many other ways, however, often through multiplicative effects similar to those observed for IQ (Dickens & Flynn, 2001). A child who lives in a stable family in a safe neighborhood might still worry about divorce and crime because he sees his friends' parents divorcing and he sees victims of crime on the news. As noted previously, changes in the divorce and crime rates lead to multiple changes in the environment, influencing media coverage, conversations between people, and protective behaviors. This "social multiplier" phenomenon may help explain why birth cohort differences are so large compared with the effects of the individual family environment.

Heritability Estimates

The existence of strong birth cohort effects suggests that hertiability estimates for personality traits are inflated. As noted earlier, a twin study that included individuals from a wider range of birth cohorts would see the overall variance in personality increase (in the case of anxiety/ neuroticism, it would increase by 20%). The absolute area of variance explained by genetics would not change, so a pie with increased variance would shrink the percentage of variance explained by genetics. For example, studies including people from only one birth cohort have found that genetics explains about 40% of the variance in anxiety. If many birth cohorts were included and 20% of variance were added, then genetics would explain only 33% of the variance instead (40 divided by 120).

Reliance on Self-Report

Many of the studies of birth cohort involve self-reports of personality traits. Thus, change over time on the scales could reflect either true shifts in personality traits or the respondents' willingness to describe themselves in different terms, perhaps due to changes in social desirability (e.g., Edwards, 1957). This limitation cannot be completely overcome; it is difficult to study personality without relying on self-report (especially in a meta-analysis, which must gather the available data). This concern can also be addressed in several ways. First, it is unlikely that any large discrepancy between self-reported and actual personality would remain that way for long; the experienced self will likely change to meet the expressed self (Tice, 1994). It is also difficult to believe that the social environment could have changed so radically between the 1930s and 1990s without having any effect on personality traits. Last, both explanations suggest that social change has occurred. For example, it could be that women actually are more assertive now or that they are more willing to describe themselves as assertive (or a combination of both). In their own ways, both are personality changes.

The Importance of the Childhood Environment

In several of the studies presented, the influence of the larger environment was strongest during childhood. For example, in exploring changes in women's assertiveness, I found (2001b) that college women's assertiveness scores were most highly correlated with indicators of women's status from 10 years before (when the college-aged women were children). Apparently, the behavior of adult women created an environment and an expectation for female behavior that affected the development of girls' personalities. I found similar results for anxiety (Twenge, 2000); environmental dangers and social connections during the childhood years were the best predictors of anxiety at college age.

These results have several implications. First, they suggest that the environment is causing personality change, rather than vice versa, because the environmental changes precede the personality changes (e.g., Ryder, 1965). This finding complements the results of many personality researchers, who find stability in personality traits after late adolescence (e.g., Conley, 1984; Costa & McCrae, 1988; Costa et al., 1980; Finn, 1986; Kelly, 1955). It is also consistent with the views of researchers who argue that childhood is the critical time for personality development (e.g., Bengtson et al., 1974; Elder, 1974, 1981a, 1981b; Lambert, 1972; Ryder, 1965; Stewart & Healy, 1989). Personality is by far the most malleable during childhood and remains relatively stable after that time.

The second implication is the importance of the larger social environment for children's development. One might have assumed that children would be affected mainly by family influences, whereas adults would be affected by broader social trends. However, these results suggest the opposite: that childhood is the time of the greatest societal influence. Children are not isolated within their families and communities, but instead readily absorb the influences of the world around them. Theories of personality development may benefit by incorporating some understanding that children live in the society as a whole rather than in a narrow, circumscribed world.

The Interplay of Social Forces

In presenting the empirical data on birth cohort change, I grouped the studies into sections on dysphoria and individualism. The history of the past five decades clearly suggests a rise in dysphoria, as well as a rise in individualism. These two trends are a trade-off: Put simply, freedom can lead to depression (e.g., Seligman, 1988, 1990). For one thing, self-determination is anxiety producing: Your fate, presumably, lies solely in your own hands. These choices are not easy to make, and once they are made there is no one else to blame if you are a failure (Schwartz, 2000). Your self must carry the weight of responsibility for all aspects of your life. No wonder we have higher self-esteem—we need a foundation of concrete and steel to hold the weight of our destinies. All too often, however, the weight is too great to bear, and we become anxious and depressed. This is not entirely surprising: People who make internal attributions for failure are more likely to be depressed (Abramson, Seligman, & Teasdale, 1978; Seligman, 1990).

In addition, being an individual can be a lonely enterprise—you must move away from your family, find a mate on your own, and perhaps deal with the consequences when your mate exercises the individualistic prerogative to dump you for someone better. This is also an obvious formula for depression (e.g., Baumeister & Leary, 1995); for example, unmarried people show higher rates of mental disorders than married people (e.g., Williams, Takeuchi, & Adair, 1992). Our greater autonomy may lead to increased challenges and excitement, but it also leads to greater isolation from others, more threats to our bodies and minds, and thus higher levels of dysphoria. The psychological history of the past few decades shows that the completely autonomous and fulfilled individual, held up as the ideal by the 1970s human potential movement, is probably a myth.

The Cycle of Change

Many questions about the environment and individual personality are still unanswered, however. If social change is to occur, there must be an interplay between environment and personality. The influence cannot be completely one-way, or societies would never change. This seeming paradox is illustrated by the example of women's assertiveness. Women's status apparently creates an environment that is internalized by the younger generation, producing the "appropriate" personality (assertive, nonassertive, or somewhere in between). This creates a self-perpetuating cycle: Women have lower status, and girls acquire personalities typical of people with lower status. When women move into higher status roles, girls grow up to be more assertive.

But how did women move into these higher status roles in the first place? How social change occurs at this macroscopic level is an open question. If we absorb the messages of the larger culture, how did the baby boomer women who were children in the conservative 1950s begin the radical social change in women's roles during the late 1960s and early 1970s? These are fascinating yet perplexing questions, and we currently lack a coherent model of how social change actually occurs at the societal level (although there has been some work; see, e.g., Nowak & Vallacher, 1998, Chapter 8). This is an area that requires more research and thinking. What is clear, however, is that personality can be shaped by broad cultural forces, in addition to genetic endowments and individual family experiences.

REFERENCES

Abramson, L. Y., Seligman, M. E. P., & Teasdale, J. (1978). Learned helplessness in humans: Critique and reformulation. *Journal of Abnormal Psychology, 87,* 49–59.

Baltes, P. B., & Nesselroade, J. R. (1972). Cultural change and adolescent personality development. *Developmental Psychology, 7,* 244–256.

Barlow, D. H. (1988). *Anxiety and its disorders: The nature and treatment of anxiety and panic.* New York: Guilford Press.

Baumeister, R. F. (1987). How the self became a problem: A psychological review of historical research. *Journal of Personality and Social Psychology, 52,* 163–176.

Baumeister, R. F., & Leary, M. R. (1995). The need to belong: Desire for interpersonal attachments as a fundamental human motivation. *Psychological Bulletin, 117,* 497–529.

Baumeister, R. F., & Tice, D. M. (1990). Anxiety and social exclusion. *Journal of Social and Clinical Psychology, 9,* 165–195.

Bendig, A. W. (1960). Age differences in the interscale factor structure of the Guilford-Zimmerman Temperament Survey. *Journal of Consulting Psychology, 24,* 134–138.

Bengtson, V. L., Furlong, M. J., & Laufer, R. S. (1974). Time, aging, and the continuity of social structure: Themes and issues in generational analysis. *Journal of Social Issues, 30,* 1–30.

Bergeman, C. S., Plomin, R., McClearn, G. E., Pedersen, N. L., & Friberg, L. T. (1988). Genotype-environment interaction in personality development: Identical twins reared apart. *Psychology and Aging, 3,* 399–406.

Buss, A. R. (1974). Generational analysis: Description, explanation, and theory. *Journal of Social Issues, 30,* 55–71.

Caspi, A. (1987). Personality in the life course. *Journal of Personality and Social Psychology, 53,* 1203–1213.

Choi, I., Nisbett, R. E., & Norenzayan, A. (1999). Causal attribution across cultures: Variation and universality. *Psychological Bulletin, 125,* 47–63.

Clarey, J. H., & Sanford, A. (1982). Female career preference and androgyny. *Vocational Guidance Quarterly, 30,* 258–264.

Cohen, S., & Wills, T. A. (1985). Stress, social support, and the buffering hypothesis. *Psychological Bulletin, 98,* 310–357.

Conley, J. J. (1984). The hierarchy of consistency: A review and model of longitudinal findings in adult individual differences in intelligence, personality and self-opinion. *Personality and Individual Differences, 5,* 11–26.

Costa, P. T., & McCrae, R. R. (1988). Personality in adulthood: A six-year longitudinal study of self-reports and spouse ratings on the NEO Personality Inventory. *Journal of Personality and Social Psychology, 54,* 853–863.

Costa, P. T., McCrae, R. R., & Arenberg, P. (1980). Enduring dispositions in adult males. *Journal of Personality and Social Psychology, 38,* 793–800.

Costa, P. T., McCrae, R. R., Zonderman, A. B., Barbano, H. E., Lebowitz, B., & Larson, D. M. (1986). Cross-sectional studies of personality in a national sample: 2. Stability in neuroticism, extraversion, and openness. *Psychology and Aging, 1,* 144–149.

Dickens, W. T., & Flynn, J. R. (2001). Heritability estimates versus large environmental effects: The IQ paradox resolved. *Psychological Review, 108,* 346–369.

Diekman, A. B., & Eagly, A. H. (2000). Stereotypes as dynamic constructs: Women and men of the past, present, and future. *Personality and Social Psychology Bulletin, 26,* 1171–1188.

Durkheim, E. (1951). *Suicide* (J. A. Spaulding & G. Simpson, Trans.). New York: Free Press. (Original work published 1897)

Dyer, E. D. (1987). Ten-year differences in level of entering students' profile on the California Psychological Inventory. *Psychological Reports, 60,* 822.

Eagly, A. H. (1983). Gender and social influence: A social psychological analysis. *American Psychologist, 38,* 971–981.

Eagly, A. H. (1987). *Sex differences in social behavior: A social-role interpretation.* Hillsdale, NJ: Erlbaum.

Edwards, A. L. (1957). *The social desirability variable in personality assessment and research.* New York: Dryden Press.

Egeland, J. A., & Hostetter, A. M. (1983). Amish study: I. Affective disorders among the Amish, 1976–1980. *American Journal of Psychiatry, 140,* 56–61.

Egeland, J. A., Hostetter, A. M., & Eshleman, S. K. (1983). Amish study: III. The impact of cultural factors on diagnosis of bipolar illness. *American Journal of Psychiatry, 140,* 67–71.

Ehrenreich, B., & English, E. (1978). *For her own good: 150 years of the experts' advice to women.* New York: Doubleday.

Elder, G. H. (1974). *Children of the Great Depression: Social change and life experience.* Chicago: University of Chicago Press.

Elder, G. H. (1979). Historical change in life patterns and personality. In P. Baltes & O. Brim (Eds.), *Life-span development and behavior* (Vol. 2). New York: Academic Press.

Elder, G. H. (1981a). History and the life course. In D. Bertaux (Ed.), *Biography and society: The life history approach in the social sciences* (pp. 21–39). Beverly Hills, CA: Sage.

Elder, G. H. (1981b). Social history and life experience. In D. H. Eichorn, J. A. Clausen, N. Haan, M. P. Honzik, & P. H. Mussen (Eds.), *Present and past in middle life* (pp. 181–203). New York: Academic Press.

Eysenck, H. J., & Eysenck, S. B. G. (1975). *Manual of the Eysenck Personality Questionnaire.* San Diego, CA: EDITS.

Eysenck, S. B. G., & Eysenck, H. J. (1969). Scores on three personality variables as a function of age, sex, and social class. *British Journal of Social and Clinical Psychology, 8,* 69–76.

Finn, S. E. (1986). Stability of personality self-ratings over 30 years: Evidence for an age/cohort interaction. *Journal of Personality and Social Psychology, 50,* 813–818.

Flynn, J. R. (1987). Massive gains in 14 nations: What IQ tests really measure. *Psychological Bulletin, 101,* 171–191.

Frum, D. (2000). *How we got here: The 70s, the decade that brought you modern life (for better or worse).* New York: Basic Books.

Fukuyama, F. (1999). *The great disruption: Human nature and the reconstitution of social order.* New York: Free Press.

Gergen, K. J. (1973). Social psychology as history. *Journal of Personality and Social Psychology, 26,* 309–320.

Gough, H. (1991, August). *Scales and combinations of scales: What do they tell us, what do they mean?* Paper presented at the annual convention of the American Psychological Association, San Francisco.

Gutman, G. M. (1966). A note on the MPI: Age and sex differences in extraversion and neuroticism in a Canadian sample. *British Journal of Social and Clinical Psychology, 5,* 128–129.

Hagnell, O., Lanke, J., Rorsman, B., & Ojesjo, L. (1982). Are we entering an age of melancholy? Depressive illnesses in a prospective epidemiological study over 25 years: The Lundby Study, Sweden. *Psychological Medicine, 12,* 279–289.

Heine, S. J., & Lehman, D. R. (1997). Culture, dissonance, and self-affirmation. *Personality and Social Psychology Bulletin, 23,* 389–400.

Jones, L. Y. (1980). *Great expectations: America and the Baby Boom generation.* New York: Coward, McCann, & Geoghegan.

Kelly, E. L. (1955). Consistency of the adult personality. *American Psychologist, 10,* 659–681.

Klerman, G. L. (1978). Affective disorders. In M. Armand & M. D. Nicholi, Jr. (Eds.), *The Harvard guide to modern psychiatry* (pp. 253–281). Cambridge, MA: Belknap Press.

Klerman, G. L., & Weissman, M . M. (1989). Increasing rates of depression. *Journal of the American Medical Association, 261,* 2229–2235.

Lambert, T. A. (1972). Generations and change: Toward a theory of generations as a force in historical process. *Youth and Society, 4,* 21–46.

Langinvaionio, H., Kaprio, J., Koskenvuo, M., & Lonngvist, J. (1984). Finnish twins reared apart: 3. Personality factors. *Acta Geneticae Medicae of Gemellogiae, 33,* 259–264.

Levitt, E. E. (1959). A comparison of parental and self-evaluations of psychopathology in children. *Journal of Clinical Psychology, 15,* 402–404.

Lewinsohn, P., Rohde, P., Seeley, J., & Fischer, S. (1993). Age-cohort changes in the lifetime occurrence of depression and other mental disorders. *Journal of Abnormal Psychology, 102,* 110–120.

Loehlin, J. C. (1989). Partitioning environmental and genetic contributions to behavioral development. *American Psychologist, 44*, 1285–1292.

Loehlin, J. C. (1992). *Genes and environment in personality development.* Newbury Park, CA: Sage.

Mannheim, K. (1952). The problem of generations. In K. Mannheim (Ed.), *Essays on the sociology of knowledge.* London: Routledge & Kegan Paul. (Original work published 1928)

Matthews, G., & Deary, I. (1998). *Personality traits.* Cambridge, UK: Cambridge University Press.

McCrae, R. R., & Costa, P. T. (1996). Toward a new generation of personality theories: Theoretical contexts for the five-factor model. In J. S. Wiggins (Ed.), *The five-factor model of personality: Theoretical perspectives* (pp. 51–87). New York: Guilford Press.

McCrae, R. R., & Costa, P. T. (1999). A Five-Factor theory of personality. In L. A. Pervin & O. P. John (Eds.), *Handbook of personality: Theory and research* (2nd ed., pp. 139–153). New York: Guilford Press.

McCrae, R. R., Costa, P. T., Ostendorf, F., Angleitner, A., Hrebickova, M., Avia, M. D., Sanz, J., Sanchez-Bernardos, M. L., Kusdil, M. E., Woodfield, R., Saunders, P. R., & Smith, P. B. (2000). Nature over nurture: Temperament, personality, and life span development. *Journal of Personality and Social Psychology, 78*, 173–186.

Miller, J. B. (1986). *Toward a new psychology of women* (2nd ed.). Boston: Beacon Press.

Nesselroade, J. R., & Baltes, P. B. (1974). Adolescent personality development and historical change, 1970–1972. *Monographs of the Society for Research in Child Development, 39*(1, Serial No. 154).

Nisbett, R. E., & Cohen, D. (1996). *Culture of honor: The psychology of violence in the South.* Boulder, CO: Westview Press.

Nowak, A., & Vallacher, R. R. (1998). *Dynamical social psychology.* New York: Guilford Press.

Plomin, R., & Daniels, D. (1987). Why are children in the same family so different from one another? *Behavioral and Brain Sciences, 10*, 1–16.

Putnam, R. D. (2000). *Bowling alone: The collapse and revival of American community.* New York: Simon & Schuster.

Remley, A. (1988, October). From obedience to independence. *Psychology Today*, 56–59.

Roberts, B. W., & Helson, R. (1997). Changes in culture, changes in personality: The influence of individualism in a longitudinal study of women. *Journal of Personality and Social Psychology, 72*, 641–651.

Robins, L. N., Helzer, J. E., & Weissman, M. M. (1984). Lifetime prevalence of psychiatric disorders in three communities, 1980–1982. *Archives of General Psychiatry, 41*, 959–967.

Rosen, B. C. (1998). *Winners and losers of the information revolution: Psychosocial change and its discontents.* Westport, CT: Praeger.

Rowe, D. C. (1990). As the twig is bent? The myth of child-rearing influences on personality development. *Journal of Counseling and Development, 68*, 606–611.

Ryder, N. B. (1965). The cohort as a concept in the study of social change. *American Sociological Review, 30,* 843–861.

Schaie, K. W. (1965). A general model for the study of developmental problems. *Psychological Bulletin, 64,* 92–107.

Schwartz, B. (2000). Self-determination: The tyranny of freedom. *American Psychologist, 55,* 79–88.

Seligman, M. E. P. (1988). Boomer blues. *Psychology Today, 22*(10), 50–53.

Seligman, M. E. P. (1990). Why is there so much depression today? The waxing of the individual and the waning of the commons. In R. E. Ingram (Ed.), *Contemporary psychological approaches to depression* (pp. 50–76). New York: Plenum.

Seligman, M. E. P. (1995). *The optimistic child.* New York: Harper.

Shields, J. (1962). *Monozygotic twins brought up apart and together.* London: Oxford University Press.

Slater, P. E. (1970). *The pursuit of loneliness: American culture at the breaking point.* Boston: Beacon Press.

Smith, T. W. (1997). Factors relating to misanthropy in contemporary American society. *Social Science Research, 26,* 170–196.

Spence, J. T., & Hahn, E. D. (1997). The attitudes toward women scale and attitude change in college students. *Psychology of Women Quarterly, 21,* 17–34.

Spielberger, C. D., & Rickman, R. L. (1990). Assessment of state and trait anxiety. In N. Sartorius, V. Andreoli, G. Cassano, L. Eisenberg, P. Kielkolt, P. Pancheri, & G. Racagni (Eds.), *Anxiety: Psychobiological and clinical perspectives* (pp. 69–83). New York: Hemisphere.

Stewart, A. J., & Healy, J. M. (1989). Linking individual development and social changes. *American Psychologist, 44,* 30–42.

Suh, E., Diener, E., Oishi, S., & Triandis, H. C. (1998). The shifting basis of life satisfaction judgments across cultures: Emotions versus norms. *Journal of Personality and Social Psychology, 74,* 482–493.

Swann, W. B. (1996). *Self-traps: The elusive quest for higher self-esteem.* New York: Freeman.

Swindle, R., Heller, K., Pescosolido, B., & Kikuzawa, S. (2000). Responses to nervous breakdowns in America over a 40-year period: Mental health policy implications. *American Psychologist, 55,* 740–749.

Tanaka-Matsumi, J., & Kameoka, V. A. (1986). Reliabilities and concurrent validities of popular self-report measures of depression, anxiety, and social desirability. *Journal of Consulting and Clinical Psychology, 54,* 328–333.

Taylor, S. E., & Brown, J. D. (1988). Illusion and well-being: A social psychological perspective on mental health. *Psychological Bulletin, 103,* 193–210.

Tellegen, A. (1985). Structures of mood and personality and their relevance to assessing anxiety, with an emphasis on self-report. In A. H. Tuma & J. D. Maser (Eds.), *Anxiety and the anxiety disorders* (pp. 681–706). Hillsdale, NJ: Erlbaum.

Tice, D. M. (1994). Pathways to internalization: When does overt behavior change the self-concept? In T. M. Brinthaust & R. P. Lipka (Eds.), *Changing the self: Philosophies, techniques, and experience* (pp. 229–250). Albany, NY: State University of New York Press.

Twenge, J. M. (1997). Changes in masculine and feminine traits over time: A meta-analysis. *Sex Roles, 36,* 305–325.

Twenge, J. M. (2000). The age of anxiety? Birth cohort change in anxiety and neuroticism, 1952–1993. *Journal of Personality and Social Psychology, 79,* 1007–1021.

Twenge, J. M. (2001a). Birth cohort changes in extraversion: A cross-temporal meta-analysis, 1966–1993. *Personality and Individual Differences, 30,* 735–748.

Twenge, J. M. (2001b). Changes in women's assertiveness in response to status and roles: A cross-temporal meta-analysis, 1931–1993. *Journal of Personality and Social Psychology, 81,* 133–145.

Twenge, J. M., & Campbell, W. K. (2001). Age and birth cohort differences in self-esteem: A cross-temporal meta-analysis. *Personality and Social Psychology Review, 5,* 321–344.

Wertheim, E. G., Widom, C. S., & Wortzel, L. H. (1978). Multivariate analysis of male and female professional career choice correlates. *Journal of Applied Psychology, 63,* 234–242.

Whyte, W. H. (1956). *The organization man.* New York: Simon & Schuster.

Williams, D. R., Takeuchi, D. T., & Adair, R. K. (1992). Marital status and psychiatric disorders among blacks and whites. *Journal of Health and Social Behavior, 33,* 140–157.

Wilson, K., & Gallois, C. (1993). *Assertion and its social context.* New York: Pergamon Press.

Woodruff, D. S., & Birren, J. E. (1972). Age changes and cohort differences in personality. *Developmental Psychology, 6,* 252–259.

Yankelovich, D. (1981). *New rules.* New York: Bantam.

CHAPTER 9

Looking Backward
Changes in the Mean Levels
of Personality Traits from 80 to 12

PAUL T. COSTA, JR.
ROBERT R. McCRAE

[N]owhere can we find more solid ground for daring
anticipations of [understanding] human development during
the next one thousand years, than by "Looking Backward"
upon the progress of the last one hundred.
—EDWARD BELLAMY (1888)

We borrowed our title from a utopian novel set in the distant future: The
Year 2000. That date has come and gone, and—aside from credit cards—
few of the specific predictions Edward Bellamy made have proven correct. Still, we believe his basic strategy was well chosen: We can best antici-
pate the future by reviewing the past. And in our case, we have the
advantage of hindsight, whereas he could look backward only from the
vantage point of his imagination.

In this chapter we sketch out what we have learned in the past quarter century about personality development—specifically, maturational
trends in the mean levels of personality traits across the lifespan. It is a
curious history in one respect: It has proceeded backward, from full adulthood and old age to college age, and most recently to early adolescence.
Links to infant temperament are now tantalizingly close.

The focus of this chapter is on mean levels of traits, in contrast to
the stability of individual differences (Roberts & DelVecchio, 2000). Mean

levels summarize the general direction of maturational trends and have obvious social import: Should we prepare for an epidemic of depression as baby boomers reach retirement? Should the legal age for driving be raised from 16 to 18 to reduce the dangers of joyriding? In addition, the study of age changes across the lifespan is of theoretical significance, because aging can be viewed as a set of natural experiments. From the direction and timing of trait level changes we may be able to make inferences about the influences of social norms, life events, and biological processes on personality development.

We began our collaboration at the Normative Aging Study (Bell, Rose, & Damon, 1972) in Boston, where we focused on age and personality. At that time there were many theories—classic theories such as Erikson's (1950), contemporary theories such as Levinson's (Levinson, Darrow, Klein, Levinson, & McKee, 1978), and popular accounts such as Sheehy's (1976) *Passages*. There were also dozens of cross-sectional studies measuring dozens of traits, but no one really knew how to organize them into an intelligible body of knowledge. Neugarten's (1977) comprehensive review concluded that the only consistent trend was a slight decrease in Extraversion. But most gerontologists at the time were convinced that only longitudinal studies would give real insight into personality development, and few longitudinal studies had yet begun to yield results.

All of that changed quickly and dramatically as results from Durham (Siegler, George, & Okun, 1979), Baltimore (Douglas & Arenberg, 1978), and Boston (Costa & McCrae, 1978) were published in the late 1970s. Much to everyone's surprise, the answer to "what changes in adulthood?" appeared to be "nothing." Middle-aged men did not have midlife crises; postmenopausal women did not become masculine; old age did not bring depression or withdrawal or rigidity. We wrote a chapter called "Still Stable After All These Years" to announce these findings (Costa & McCrae, 1980).

That chapter also included a spirited defense of personality traits, which, at the time, were desperately in need of defending. We argued that they were real and important, and that they could be organized in terms of a few broad factors. Neuroticism, Extraversion, and Openness appeared to be the most pervasive factors, and we had developed the NEO Inventory to assess them.

Within a few years, however, we had expanded this model and merged it with an older, lexical tradition to form the Five-Factor Model (FFM) that we continue to use today. The FFM has been widely adopted as a framework for literature reviews that examine personality traits (e.g., DeNeve & Cooper, 1998; Feingold, 1994). It can also be used to summarize developmental trends. Figure 9.1 shows what we thought we knew

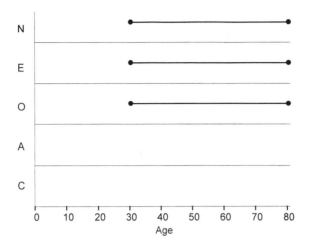

FIGURE 9.1. Schematic representation of mean levels of Neuroticism (N), Extraversion (E), and Openness to Experience (O) from age 80 to age 30, as understood circa 1980. Developmental trends for Agreeableness (A) and Conscientiousness (C) were unknown.

about personality as of 1980, at the level of the five broad factors of Neuroticism (N), Extraversion (E), Openness to Experience (O), Agreeableness (A), and Conscientiousness (C). The figure consists of five horizontal panels, each with a line that represents the mean level of one of the factors at each age. Figure 9.1 suggests that after age 30, N, E, and O are stable, neither increasing nor decreasing on average.

Today, even those adult developmentalists most committed to models of change (e.g., Helson, 1993) would probably concede that stability is the predominant trend in this age range, and it is hard to convey how radical a position it was in 1980. Perhaps the most telling evidence is that we were once introduced at a symposium as "the Antichrists of adult development." Our position has been modified a bit by subsequent data, and new data on different portions of the lifespan show more interesting curves, but it is instructive to view maturational change in the context of the remarkable stability of personality traits in adulthood. Menopause, the empty nest, grandparenthood, retirement, failing health, sensory loss, and bereavement seem to have no systematic effects on mean levels of these three broad trait factors.

Although the key evidence for stability came chiefly from longitudinal studies, perhaps the most dramatic support came from a cross-sectional study of 10,000 adults aged 35–84 from a national probability sample, the NHANES Follow-Up (Costa et al., 1986). When plotted decade by decade or even year by year, the age curves were nearly flat, and this was true for men and women, blacks and whites (see Figure 9.2). There were no spikes at midlife, no precipitous declines in old age. A close examination of the plots revealed small downward slopes, corresponding to correlations between age and the three personality traits ranging from −.12 to −.19. In 1986 we didn't take these small correlations seriously, because they might well have been attributable to birth cohort effects, age differences in response tendencies, or any number of other artifacts. Looking backward, however, we now believe they represent real maturational changes (see Figure 9.3). In a recent analysis (Costa, Herbst, McCrae, & Siegler, 2000) of longitudinal changes over a 9-year interval in a large group initially about age 40, there were significant declines in N, E, and O scores, amounting to about one *T*-score point (or one tenth *SD*). At

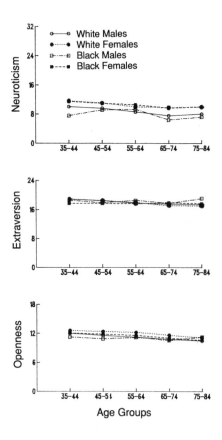

FIGURE 9.2. Mean levels of Neuroticism, Extraversion, and Openness in a nationally representative sample. Adapted from Costa et al. (1986).

that rate, these three traits would decline about one half standard deviation over the full adult lifespan.

We began collecting data on the two new factors, A and C, in 1983 and had some 3-year retest data by 1986 (Costa & McCrae, 1988). Different analyses led to different conclusions: Cross-sectional analyses of self-reports suggested an increase in A, whereas longitudinal and cross-sequential analyses suggested a decline. Longitudinal and cross-sequential analyses of C pointed to a decline, whereas cross-sectional analyses of spouse ratings showed an increase with age. Taken together, the most parsimonious conclusion appeared to be that there were no maturational effects on A and C (Costa & McCrae, 1982). Curiously, that remains an unresolved issue today. Several cross-sectional studies (e.g., Costa & McCrae, 1992) suggest a small increase in A and C with age, but a recent, large-scale longitudinal study of midlife (Costa, Herbst, et al., 2000) showed no change in A over 6 years and a small but significant *decrease* in C. It still seems parsimonious to conclude that there is no change in A and C from age 30 on. Figure 9.3 summarizes the status of the five factors in full adulthood.

FROM MIDLIFE TO COLLEGE AGE

In 1978 we joined the Baltimore Longitudinal Study of Aging and continued our research on adult samples. In contrast to the usual academic

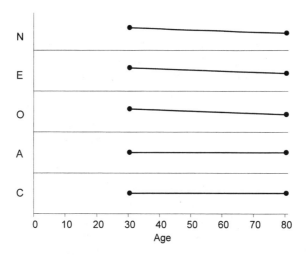

FIGURE 9.3. Schematic representation of mean levels of five personality factors from age 80 to age 30.

practice, until the late 1980s we had never conducted research on college students. When the NEO Personality Inventory was first published (Costa & McCrae, 1985), we heard from psychologists around the country who thought there was something wrong with our norms, because their student samples were far from average. Colleagues generously provided data from students at two West Coast universities, one East Coast, and one Southern university. A comparison of these data showed several striking effects: All the students differed substantially from our adult norms; all the subsamples showed very similar patterns; and men and women had parallel age trends (Costa & McCrae, 1989). The implication was that college students differed systematically from adults in the mean levels of many traits.

That conclusion was reinforced a few years later when other generous colleagues provided student data on the Revised NEO Personality Inventory (Costa & McCrae, 1992), an instrument that yields scores for the five factors and for six specific traits, or facets, related to each. The same age differences were seen in these groups, which included university students from the American South and from Canada. Perhaps even more informative was a study conducted on Navy recruits in the age range of 17 to 21 (J. Holland, personal communication, February 15, 1989). The recruits were less well educated and less academically inclined than the typical college student, and they scored somewhat lower in O, but they showed a very similar pattern of age differences when compared with adult norms. As a result, we issued "college age" norms intended for everyone aged 18–21, and we were able to extend backward the development curves for the five factors. Results are shown in Figure 9.4.

As the figure illustrates, college students appear to be distinctly higher in N, E, and O than are adults and substantially lower in A and C. That means that late adolescents describe themselves as being more emotionally volatile and open to new possibilities than adults, but also more aggressive and disorganized. That depiction seems to square with common experience.

But there are three qualifications that must be addressed before concluding that this is an accurate depiction of personality maturation from late adolescence to adulthood. First, Figure 9.4 reports trends only for the five broad factors. At the level of specific traits, somewhat different developmental curves are seen. For example, E declines from college age to middle adulthood, but not all facets of E show the same rate of decline. E5: Excitement Seeking drops almost a full standard deviation in these few years (cf. Zuckerman, 1979), which is of course a blessing for law enforcement and medical trauma units. In contrast, E1: Warmth declines only about one quarter standard deviation in the same period.

Second, all the data on which these curves are based are cross-sectional. It is true that, in adulthood, cross-sectional and longitudinal

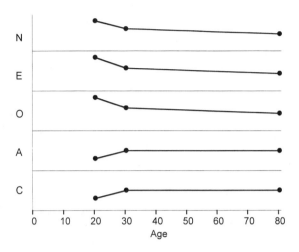

FIGURE 9.4. Schematic representation of mean levels of five personality factors in adulthood and college age.

data usually yield the same conclusions, but this need not be so in adolescence. In particular, Twenge (2000, 2001) has recently offered provocative evidence that there have been birth cohort differences in N and E over the past half century. Specifically, recent cohorts have scored substantially higher in both N and E than their age peers did in the 1950s and 1960s. If this analysis is correct, then college-age individuals may score higher than adults not because they are younger but because they were born later in the 20th century.

It will take researchers some time to evaluate Twenge's claims. Strong birth-year cohort effects are rarely seen in cross-sectional personality data in adults (Costa et al., 1986) or in sequential analyses intended to detect just such patterns (e.g., Douglas & Arenberg, 1978)—although many of the adults in these studies were born before the time span surveyed by Twenge. When Gough (1991; see Roberts & Helson, 1997) examined patterns of item endorsement in successive classes of college students, he found increases from the 1960s to the 1980s in items expressing nonconformity and individualism (perhaps related to O and low C) but not large increases in the endorsement of N- and E-related items.

In any case, the cross-sectional findings in Figure 9.4 have been corroborated by longitudinal evidence that N, E, and O actually do decline between adolescence and adulthood, whereas A and C increase. For example, Watson and Walker (1996) reported declines in negative affect in this period, and McGue, Bacon, and Lykken (1993) reported declines in absorption (which is like O) and increases in achievement (like C). And within a few years another line of evidence in support of these cross-sectional findings appeared: cross-cultural studies.

The problem with cross-sectional studies, of course, is that they confound aging with time of birth, and historical cohort effects—living through the Great Depression or coming of age in the Internet era—could account for age differences. But it is possible to deconfound age and cohort effects by comparing individuals of the same age who have had different historical experiences, and that is generally true for people in different countries. Older and younger Chinese have had life experiences vastly different from those of older and younger Americans, and if there are important formative effects of life events on subsequent adult personality, we can expect to see major differences in developmental curves of Chinese and Americans based on cross-sectional comparisons. Conversely, if the same pattern of age differences is seen in Chinese and Americans (Yang, McCrae, & Costa, 1998) and across a variety of other cultures, it is likely to reflect a universal maturational process rather than a historical artifact.

And, with a few minor exceptions, the same pattern *is* seen. Figure 9.5 presents data from Germany, Italy, Portugal, Croatia, and South Korea on mean levels of C in four age groups (McCrae et al., 1999). Note that college students—the first of the four bars in each group—are less conscientious than their elders in each case.[1] Cross-sectional studies in Russia,

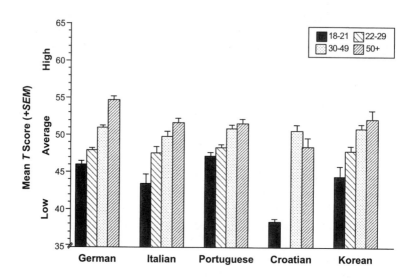

FIGURE 9.5. Mean levels of Conscientiousness in four age groups in five cultures. Note that no Croatian respondents were aged 22 to 29. Adapted from McCrae et al. (1999).

Japan, Estonia, Spain, Britain, Turkey, and the Czech Republic show similar patterns for C, and American patterns of age differences are also generally replicated for N, E, O, and A (Costa, McCrae et al., 2000; McCrae et al., 2000).

We can conclude from longitudinal and cross-cultural studies that there are true maturational changes between college age and middle adulthood somewhat along the lines depicted in Figure 9.4. However, a third reservation is still needed. These age trends are represented as straight lines, but only because they are based on two-point data. If we had data from each year between 18 and 30, we might find that most of the change occurs between 18 and 21, or between 25 and 30, or that development follows a complex zigzag pattern during the 20s. We know what happens to the average 20-year-old by age 30, but we do not yet know what path is taken to get there. This is in contrast to studies of adults, where year-by-year analyses (Costa et al., 1986) suggest simple linear trends.

Part of the answer to what happens in detail is provided in a new study by Robins and colleagues (Robins, Fraley, Roberts, & Trzesniewski, 2001). They traced 270 students through the college years using the short form of the NEO-PI-R and found a modest decline in N and increases in A and C. They also found a small increase in O. Increases in O, A, and C were also reported in another longitudinal study of college students using a different measure of the FFM (Gray, Haig, Vaidya, & Watson, 2001). These age changes during college have been added in Figure 9.6.

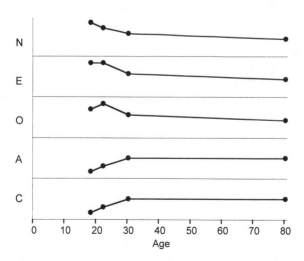

FIGURE 9.6. Schematic representation of mean levels of five personality factors in adulthood, the 20s, and during college.

Trends for N, A, and C are consistent with earlier studies contrasting college students and adults. E, however, did not change in the Robins et al. (2001) study and actually increased in Gray et al.'s (2001) results. The long-term decline in E appears to begin sometime after the end of college age. O shows an even more remarkable pattern, with increases during college preceding the eventual decline (see Sapolsky, 1998, for observations on this trend). It is possible, of course, that these increases in O are effects of higher education that would not be replicated in a noncollege sample of the same age—a possibility that should be tested in future research. However, at least within the college-educated population, O appears to show a curvilinear developmental trend, peaking some time after age 18.

ADOLESCENCE AND CHILDHOOD

The NEO-PI-R was designed for use by adults, and if the developmental curves we have been tracing depend on NEO-PI-R data, it would appear that we have reached the end of the line. It is true that some clinicians use the adult NEO-PI-R to assess adolescents, and some research has been published on adolescent samples (e.g., Fickova, 1999), but until recently we were skeptical about these applications. Would junior or senior high school students really understand the items? Would the items be relevant? Would the self-concepts of adolescents be sufficiently developed to yield reliable self-reports? Would the same personality dimensions appear in this age group? Parker and Stumpf (1998) had a unique opportunity to examine these questions because they worked with a sample of intellectually gifted children.[2] At age 12 they had a higher reading level than most adults and could certainly comprehend the items. When Parker and Stumpf administered the short form of the NEO-PI-R, the NEO Five-Factor Inventory (NEO-FFI; Costa & McCrae, 1992), to their sample, they found that it maintained its psychometric properties. Internal consistency, factor structure, and correlations with other self-report measures suggested reliability and validity. Most impressive were cross-observer correlations with parent ratings. For example, children who reported themselves to be high on N were described by their parents as *nervous, touchy, moody*, and not *confident*; those who scored high on O were described as *original, insightful, unconventional*, and *interests wide*.

When the NEO-FFI was readministered 4 years later, rather surprising results were seen (Costa, Parker, & McCrae, 2000). O increased substantially for both boys and girls, and girls showed a small increase in N. Otherwise, however, there were no changes in mean levels. Despite the volatility usually attributed to this age period (Arnett, 1999), there was no evidence of change in E, A, or C. Adolescents resembled college students on all five factors. Figure 9.7 extends developmental curves back to age 12 based on these results.

There is not a large literature on personality trait development in adolescence, but what there is appears to be consistent with this account. The increase in N among girls has parallels in cross-sectional studies of self-esteem, which declines markedly for girls from age 9 to age 13 (Robins, Trzesniewski, Tracy, Gosling, & Potter, 2000) before beginning to rise. The increase in O is seen in some cross-cultural analyses that compared 14- to 17-year-olds with college-age respondents (McCrae et al., 2000). And the general lack of mean-level changes in other factors has been reported by several investigators (Arrindell, Van Faassen, & Pereira, 1986; Graziano, Jensen-Campbell, & Finch, 1997).

A particularly interesting comparison is provided by the High School Personality Questionnaire (Cattell, Cattell, & Johns, 1984), an instrument designed for use by adolescents and administered to large samples aged 12 to 18. The authors note that "age trends were significant only for a few factors (most notably on Factor B—intelligence)" (p. 79), but they provide age corrections for boys and girls and for different forms of the test on which significant age effects were found. Among the few consistent effects was a small increase in I: Sensitivity, which is related chiefly to facets of O, especially O2: Aesthetics (Conn & Rieke, 1994).

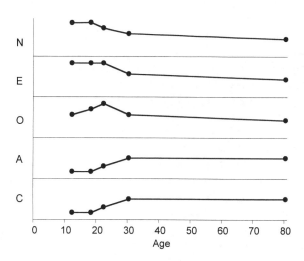

FIGURE 9.7. Schematic representation of mean levels of five personality factors in adulthood, the 20s, college age, and adolescence, as understood circa 2001.

In some respects, this seems like déjà vu. We began our careers looking for signs of adult development and found mainly stability. Examining what might be expected to be the most volatile time of life, the teenage years, we now find—mostly stability. As Figure 9.7 shows, adolescence appears to occupy a plateau before the important changes of the next decade. But there is one extremely important difference between this plateau and that seen after age 30. As Roberts and DelVeccio (2000) show, the stability of individual differences is inversely related to age. Costa, Herbst et al. (2000) studied 40-year-olds over a 6- to 9-year interval and reported a median retest correlation of .83 across the five factors. Over the 4 years of college, Robins et al. (2001) reported a substantially lower median retest correlation of .60, and the median retest for gifted 12-year-olds was only .38 (Costa, Parker, & McCrae, 2000).

What these dramatically lower stability coefficients mean is that adolescence really is a turbulent time in which the personality traits of any given individual may change considerably. But across individuals, there is no uniform trend. Some teenagers become more agreeable—more courteous, generous, and modest—as they go through junior high and high school, but an equal number become more antagonistic, belligerent, and arrogant. Similarly, individuals' shifts in N, E, and C appear to yield no net effect on mean levels at this age.

The exception is O, on which both boys and girls show systematic change in mean level. Increasing O during adolescence is perhaps understandable in part as a consequence of growth in cognitive competencies and in the scope of life experience. In turn, greater experiential openness may account in part for identity exploration (Clancy & Dollinger, 1993) and development in moral reasoning (Lonky, Kaus, & Roodin, 1984). Some aspects of adolescent rebelliousness may also be associated with Openness—indeed, many of the central developmental issues of adolescence seem to be tied to the growth of O.

Clearly, personality development at this age represents an important research opportunity for trait psychologists, and fortunately, it now appears that research need not await the development of new personality instruments. DeFruyt and colleagues (De Fruyt, Mervielde, Hoekstra, & Rolland, 2000) administered the Flemish version of the adult NEO-PI-R to a large and reasonably representative sample of schoolchildren from age 12 to age 18. Children were instructed to omit items if they did not understand them or if the items did not apply. Most children answered most items—only about 1% of all items were left blank—and De Fruyt and colleagues showed that the resulting scores were reliable and valid and yielded the same factor structure as adults', even when the data for the 12–14-year-olds were analyzed separately. It appears that the adult

NEO-PI-R can be used "as is" for research with junior and senior high school students (McCrae et al., 2001).

TOWARD INFANT TEMPERAMENT

Could the NEO-PI-R, or the briefer NEO-FFI, be validly used by grade school children? Perhaps. The Junior Eysenck Personality Inventory (Eysenck, 1965) has norms for children as young as age 7, suggesting that self-reports have some reliability and validity even at that early age. Language would certainly be a problem for the NEO-PI-R, which has a sixth-grade reading level (Schinka & Borum, 1994). One way to handle this is by providing prompts, additional material to explain the meaning of words or items. That strategy was used by Markey and colleagues (Markey, Markey, Ericksen, & Tinsley, 2001) in a sample of fifth graders. The strategy apparently worked; correlations with mothers' ratings ranged from .23 to .46 (all $p < .05$), suggesting reasonable validity.

However, most studies of children below age 12 rely on ratings by parents or teachers. Mervielde and DeFruyt have an instrument, the Hierarchical Personality Inventory for Children (HiPIC), that can be used by either parent raters or children (Mervielde & De Fruyt, 1999), and Parker and Stumpf (1998) showed validity for parent ratings of sixth graders on the observer form of the NEO-FFI. Thus, it would be possible to conduct a calibration study, administering measures to both parents and, say, their 12- to 14-year-old children. Regression analyses could be used to predict self-reported NEO-PI-R scores from parent ratings, and then parent ratings of younger children could be used to extend developmental curves further backward in the metric of the NEO-PI-R.

Such a line of research would bring us to the territory long explored by child temperament researchers and allow us to test some of the speculations about how temperament develops into the adult five factors. There have already been studies correlating temperament scales with personality factors, which have also proceeded backward. In a sample of adults, Angleitner and Ostendorf (1994) conducted a joint factor analysis of adult temperament measures and markers of the FFM and found that almost all the temperament scales could be understood as aspects of the FFM. In a sample of college students, Rothbart, Ahadi, and Evans (2000) administered their Adult Temperament Questionnaire (ATQ), together with adjective markers of the FFM. ATQ Extraversion and Negative Affect were correlated with corresponding adjective E and N factors; ATQ Effortful Attention was related to C, and ATQ Orienting Sensitivity was strongly correlated with O. Because the scales of the ATQ had been modeled on temperament research in children and infants, the authors concluded that their findings suggested "considerable convergence of lindividual differences across ages, methods, and levels of analysis" (p. 133).

Studies comparing FFM measures with assessments of temperament in children or infants have not yet been reported, but conceptual correspondences can readily be hypothesized. For example, Rothbart and Mauro (1990) argue that there are six major temperament variables in infancy: fearful distress, irritable distress, positive affect, activity level, attention span, and rhythmicity. The first two are likely related to N, the second pair to E, and the last two to C and low O, respectively. Secondary associations are also possible: For example, fearful distress in infants might also be related to low O, as it is often provoked by novelty.

The difficulty with testing these hypotheses is that it is not clear how the FFM can be assessed in infants as anything other than temperament: The same observed behavior would have to be used to infer both FFM and temperament constructs. How, then, could we meaningfully relate these variables? Proponents of a psychobiological model of temperament (e.g., Gray, 1991; Posner & Rothbart, 2000; Rothbart, Derryberry, & Posner, 1994) might argue that their equivalence could be assessed at the neurophysiological level. If the same brain circuits are activated in infants high in positive affect and in teenagers high in E, then these are arguably the same dimension. In principle, this method might be applied to chart the full developmental course: Perhaps it could be shown that some neurological structure or neurohormonal process waxes and wanes with the years to produce the rise and fall of O seen in Figure 9.7.

LOOKING FORWARD

Personality psychologists know much more about the lifespan development of traits than we did 25 years ago, but we still have a great deal to learn. We should devote more attention to changes in specific facets that define the five factors. For example, cross-cultural studies suggest that the E6: Positive Emotions declines substantially over the adult lifespan, whereas E4: Activity does not (Costa, McCrae, et al., 2000)—although longitudinal studies do show a decline in activity level in the latter half of adulthood (Costa, Herbst, et al., 2000; Douglas & Arenberg, 1978). Most facets follow the developmental curve of the factor they define, but analyses of residual scores suggest that there are also maturational trends in the specific variance associated with each facet (Costa, McCrae, et al., 2000).

Future analyses might also focus on subgroups defined by gender, class, or physical or mental health status. One of the remarkable facts that has emerged about personality development is that, in general, the same maturational trends are seen for males and females (Costa, Herbst, et al., 2000; Costa, McCrae, et al., 2000). However, there is suggestive evidence that boys and girls diverge on N as they enter adolescence (Costa, Parker, et al., 2000), and other investigators have noted special circumstances in which women's development is distinct from men's (Wink & Helson, 1993). Social class certainly has marked effects on the life course, but there is little data on whether personality traits develop differently in different social groups. Physical health status in general has little effect on personality or its stability (Costa, Metter, & McCrae, 1994), but there are predictable changes among patients with Alzheimer's disease, who increase in N and decline dramatically in C (Siegler et al., 1991). These deviations from normal stability might be useful as early signs of the disease process.

Perhaps the most interesting question remaining is the *cause* of all these changes. Our working hypothesis is that changes in trait levels are primarily governed by intrinsic, biologically based maturation. The cross-cultural universality of age differences is consistent with that view, as are intriguing observations of aging chimpanzees (King, Landau, & Guggenheim, 1998) and behavior genetic studies of age changes in personality traits (McGue et al., 1993). However, it is also possible that historical, cultural, or environmental effects are superimposed on biological programs. And, of course, it is possible that deliberate interventions, such as psychotherapy, might change the course of trait development.

The last 25 years have been extraordinarily fruitful in charting personality development; the past bodes well for the future.

NOTES

1. Figure 9.5 also shows that adults 50 and over, shown in the fourth bar, are generally more conscientious than adults 30–50. This is an example of the cross-sectional findings that suggest a continued rise in C across the lifespan.
2. The initial age of this group was erroneously reported as 13.77 in Parker and Stumpf (1998); in fact, they were sixth graders aged 10 to 12 when they completed the NEO Five-Factor Inventory.

REFERENCES

Angleitner, A., & Ostendorf, F. (1994). Temperament and the Big Five factors of personality. In C. F. Halverson, G. A. Kohnstamm, & R. P. Martin (Eds.), *The developing structure of temperament and personality from infancy to adulthood* (pp. 69–90). Hillsdale, NJ: Erlbaum.

Arnett, J. J. (1999). Adolescent storm and stress, reconsidered. *American Psychologist, 54*, 317–326.

Arrindell, W. A., Van Faassen, H. K., & Pereira, J. L. (1986). A cross-cultural study of patterns of self-reported emotional distress in Dutch and Antillean secondary-school pupils living on the Netherlands-Antilles. *Personality and Individual Differences, 6*, 725–736.

Bell, B., Rose, C. L., & Damon, A. (1972). The Normative Aging Study: An interdisciplinary and longitudinal study of health and aging. *International Journal of Aging and Human Development, 3*, 5–17.

Bellamy, E. (1888). *Looking backward: 2000–1887*. Boston: Ticknor.

Cattell, R. B., Cattell, M. D., & Johns, E. (1984). *Manual and norms for the High School Personality Questionnaire*. Champaign, IL: Institute for Personality and Ability Testing.

Clancy, S. M., & Dollinger, S. J. (1993). Identity, self and personality: I. Identity status and the five-factor model of personality. *Journal of Research on Adolescence, 3*, 227–245.

Conn, S. R., & Rieke, M. L. (Eds.). (1994). *16PF Fifth Edition technical manual*. Champaign, IL: Institute for Personality and Ability Testing.

Costa, P. T., Jr., Herbst, J. H., McCrae, R. R., & Siegler, I. C. (2000). Personality at midlife: Stability, intrinsic maturation, and response to life events. *Assessment, 7*, 365–378.

Costa, P. T., Jr., & McCrae, R. R. (1978). Objective personality assessment. In M. Storandt, I. C. Siegler, & M. F. Elias (Eds.), *The clinical psychology of aging* (pp. 119–143). New York: Plenum Press.

Costa, P. T., Jr., & McCrae, R. R. (1980). Still stable after all these years: Personality as a key to some issues in adulthood and old age. In P. B. Baltes & O. G. Brim, Jr. (Eds.), *Life span development and behavior* (Vol. 3, pp. 65–102). New York: Academic Press.

Costa, P. T., Jr., & McCrae, R. R. (1982). An approach to the attribution of age, period, and cohort effects. *Psychological Bulletin, 92*, 238–250.

Costa, P. T., Jr., & McCrae, R. R. (1985). *The NEO Personality Inventory manual*. Odessa, FL: Psychological Assessment Resources.

Costa, P. T., Jr., & McCrae, R. R. (1988). Personality in adulthood: A six-year longitudinal study of self-reports and spouse ratings on the NEO Personality Inventory. *Journal of Personality and Social Psychology, 54*, 853–863.

Costa, P. T., Jr., & McCrae, R. R. (1989). *The NEO-PI/NEO-FFI manual supplement*. Odessa, FL: Psychological Assessment Resources.

Costa, P. T., Jr., & McCrae, R. R. (1992). *Revised NEO Personality Inventory (NEO-PI-R) and NEO Five-Factor Inventory (NEO-FFI) professional manual*. Odessa, FL: Psychological Assessment Resources.

Costa, P. T., Jr., McCrae, R. R., Martin, T. A., Oryol, V. E., Senin, I. G., Rukavishnikov, A. A., Shimonaka, Y., Nakazato, K., Gondo, Y., Takayama, M., Allik, J., Kallasmaa, T., & Realo, A. (2000). Personality development from adolescence through adulthood: Further cross-cultural comparisons of age differences. In V. J. Molfese & D. Molfese (Eds.), *Temperament and personality development across the life span* (pp. 235–252). Hillsdale, NJ: Erlbaum.

Costa, P. T., Jr., McCrae, R. R., Zonderman, A. B., Barbano, H. E., Lebowitz, B., & Larson, D. M. (1986). Cross-sectional studies of personality in a national sample: 2. Stability in neuroticism, extraversion, and openness. *Psychology and Aging, 1,* 144–149.

Costa, P. T., Jr., Metter, E. J., & McCrae, R. R. (1994). Personality stability and its contribution to successful aging. *Journal of Geriatric Psychiatry, 27,* 41–59.

Costa, P. T., Jr., Parker, W. D., & McCrae, R. R. (2000, February). *Adult development: Episode I. Personality stability and change in gifted adolescents.* Paper presented at the annual meeting of the Society for Personality and Social Psychology, Nashville, TN.

De Fruyt, F., Mervielde, I., Hoekstra, H. A., & Rolland, J.-P. (2000). Assessing adolescents' personality with the NEO-PI-R. *Assessment, 7,* 329–345.

DeNeve, K. M., & Cooper, H. (1998). The happy personality: A meta-analysis of 137 personality traits and subjective well-being. *Psychological Bulletin, 124,* 197–229.

Douglas, K., & Arenberg, D. (1978). Age changes, cohort differences, and cultural change on the Guilford-Zimmerman Temperament Survey. *Journal of Gerontology, 33,* 737–747.

Erikson, E. H. (1950). *Childhood and society.* New York: Norton.

Eysenck, S. B. G. (1965). *Manual of the Junior Eysenck Personality Inventory.* London: University of London Press.

Feingold, A. (1994). Gender differences in personality: A meta-analysis. *Psychological Bulletin, 116,* 429–456.

Fickova, E. (1999). Personality dimensions and self-esteem indicators relationships. *Studia Psychologica, 41,* 323–328.

Gough, H. G. (1991, August). *Scales and combinations of scales: What do they tell us, what do they mean?* Paper presented at the annual convention of the American Psychological Association, San Francisco.

Gray, E. K., Haig, J., Vaidya, J., & Watson, D. (2001, February). *Personality stability in young adulthood.* Paper presented at the annual meeting of the Society for Personality and Social Psychology, San Antonio, TX.

Gray, J. A. (1991). The neuropsychology of temperament. In J. Strelau & A. Angleitner (Eds.), *Explorations in temperament: International perspectives on theory and measurement* (pp. 105–128). New York: Plenum Press.

Graziano, W. G., Jensen-Campbell, L. A., & Finch, J. F. (1997). The self as a mediator between personality and adjustment. *Journal of Personality and Social Psychology, 73,* 392–404.

Helson, R. (1993). Comparing longitudinal studies of adult development: Toward a paradigm of tension between stability and change. In D. Funder, R. Parke, C. Tomlinson-Keasey, & K. Widaman (Eds.), *Studying lives through time: Personality and development* (pp. 93–120). Washington, DC: American Psychological Association.

King, J. E., Landau, V. I., & Guggenheim, C. B. (1998, May). *Age-related personality changes in chimpanzees.* Paper presented at the annual convention of the American Psychological Society, Washington, DC.

Levinson, D. J., Darrow, C. N., Klein, E. B., Levinson, M. L., & McKee, B. (1978). *The seasons of a man's life.* New York: Knopf.

Lonky, E., Kaus, C. R., & Roodin, P. A. (1984). Life experience and mode of coping: Relation to moral judgment in adulthood. *Developmental Psychology, 20,* 1159–1167.

Markey, C. N., Markey, P. M., Ericksen, A. J., & Tinsley, B. J. (2001, February). *Personality and risk behavior among early adolescents.* Paper presented at the annual meeting of the Society for Personality and Social Psychology, San Antonio, TX.

McCrae, R. R., Costa, P. T., Jr., Lima, M. P. d., Simões, A., Ostendorf, F., Angleitner, A., Marušić, I., Bratko, D., Caprara, G. V., Barbaranelli, C., Chae, J.-H., & Piedmont, R. L. (1999). Age differences in personality across the adult life span: Parallels in five cultures. *Developmental Psychology, 35,* 466–477.

McCrae, R. R., Costa, P. T., Jr., Ostendorf, F., Angleitner, A., Hřebíčková, M., Avia, M. D., Sanz, J., Sánchez-Bernardos, M. L., Kusdil, M. E., Woodfield, R., Saunders, P. R., & Smith, P. B. (2000). Nature over nurture: Temperament, personality, and lifespan development. *Journal of Personality and Social Psychology, 78,* 173–186.

McCrae, R. R., Costa, P. T., Jr., Parker, W. D., Mills, C. J., De Fruyt, F., & Mervielde, I. (2001). *Personality trait development from 12 to 18: Longitudinal, cross-sectional, and cross-cultural analyses.* Unpublished manuscript, National Institute on Aging, Baltimore, MD.

McGue, M., Bacon, S., & Lykken, D. T. (1993). Personality stability and change in early adulthood: A behavioral genetic analysis. *Developmental Psychology, 29,* 96–109.

Mervielde, I., & De Fruyt, F. (1999). Construction of the Hierarchical Personality Inventory for Children. In I. Mervielde, I. Deary, F. De Fruyt, & F. Ostendorf (Eds.), *Personality psychology in Europe: Proceedings of the Eighth European Conference on Personality Psychology* (pp. 107–127). Tilburg, The Netherlands: Tilburg University Press.

Neugarten, B. L. (1977). Personality and aging. In J. E. Birren & K. W. Schaie (Eds.), *Handbook of the psychology of aging* (pp. 626–649). New York: Van Nostrand Reinhold.

Parker, W., & Stumpf, H. (1998). A validation of the Five-Factor Model of personality in academically talented youth across observers and instruments. *Personality and Individual Differences, 25,* 1005–1025.

Posner, M. I., & Rothbart, M. K. (2000). Developing mechanisms of self-regulation. *Development and Psychopathology, 12,* 427–441.

Roberts, B. W., & DelVecchio, W. F. (2000). The rank-order consistency of personality traits from childhood to old age: A quantitative review of longitudinal studies. *Psychological Bulletin, 126,* 3–25.

Roberts, B. W., & Helson, R. (1997). Changes in culture, changes in personality: The influence of individualism in a longitudinal study of women. *Journal of Personality and Social Psychology, 72,* 641–651.

Robins, R. W., Fraley, R. C., Roberts, B. W., & Trzesniewski, K. H. (2001). A longitudinal study of personality change in young adulthood. *Journal of Personality, 69,* 617–640.

Robins, R. W., Trzesniewski, K. H., Tracy, J. L., Gosling, S. D., & Potter, J. (2000). *Self-esteem across the lifespan.* Unpublished manuscript, University of California, Davis.

Rothbart, M. K., Ahadi, S. A., & Evans, D. E. (2000). Temperament and personality: Origins and outcomes. *Journal of Personality and Social Psychology, 78,* 122–135.

Rothbart, M. K., Derryberry, D., & Posner, M. I. (1994). A psychobiological approach to the development of temperament. In J. E. Bates & T. D. Wachs (Eds.), *Temperament: Individual differences at the interface of biology and behavior* (pp. 83–116). Washington, DC: American Psychological Association.

Rothbart, M. K., & Mauro, J. A. (1990). Questionnaire approaches to the study of infant temperament. In J. W. Fagen & J. Colombo (Eds.), *Individual differences in infancy: Reliability, stability and prediction* (pp. 411–429). Hillsdale, NJ: Erlbaum.

Sapolsky, R. M. (1998, March 30). Open season: When do we lose our taste for the new? *New Yorker,* 57–58, 71–72.

Schinka, J. A., & Borum, R. (1994). Readability of normal personality inventories. *Journal of Personality Assessment, 62,* 95–101.

Sheehy, G. (1976). *Passages: Predictable crises of adult life.* New York: Dutton.

Siegler, I. C., George, L. K., & Okun, M. A. (1979). Cross-sequential analysis of adult personality. *Developmental Psychology, 15,* 350–351.

Siegler, I. C., Welsh, K. A., Dawson, D. V., Fillenbaum, G. G., Earl, N. L., Kaplan, E. B., & Clark, C. M. (1991). Ratings of personality change in patients being evaluated for memory disorders. *Alzheimer Disease and Associated Disorders, 5,* 240–250.

Twenge, J. M. (2000). The Age of Anxiety? Birth cohort change in anxiety and neuroticism, 1952–1993. *Journal of Personality and Social Psychology, 79,* 1007–1021.

Twenge, J. M. (2001). Birth cohort changes in extraversion: A cross-temporal meta-analysis, 1966–1993. *Personality and Individual Differences, 30,* 735–748.

Watson, D., & Walker, L. M. (1996). The long-term stability and predictive validity of trait measures of affect. *Journal of Personality and Social Psychology, 70,* 567–577.

Wink, P., & Helson, R. (1993). Personality change in women and their partners. *Journal of Personality and Social Psychology, 65,* 597–605.

Yang, J., McCrae, R. R., & Costa, P. T., Jr. (1998). Adult age differences in personality traits in the United States and the People's Republic of China. *Journal of Gerontology: Psychological Sciences, 53B,* P375–P383.

Zuckerman, M. (1979). *Sensation seeking: Beyond the optimal level of arousal.* Hillsdale, NJ: Erlbaum.

PART III

PERSONALITY AS
A COMPLEX SYSTEM
Social-Cognitive
and Affective Dynamics

CHAPTER 10

What Remains Invariant?
Finding Order within
a Person's Thoughts, Feelings,
and Behaviors across Situations

YUICHI SHODA
SCOTT LEETIERNAN

One long-standing goal of personality psychology is to identify the co-herence and stability that underlie individuals' thoughts, feelings, and behaviors. Attempts to do so, however, inevitably require confronting the challenge of bringing together change and variation with endurance and stability. People's behaviors vary widely across situations in ways that are seemingly inconsistent, yet the core mission of personality psychology and our intuition compel us to seek an enduring set of characteristics that define the person across situations and over time. How does one reconcile be-havioral variation with the notion that each individual is characterized by stable and distinctive qualities? What remains invariant through the changing stream of thoughts, feelings, and behaviors, and how might one capture what is constant? Addressing these questions is the basic challenge to any conception of personality.

To illustrate this challenge, imagine tracing any aspect of an indi-vidual's experience, mood, the salience of a particular type of thought, or a particular type of behavior, over time and across situations. The result is likely to resemble Figure 10.1, showing a wide variation in thoughts, feelings, and behaviors within the same individual.

Perhaps all this variation is random fluctuation, and we should re-move it by averaging across these situations. But if we do so we may be

Person 1

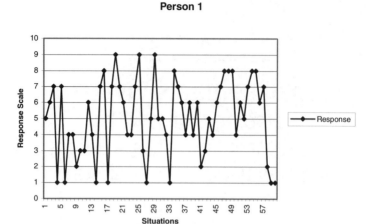

FIGURE 10.1. Example response pattern to 60 situations.

losing some important information. Besides, that may amount to accepting the possibility that personality accounts for only that small portion of behavioral variance represented by *average* behavioral tendencies and that the usefulness of the personality construct is limited to predicting the location of an individual as a point on a continuum. On the other hand, if one is not to give up on understanding intraindividual variation, one needs to ask: Are there any patterns and regularities here? Could important information about a person, and how that person's mind works, be discovered by looking for regularities in what may appear to be random fluctuations? That these "random fluctuations" *do* contain regularities that reflect personality is the fundamental assumption of our approach to the science of personality.

We propose that within the patterns of intraindividual variation, there may be a discernible order, a stable pattern that is unique to each individual. The thoughts, feelings, and behaviors of an individual may vary considerably, and on the surface, this may appear to go against the central tenet of the construct of personality—that personality is invariant or consistent over time and across situations. But when we look beyond the surface and focus on how it varies and on what external and internal situations it depends, we may find a regular pattern that is distinctive for each individual and that transcends the surface level variation.

To this end, this chapter has three goals. First, we summarize evidence that this intraindividual variation is indeed more than random fluctuation, that there is an order there that can be measured and even predicted.

Specifically, our first goal is to show that behavior variation across situations is systematic and that the patterns of variation are stable over time, reflecting the unique and stable characteristics of each individual. Our approach to finding order amid the variation is to adopt an information processing model of personality, to think of personality as a system operating in continual concert with the social environment. There are two components to this approach: defining the social environment as configurations of features that are psychologically meaningful and measuring and modeling the unique way individuals process those features in producing behaviors. Exploring these two components are our second and third goals for this chapter. Specifically, we present a method for finding these features and determining the degree to which they are present in social situations. We then illustrate two methods for modeling the unique way individuals process these features.

VARIATIONS IN BEHAVIOR ARE NOT ALWAYS RANDOM

Some evidence that not all intraindividual variation in behavior is random fluctuation comes from recent studies of the meaningful temporal patterning of behavior variation. Although still relatively few, the number of investigators focusing on and finding such stable intraindividual patterning is increasing (e.g., Eizenman, Nesselroade, Featherman, & Rowe, 1997; Fleeson, 2001; Rhodewalt & Morf, 1998, Zelenski & Larsen, 2000). Encouraging evidence is coming from studies using new tools such as spectral analysis (Larsen, 1987), which identifies discernible cyclic patterns embedded in what may first appear as random fluctuations. With these techniques, Larsen and Kasimatis (1990) found that some individuals' affective experiences clearly follow a 7-day weekly cycle, whereas others do not show such a pattern. Similarly, Brown and Moskowitz (1998) showed that some individuals have discernible daily cycles in their interpersonal behaviors, such as dominance–submissiveness and agreeableness–quarrelsomeness, whereas others do not, and Rusting and Larsen (1998) found that an "evening-worse" pattern was associated with neuroticism, depression, and anxiety, as well as with a cognitive style indicative of hopelessness. In the same vein, multilevel analyses (e.g., Bolger & Zuckerman, 1995) identify the functional situation–behavior relationships that characterize different individuals or types (e.g., Bolger & Zuckerman, 1995).

Other evidence comes from studies of systematic covariation patterns among behaviors and subjective experiences. Cote and Moskowitz (1998), for example, found that individuals who score high on a given interpersonal trait (e.g., agreeableness) exhibit a stronger pattern of covariation (called "behavioral concordance" by Cote & Moskowitz) between the level of pleasant affect they feel in a given interpersonal interaction and the agreeableness of their behavior in that interaction. In contrast, those who score low on such a trait do not show such correspondence as strongly. Larsen and Cutler (1996) defined a measure of affect complexity as the number of intraindividual factors needed to account for a given amount of variance in daily mood. Carstensen, Pasupathi, Mayr, and Nesselroade (2000) examined age differences in the patterns of intraindividual variation in daily emotional experience and found that older adults' emotional experiences were more highly differentiated than those of younger adults. In addition, among older people periods of highly positive emotional experience were more likely to endure and periods of highly negative emotional experience were less stable. Feldman (1995) found that individual differences in attention to the hedonic versus arousal components of affective experience were related to intraindividual correlations between specific affective elements, such as anxious and depressed mood and negative and positive affects.

LOOKING FOR REGULARITIES (AND PERSONALITY) IN SITUATION–BEHAVIOR RELATIONS

Sometimes, however, regularities in the stream of behaviors contain more information than just the periodicity or patterns of covariation among behaviors. Behaviors do not occur in a vacuum; they occur in specific situations. Therefore, it may be possible to identify the regularities that characterize the stream of an individual's behavior in relation to the characteristics of the situations. When the situation changes, so do the behaviors, but the relationship between the situations and behaviors may be stable and may express an individual's distinctive cognitive, behavioral, and affective response characteristics. Identifying the situation features that covary with behaviors is important because it can lead to making predictions of an individual's behavior in response to novel situations. It may lead to answers to questions such as: What kind of advising style would help a particular graduate student flourish? Which school should a child attend? Which of multiple job offers should a person accept? Or whom should one marry?

Some situation–behavior relations are obvious. After all, most people are happier at weddings than at funerals. But are there regularities at an individual level, so that it is possible to identify for each individual a distinctive and stable pattern of situation–behavior relationships? Many years of systematic observation of social behavior, ranging from honesty, conscientiousness, friendliness, and aggressiveness, seem to support such a possibility. For example, Shoda, Mischel, and Wright (1994) followed aggressive behaviors of children at a summer camp over an entire summer, some of which had serious consequences (e.g., a camper hitting a counselor on the head with a flashlight). Children's aggressiveness varied across situations, such as when warned by an adult or when teased by a peer, and such variations remained even after the differences among situations in the average aggressiveness of children in general were statistically removed. One child was substantially more aggressive than other children when warned by an adult. But the same child may be substantially less aggressive than other children when teased by a peer.

Of course, such variations may be due to chance. Therefore, more than 150 hours of observations per individual were averaged to form a reliable measure of how each camper responded to each type of situation. Most campers still showed substantial variability across situations. That is, reliable intraindividual variations across situations remained even after the normative levels of behavior in each situation were controlled for. Most important, when the pattern of intraindividual variation for each child observed during one half of the summer was compared with the pattern during the other half of the summer, the patterns resembled each other. If the pattern of variation reflected chance fluctuations, one would not expect it to be repeated. But for a sizable and statistically highly significant majority of the campers, the pattern from one time sample predicted that from the other. Thus, for example, if in one half of the summer a child was distinctively more aggressive than other children in response to adult warning but less aggressive than others in response to peer teasing, in the other half of the summer the child would show a similar pattern.

Data from this and other studies (e.g., Vansteelandt & Van Mechelen, 1998) have begun to establish that it is a rule, rather than an exception, that such reliable patterns of behavior variability distinctively characterize each individual. We have been referring to these patterns as an individual's *behavioral signature* to emphasize the fact that they distinctively and stably characterize each individual. Stability and distinctiveness in an individual's behaviors were found in an unexpected place: the pattern of variation itself.

IDENTIFYING PSYCHOLOGICAL FEATURES
OF SOCIAL SITUATIONS

Like their handwritten counterparts, these behavioral signatures can be seen as identifying the individual, as an expression of individuality. Do behavioral signatures have a meaning that can be understood and that can help us generalize and predict behaviors in a different context? Can they also be used to predict future behaviors in new situations? We believe answering these questions requires going beyond the "nominal" definition of situations to identifying their psychological features. A nominal definition identifies situations by name, such as "canoeing at Camp Caribou," or "being teased by Joey." These are valid and reliable definitions and are perfectly suitable for assessing cross-situational consistency of behaviors. But they do not tell us just what about each situation is responsible for the observed pattern of behavior variation, therefore limiting our ability to make predictions in new situations. For example, if a child is repeatedly observed as being unkind to friends while canoeing but not while horseback riding, can one predict what she will be like when she goes for a swim with friends or when she goes to an amusement park? The challenge at hand is analogous to one faced by an allergy specialist. Suppose a patient has reliably identified that he has an allergic reaction every time he eats breakfast cereal brands A and E but that he can eat brands B, C, and D without any problems. Note that the "situations," the brands of cereal, are defined *nominally*. The pattern of variation in the patient's reactions across the situations (brands of cereal) is reliable and reflects some stable characteristics of his immune system— it is his "allergy signature." But to go beyond it and to predict whether or not he can safely eat brand X, a new brand he has not tried before, it would be necessary to identify just what it is about brands A and E that cause the allergic reaction. How, then, might one identify the critical ingredient(s) of social situations?

The approach we have been pursuing draws on George Kelly's personal construct theory (Kelly, 1955), with some key variations. Like Kelly's, our general strategy starts with identifying the nominal units of situations; then we seek to identify their psychological ingredients by comparing and contrasting functionally similar and dissimilar sets of situations. For Kelly, whose primary goal was clinical intervention, the "situations" were specific individuals who played significant roles in a particular client's life. In his "role repertory test" procedure, he had clients identify ways in which two of these people in their lives were more similar to each other than to a third person. The result of this procedure was a set of personal constructs, which constituted the most salient dimensions in which the significant individuals were perceived, constituting the structure of the client's subjective social world.

Kelly's procedure was highly effective for understanding a particular individual's subjective world. However, it was not intended to provide results that could be readily applicable to other individuals. There were two aspects of this procedure that contributed to this idiographic focus. First, the "situations" presented to his clients were the specific individuals in the client's life, and therefore it was unlikely that they were a part of any other client's life. Second, the personal constructs an individual identifies may be idiosyncratic and may differ qualitatively from those employed by another individual.

The goal of our approach, in contrast, was to find a set of situation features that allows generalization across situations and individuals. For that purpose, we first select a representative set of situations that *all* individuals in a sample are asked to consider. We then seek to identify the psychological features that seem to be salient, not for just one but for at least a nontrivial portion of the population. The goal is to identify a set of situation features, a subset of which are expected to be salient for any given individual. For example, for one individual, features *a*, *c*, and *d* may be salient characteristics differentiating the set of situations, whereas for another individual, features *b*, *c*, and *e* may be salient. The union of these sets, *a*, *b*, *c*, *d*, and *e*, will provide a set of finite (and hopefully small number of) features that are likely to be salient to at least some of the individuals. This set provides a nomothetic *language* with which to characterize situations. Individual differences can then be captured by identifying the subset of the common situation features that are salient for a given individual.

The logic of our procedure for identifying the critical features, however, is the same as Kelly's. We seek those features that distinguish functionally equivalent sets of situations. More concretely, we first have individuals "experience" each situation, while asking them to indicate how they might respond to each situation. They are then asked to report the features that seemed to distinguish those situations to which they responded in one way from those to which they responded in another way. Again, we do *not* expect that any given participant is necessarily able to provide a complete account of the features that underlie the psychological meaning of these situations. Instead, our procedure seeks to identify *some* of the features used by each individual, with the hope that, collectively, the total set of features will cover most of the aspects of these situations that are psychologically significant to at least some of the individuals.

There are a few critical requirements for this approach. One is that there be enough situations through which to see a *systematic* pattern of variation in a person's responses. Just as one cannot reliably diagnose what one is allergic to by just a few instances of allergic reactions, separating the factors with which an individual's behavior systematically varies from chance associations requires a large enough number of observations. In short, the number of *situations* is the relevant N. We are used to thinking of the N as the number of participants. Very few psychologists would consider a sample of only 5 individuals to be sufficient to draw a reliable conclusion. Similarly, when the goal of a study is to discover reliable patterns of covariation between an individual's behavior and the features of the situations, the number of situations sampled, the N, must be large enough.

Second, in order for the findings to be relevant beyond the specific sample of situations chosen for the study, the situations must reflect types of social situations people encounter regularly. Finally, in order to study responses to enough situations in a reasonable amount of time, we needed a mechanism for collecting many responses from each participant quickly. For this purpose, we created a laboratory-based paradigm that would allow us to collect responses to systematically chosen sets of situations in an hour or so, as we describe next.

THE "SIMULATED SITUATIONS" PARADIGM

In this paradigm participants experience and respond to a set of simulated situations presented on a computer. Each simulated situation consists of an audio clip of another person speaking to the participant, and, when relevant, the audio clip is accompanied by a photograph of the person "talking to" the participant. Typically, participants respond to 60 simulated situations per session and complete either one or two experimental sessions, yielding a behavioral signature for intraindividual response variation across the set of situations as measured at either one or two points in time.

Our simulated situations were implemented in two ways. One is the "guided imagination" format, in which participants listen to audio clips told in the second person, and the participant is instructed to imagine being in the situation. We used the "guided imagination" format to collect responses to situations previously identified as stressful to college student populations (e.g., "It is finals week. You have two exams on the same day and a paper due. . . .").

The second type of implementation simulates interpersonal interactions. In each situation, participants see a photograph of a person and hear an audio clip of the person speaking to the participants (e.g., "Would you loan me your class notes? I had to miss class because . . ."). Participants respond by indicating what they would do or how the situation would make them feel. Participants respond to 60 different versions of the same general "scenario" (e.g., 60 different people asking in their own words to borrow class notes). Thus the situations differed in the characteristics associated with the person enacting the scenario (e.g., the tone of voice, facial expression, level of confidence). It should be noted that our choice to hold the general scenario (e.g., asking to lend class notes) constant across 60 situations is deliberate and crucial for the interpretation of the results. Imagine that a biologist is interested in testing the effect of various soil conditions on the rate of plant growth by planting in soil from a variety of areas. It is easy to appreciate the importance of holding other factors, such as the amount of water, temperature, and sunlight, constant, not to mention making sure to plant the same plant. Otherwise, the experiment does not have a hope of reaching any reliable conclusion about the effect of soil type, unconfounded by other factors. Similarly, if we did not hold the scenario constant, and if the situations varied in any unconstrained way, with only 60 situations we would not be able to identify any situation feature reliably. For example, we generally would not know whether the observed variation reflects differences among the scenarios or variations in the stimulus persons in the scenarios. By holding the scenario constant but varying the stimulus persons drawn from the population of students, therefore, this study seeks to find those psychological features of situations that make up important ways in which social situations differ as a function of the individuals who are in them. (Of course, one could hold the stimulus person constant, while varying the scenario. In that case, the analysis would be seeking to find psychological features important in differentiating among the sample of scenarios. We have explored this possibility in a study of scenarios sampled from a set of situations that have been nominated as the most stressful by college students, as described later).

In summary, in order to identify the person factors important in our interpersonal situations, we presented sets of situations in which the scenario was held constant (e.g., "Would you loan me your class notes?"), and the differences across the 60 situations were due entirely to the person in the situation. In this way, the "stimulus" person—his or her looks, voice, friendliness, word choice, and so forth—is what differentiates one situation from another.

Stability and Uniqueness of Behavioral Signatures in the Simulated Situations Paradigm

A first research question we asked using this approach is whether the pattern of intraindividual variation observed across the simulated situations, the behavioral signature, was stable over time. If a person experienced the same set of situations on multiple occasions, would their behavioral signature look similar? To test for stability over time, we collected responses using the "simulated situations" paradigm from the same participants on two occasions, separated by either 1 or 2 weeks. Each participant responded to the same set of situations presented in different sequences at both experimental sessions. The level of stability in the behavioral signature was defined by the correlation between response patterns—or signatures—at the two experimental sessions, computed within each person.

From the perspective of a participant in one of these experiments, he or she came into our lab, was seated in front of a computer, and responded to 60 instances of the same scenario. For example, in one of the experiments, a participant responded to 60 different people asking in their own words to borrow a dollar to make photocopies (e.g., one phrased the question "Um, excuse me, I totally forgot my wallet. Could I borrow a dollar? I promise I'll pay you right back," while another phrased it "I hate to bother you, but I forgot my wallet at home. Could I possibly borrow a dollar and pay you back somehow?"). Each of these is a "situation," defined by the person doing the asking, his or her appearance, tone of voice, and the words chosen. Participants were students and were instructed to imagine being approached by another student they had "seen around in one of their classes" at the photocopy center in the library. They responded on a 9-point Likert scale with the likelihood that they would loan the person the dollar. This procedure was completed on two occasions separated by 1 week so that the response patterns to the 60 situations from each experimental session could be correlated to assess the stability of the response profile over time.

In an initial study, 7 participants completed this procedure, responding on two occasions to the "dollar loaning" set of 60 situations, presented in random order on each occasion. For each person, responses to the situations were quite varied, with most people using close to or the entire response scale. Each person's response signatures (see Figure 10.2a for an example response signature) from the two experimental sessions were then correlated. Across the 7 participants, the median correlation was .62, indicating relative stability in the response pattern from 1 week to the next.

Correlations between response patterns, however, do not necessarily reflect the stability of the *unique* way a person responds to the situations. It is possible that the stability over time is due simply to situational factors to which all individuals would respond similarly and consistently. Therefore, in order to address individual differences, we also tested the stability in the unique way each person responded to the situations. First, we created unique response signatures (see Figure 10.2b) for each person by subtracting the normative response to each situation (i.e., average of all participants' responses to a given situation) from that person's response. Note that, as a result, the scale on the y-axis is now centered on 0, indicating whether this person's response was above or below the typical, or normative, response to each situation. Unique response signatures were computed for each participant.

Participant 6

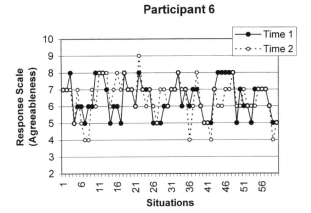

FIGURE 10.2a. Response signatures of Participant 6 at time 1 and time 2. In each of the 60 situations, a different person asked to borrow money for photocopies. The correlation between the two signatures was .62.

Participant 6

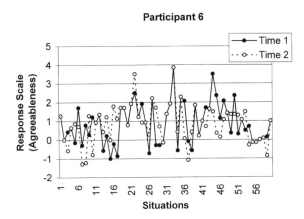

FIGURE 10.2b. Unique response signatures of Participant 6 at time 1 and time 2. In each of the 60 situations, a different person asked to borrow money for photocopies. The correlation between the two signatures was .57.

Correlations between unique responses reflected the degree of stability in the unique response pattern over time. As expected, removing systematic variance due to responses normative for each situation reduced the degree of stability over time, and the correlations were lower than their nonunique counterparts. Nonetheless, the median correlation between each person's unique response signatures at time 1 and time 2 was .55, indicating stability in the unique way each person responded to the situations.

Replication

In a second study, we repeated the procedure with 53 more participants. In addition, to assess the generality of the findings, the same procedure was repeated with different scenarios. For example, instead of encountering 60 different people asking to borrow a dollar in a library to make photocopies, one group of participants encountered 60 people asking, in their own words and voice, if they would like to come to a free swing dancing lesson. Table 10.1 shows these scenarios (first and second columns), the number of participants (third column) and the median stability of their behavioral signatures (fourth and fifth columns). The scenarios were chosen to represent a variety of social behaviors widely regarded as relevant to personality in the field, namely, agreeableness and openness to experience, as well as situations that are relevant for eliciting positive or negative emotional reactions. For the latter, participants indicated the degree to which each situation made them feel good or bad, whereas for the other situation sets they indicated the likelihood that they would engage in the relevant behavior (e.g., the likelihood of trying the dance lessons in the "swing dance" situation set). All participants returned after 1 week to respond again to the same situation set presented in a new sequence. After completing the procedure a second time, participants listed the "aspects of the situations" they felt were instrumental in determining their responses.

Like our first group of 7 participants, all response signatures contained considerable variation across the situations, with many participants' responses ranging from the lowest to the highest point on the scale. The two response patterns were then correlated to produce a stability coefficient for each participant. The results in Table 10.1, column 4, show median correlation coefficients. With median correlation coefficients ranging from .47 to .83, participants responding to the interpersonal situation sets were highly stable over time in their behavioral response signatures. Unique response signatures were computed for each person, again by subtracting a person's responses from the average over all participants. Correlating unique response signatures at times 1 and 2 reveals that across all the situation domains participants' unique response patterns were stable over time, with correlation coefficients ranging from .37 to .58 (Table 10.1, column 5).

To further test the generality of these findings, in a third study, a new group of participants responded to a set of situations identified as highly stressful to college students. These were 22 stressful situations that were selected from a set of 123 situations listed by a different group of participants as one of the two most stressful situations they had experienced in the previous 3 months. Participants provided 16 responses to each situation: the degree to which they would experience each of eight emotions and the degree to which they would react with each of eight coping behaviors (Folkman & Lazarus, 1985). Participants returned after 2 weeks to provide all 16 responses to each of the 22 stressful situations, presented in a new, randomly chosen sequence. On both occasions, participants' responses varied considerably across the situations, again with many participants' responses ranging from the lowest to the highest points on the scales. For each participant, responses with regard to each emotion and coping behavior were separately plotted against the 22 situations, yielding 16 situation-response profiles for each participant. The same procedure was applied to the time 2 data, and the stability of the profiles was assessed by computing a correlation coefficient between corresponding situation-response profiles from time 1 and time 2, yielding 16 stability coefficients for each participant. Table 10.2 presents median stability coefficients for each of the response categories, with a "grand" median stability correlation coefficient of .44.

The percentage of participants with positive correlations (Table 10.2) gives a sense of the likelihood of positively correlated stability coefficients. For the majority of response categories, close to 90% or more of participants' stability coefficients were positive. A typical participant showed a positive stability coefficient for 14 or 15 out of their 16 response signatures.

Similar to the analysis of responses to the interpersonal interactions, for each participant, 16 unique response signatures were calculated by subtracting from each individual's responses the average of the responses given by the entire sample of participants. For the unique response signatures, correlation coefficients for the stressful situations ranged from .12 to .41. The percentages of participants with positive stability coefficients for each of the 16 responses to the stressful situations dropped only slightly in comparison with percentages for nonunique responses. The slight drop is expected if we assume that the shared variance (i.e., common pattern of variability across the situations) removed in the conversion to unique scores is stable over time.

TABLE 10.1. Median Correlations between Response Patterns to the Agreeableness, Openness, and Affective Response Situations from the First and Second Experimental Sessions

Situation set	Scenarios used to create the 60 situations in each situation set	Number of participants	Stability of behavioral signatures	
			Raw response pattern	Unique response pattern
Agreeableness				
Photocopies	You are at the library and someone you have seen around approaches you and asks to borrow a dollar to make photocopies.	7	.62	.55
Class notes	After class one day, another student approaches you and asks to borrow your notes because he or she had to miss a week of class.	7	.47	.43
Bookstore	After class one day another student asks you to pick up a book from the bookstore for him or her because he or she does not have time.	5	.59	.47
Openness to experience				
Swing dance	Another student whom you have seen around approaches you one day and asks if you would like to try free swing dancing lessons going on in the H.U.B. [the student union building].	6	.56	.45

Movie extra	Another student whom you have seen around approaches you one day and asks if you would like to try out to be an extra in a movie being filmed here on campus.	7	.61	.37
Drum demo	Another student whom you have seen around approaches you one day and asks if you would like to try a free demo of African drumming that's being offered in Red Square [on campus].	7	.60	.48
Affect inducing				
Psych class	Another student you have seen around in your psych class approaches you one day and says how tough the class is but that you seem to know your stuff.	7	.62	.58
Save seat	You are in a crowded movie theater waiting for the film to start. Another person, someone you recognize from campus, says that you look nice enough to hold his or her seat while he or she goes for popcorn.	6	.83	.52
Tailgating	You are driving and when stopped at a light someone in the car next to you, whom you have seen around campus, yells at you that you were tailgaiting him or her, which is dangerous, and that you really shouldn't do it.	7	.70	.51

TABLE 10.2. Median Correlations between Response Patterns to the Stressful Situations from the First and Second Experimental Sessions

	Response patterns		Unique response patterns	
	Median correlation	Percentage of participants with positive correlations	Median correlation	Percentage of participants with positive correlations
Emotional responses				
Angry	.50	94	.31	75
Confident/hopeful/ eager	.23	88	.12	75
Disappointed	.43	94	.24	94
Disgusted	.31	88	.25	88
Guilty	.62	94	.33	81
Sad	.57	94	.36	100
Stressed	.58	100	.39	100
Worried/fearful/ anxious	.49	94	.34	94
Behavioral responses				
Avoid people	.41	81	.36	81
Blame self	.51	100	.27	75
Blame others	.48	94	.20	81
Daydream	.20	75	.21	63
Focus on good things	.43	100	.32	81
Keep mind off problem	.39	75	.31	69
Think of solution	.42	88	.41	81
Seek support	.28	94	.15	81

IDENTIFYING THE PSYCHOLOGICAL FEATURES OF SITUATIONS

The stability in the unique response signatures indicates that there is regularity in each person's responses. We wanted to understand this regularity in such a way as to go beyond any given situation and predict responses to novel situations. In order to do so, it was necessary to understand what it was about the situations that made each person respond in his or her characteristic manner. As discussed earlier, features of situations may be conceptualized at two different levels (Shoda et al., 1994). At one level are the nominal features, units of situations that are dictated by the particular logistics and ecology of research setting. In the dollar-loaning situation, for example, the nominal units of situations would be each of the

60 simulated situations, consisting of a unique configuration of the appearance and voice of a particular person asking for a dollar and the way the request was phrased. Nominal situations have limited generalizability because individual differences in relation to a specific nominal situation, even if highly stable, cannot help predict responses to other nominal situations. For example, if we observe that a given participant was reliably reluctant to loan a dollar to John but reliably more willing to do so to David, would we expect the same participant to be more willing to agree to the same request from a third person, Michael, than to a request from Paul? Because David and John are nominal situations, we are unable to generalize to the situations with Michael or Paul. To make predictions beyond the original set of nominal situations in which the behaviors were already observed (i.e., "John" and "David") to new nominal situations (e.g., "Michael" and "Paul"), one needs to understand the psychological meaning of John, David, Michael, and Paul. This requires analyzing situations at a deeper level, at which situations may be defined to capture basic *psychological features* or ingredients that occur in many different nominal situations. Just as individuals' responses to particular medications can be understood more fundamentally by considering the specific active ingredients rather than brand names, our analysis of situations focuses on the psychologically active features of situations.

Nominal situations are highly complex and contain a wide array of different psychological features. The challenge, therefore, is to capture those features that are encoded distinctively by perceivers and that activate other relevant cognitive–social person variables (e.g., expectancies, values) in the mediating process. Because in our situation sets the general scenario (e.g., someone asking to borrow a dollar to make photocopies) was held constant, variations in responses to the different situations were due almost entirely to reactions to different combinations of features regarding the stimulus person's appearance, tone of voice, and the words spoken. For example, in the study of agreeing to a request for money, we hypothesized that psychological features would include features such as how forceful a requester's voice was, the confidence in his or her manner, and how "cool" the requester appeared.

In short, one way to understand the regularity in a person's response pattern—and to predict responses to novel situations—is to characterize situations in terms of configurations of psychologically meaningful features of situations and to analyze the pattern of variation in the individual's behavior as a function of responses to those features. If a person responds in a particular way to a certain configuration of psychological situation features, then we should be able to predict that person's response to a new situation containing a similar configuration of features.

Recall that after participants completed the experimental procedure for the second time, they listed as many aspects of the situations as they felt influenced their responses. Combining responses from all participants, this procedure produced a relatively comprehensive list of features relevant to the situation sets. This list was content analyzed to eliminate duplicates, and to combine features that were highly similar in order to produce a final set of relevant features. To date we have focused most of our efforts on the interpersonal interaction situations, in particular the "would you lend me a dollar?" scenario. For those situations we identified 17 situation features (see Table 10.3 for a complete list), including, for example, "the person seemed sincere," "the person seems to lack confidence," "the person seems intelligent," and "the person is well dressed."

We asked an independent group of judges to rate each situation for the degree to which it contained each of the features, in order to characterize each situation in terms of its "feature makeup" with reasonable certainty. For each of the 17 features, six to nine raters rated the degree to which the feature was present in each of the "dollar loaning" situation 3. For each feature, interrater reliability was assessed with Cronbach's alpha (Table 10.3); 16 of the 17 features received reliability scores of $\alpha >$ .70 and were considered reliably rated. For the 16 reliably rated features, we took average ratings to derive final situation feature ratings for each

TABLE 10.3. List of Situation Features for Agreeableness Situations

Situation feature	α
Attractiveness of other person	.76
Confidence of other person	.81
How considerate was the other person?	.79
How "cool" was the other person?	.70
How well dressed was the other person?	.85
Eloquence of the other person	.82
How excited to talk to you was the person?	.74
Did the person make you feel comfortable?	.75
Friendliness of the other person	.80
Genuineness of the other person	.59
Intelligence of the other person	.78
Pleasantness of the other person	.72
Politeness of the other person	.73
Rudeness of the other person	.83
Sincerity of the other person	.72
Did the person have a nice tone of voice?	.77
Did the person have a warm face?	.93

of the 60 situations in the set. Using these ratings, each situation could then be described in terms of the degree to which it possessed each situation feature.

FROM SITUATION FEATURES
TO BEHAVIORAL SIGNATURES

Ultimately the goal is to characterize a given person by the "if . . . then . . ." regularities in which the "if" refers to psychological features of situations (e.g., if approached by a friendly and confident person, then person X responds agreeably). We hypothesized that the response signatures would reflect the unique social information processing system each person employs to determine responses to social situations. If each person processes the different situation features uniquely and stably, the characteristics of the processing system should be reflected in the response signatures.

As an example, consider the responses from a participant in an additional study in which 53 people responded to the "dollar loaning" situation set, shown in Figure 10.3. The dark circles in this graph are the situations in which the person asking to make a copy was rated as looking very sincere. Note that in all situations involving a sincere-sounding per-

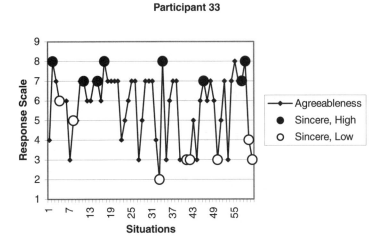

FIGURE 10.3. Responses by Participant 33, with the situations rated high or low in sincerity indicated. Note that sincerity in the person asking was a critical situation feature to this participant.

son asking for a favor, this participant was agreeable, accounting for some of the peaks of the agreeable responses. We also found that situations in which the person asking for a favor was independently judged to be low in sincerity, indicated by open circles, invariably led to less-than-average agreeableness and accounted for the valleys in the zigzag graph.

But does this reflect what is unique about Participant 33, or does it reflect a pattern that is common to all individuals? To test this, we repeated a similar analysis with other participants. Figure 10.4a shows the response pattern for a different participant—Participant 38—whose agreeableness also varied widely across situations but whose pattern of variation is quite different from that of Participant 33. The dark circles show the same situations involving a sincere-sounding person, and yet Participant 38's agreeableness in such situations is somewhere in the middle. The open circles indicate the situations involving an insincere-sounding person. Again, there is no correspondence between sincerity in the person asking for money and Participant 38's responses. So sincerity of the requester does not help account for Participant 38's pattern.

Instead, we found that a different feature explains person 38's response pattern. When looking at situations involving how well dressed the requester was (Figure 10.4b), Person 38's behavior variation begins to make a lot of sense. Like "sincerity" for Person 33, how well dressed a person is, as reliably rated by an independent group of people, can account for some of the peaks and valleys of Person 38's response signature.

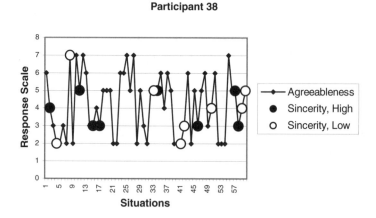

FIGURE 10.4a. Responses by Participant 38, with the situations rated high or low in sincerity indicated. Note that sincerity of the person asking for money does not account for this person's response pattern.

Participant 38

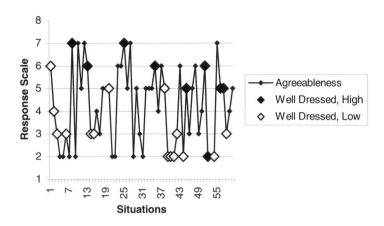

FIGURE 10.4b. Responses by Participant 38, with the situations rated high or low in how well dressed the person in each situation was. Note that the feature "well dressed" accounted for Participant 38's response pattern reasonably well.

CHARACTERIZING EACH PERSON BY A SET OF WEIGHTS REFLECTING SENSITIVITY TO EACH SITUATION FEATURE

We needed a systematic method for determining the weightings each person gives the situation features. To obtain such weights, we returned to the 7 participants in the original study and regressed the participant's responses to the situations from each time sample on the situation feature ratings. This yielded two sets of weights given to each feature for each participant. To test for stability, for each person the weight sets from each session were correlated. A median correlation across the 7 people of .75 indicated the weight sets were reliable. Table 10.4 shows three individuals. Importantly, the feature weightings were unique to each individual. Notice the differences in the weightings these three people gave to the attractiveness of the person asking to borrow money. Persons 2 and 4 actually weight attractiveness negatively, whereas Person 6 weights attractiveness positively. Politeness is also weighted negatively for Person 2 but positively for persons 4 and 6.

The primary goal of identifying an individual's behavioral signature in terms of active ingredients of situations is to go beyond the situations in which the person's behavior was observed to predict behavior in new situations. The true test of this approach, therefore, is to see whether the weightings can predict a person's responses in an entirely new set of situations. We tested this by first creating a reliable response profile for each

TABLE 10.4. Regression Weights for Predicting Response Variations from Situation Features

Feature	Person 2		Person 4		Person 6	
	Time 1	Time 2	Time 1	Time 2	Time 1	Time 2
Attractiveness	−0.76	−0.25	−0.50	−0.19	0.33	0.37
Make comfortable	1.36	1.15	−0.03	−0.50	0.62	0.31
Confidence	−0.08	0.07	−0.22	−0.48	−0.96	−0.71
Considerate	−0.44	−0.80	0.28	0.51	−0.86	−0.86
Cool	0.76	0.87	0.30	−0.01	−0.20	−0.27
Eloquent	0.20	0.12	−0.26	−0.15	0.17	0.6
Excited to talk	0.27	−0.02	0.32	0.57	−0.20	−0.05
Friendly	0.47	0.51	−0.14	−0.54	0.40	0.51
Intelligent	0.55	0.18	0.82	0.39	0.30	−0.19
Pleasant	0.02	−0.43	0.20	0.62	0.44	−0.05
Pleasant voice	−0.13	0.15	0.65	0.34	0.12	0.20
Polite	−1.96	−0.93	0.21	0.28	0.72	0.41
Rude	0.02	0.54	−0.89	−1.05	0.60	0.65
Sincere	0.19	0.50	−0.29	−0.25	−0.08	0.52
Warm face	0.00	−0.03	0.03	0.00	−0.04	−0.03
Well dressed	−0.36	−0.30	−0.34	−0.05	0.03	0.14
Stability (correlation between time 1 and time 2)	.84		.79		.79	

of the 7 participants by simply averaging each participant's responses at time 1 and time 2. From each person's average response profile, we then regressed responses to the first 30 of the 60 situations on the feature ratings for those situations to generate a set of feature weights for each person. This yielded a set of weights that each person gave to the 16 situation features. The fact that the regression weights were based on only the first 30 (of 60) situations is critical. This allowed the second set of 30 situations to effectively serve as a new set of situations to which we could predict responses using our models. The goal is to predict not just how agreeable on average a given participant is likely to be in a new set of situations, but also, and importantly, how their behavior will *vary* across the new set of situations. For each of the remaining 30 situations we generated predicted responses for each participant by applying the regression equation based on each person's responses to the first 30 situations (i.e., situation feature rating of each of the second 30 situations were multiplied by each person's feature weight obtained in the first 30 situations and then summing each term and the intercept). The resulting 30 predicted responses were then correlated with the person's actual responses as an index of the degree to which the weight set captured that person's behavioral signature. At the median, the correlation across these 7 people was .53.

As mentioned earlier in a separate study, 53 additional participants responded to the "dollar loaning" situation set. Again we generated feature weights for each participant based on responses to 30 of the 60 situations, and then predicted responses to the remaining 30 by applying each person's weight set. On average, across the 53 participants, the predicted responses correlated .42 with the actual responses.

How much of the predictability is due to the weight sets' ability to capture each person's unique processing system? To address this question, we computed the correlations between each person's actual responses and every other person's predicted responses. With 52 other individuals to compare with, this is similar to asking how much the average or typical feature weighting can predict any one person's responses. Across all participants, the average correlation between any one person's actual responses and all other people's predicted responses was .31. Thus the typical weight set explained about 9% of the variance in the second set of 30 situations, and the unique weight sets explained an *additional* 7% of the variance. This more than 75% gain in variance explained represents information that uniquely defines the way each individual translates the situation features into responses.

In addition to regression, we also tried a second approach to modeling and predicting responses to our simulated situations: back-propagation neural networks (for more on neural networks and social and personality psychology, see Smith, 1996, and Read & Miller, 1998). A back-propagation neural network was created for each person using the situation feature ratings as inputs and that person's responses to 30 of the situations as outputs. In addition to the 16-unit input and single unit output layers, our back-prop networks also had a 7-unit hidden layer. Thus in the neural network model, a weight set is assigned to an initial processing of the situation features and also to a secondary processing, mapping the nodes in the hidden layer to the output layer.

Similar to the regression analysis, we used each person's back-propagation network that had been trained on the first 30 responses to predict responses to the remaining 30 situations. In this case, on average across all participants, the predicted responses correlated .50 with the actual responses, explaining 25% of the response variance. Like the regression analysis, each person's network was used to predict every other person's responses. Each person's actual responses were then correlated with the responses predicted by every other person's network, with an average correlation of .39, explaining about 15% of the variance in responses to the second set of 30 situations. Thus with the back-propagation models, we were able to capture enough information about idiosyncratic processing of situation features to add 10% of the total variance for predicting responses to new situations.

In summary, in the studies described herein, we first established that responses to the simulated social situations we observed in the laboratory followed a pattern of cross-situational variation that was unique to each individual and stable over time, constituting a *behavioral signature* (Shoda et al., 1994). We then identified a representative set of possible situation features. It was possible to reliably rate the degree to which each situation contains each feature and then to model the pattern of variability in the participants' responses across the situations that were psychologically "active," or meaningful, to participants.

An effort to model individuals' behavioral signatures requires a mechanism for describing a situation. Characterizing situations in terms of their psychologically meaningful features is one way to achieve that goal. The weights we computed to describe the sensitivity of a person's behavior as a function of each situation feature may in turn provide a glimpse into how the relevant social situational information was uniquely translated into subjective meaning by each person, leading to his or her response signature.

DIRECTIONS

A number of next steps are apparent, and undoubtedly many more have yet to be discovered. One direction is generalizing to new types of situations. As we move into different situational domains, we will start to get a sense of whether the psychological situation features reported here as relevant to the "agreeableness" scenario generalize to different situations. Currently we are working on finding features and modeling responses to the situations involving openness to experience, as well as those eliciting both positive and negative affective responses. As the feature sets for each additional situation domain become available, we move closer to a set of comprehensive features from which a subset can be used to describe any situation type.

Systematic expansion of this approach to personality research into new situational domains would benefit greatly from a situation typology. For example, interdependence theory (Thibaut & Kelley, 1959; Kelley & Thibaut, 1978) provides a typology of dyadic interpersonal situations, such as *chicken* and *prisoner's dilemma*, that might provide a situational structure in which to grow this situation feature processing approach to personality. Kelley (2000) has made a call to extend the interdependence theory situation typology to include all situations of interdependence, and indeed a set of prototypical interdependence situations may soon be available (Kelley, 2000).

We see another future direction for laboratory-based studies that should help measure more precisely the variations in situation features that result in changes in response behavior or affect. The features of simulated situations such as those we used can be systematically manipulated via software (Pelachaud, Badler, & Steedman, 1996; Mendoza-Denton, 1999). For example, if a visual feature such as skin color is heavily weighted by a given person, changing the skin color should induce a corresponding behavioral or affective response change. Because the rest of the features are held constant (e.g., facial expression, clothing, tone of voice remain the same) we can measure the effect of skin color on the respondent's behavior or affect.

Responses to situations using the simulated situations paradigm may predict or be predicted by other measures or constructs. For example, individuals' weights for skin color and other features associated with race may be predicted by measures of automatic associations among concepts, such as the Implicit Association Test (Greenwald, McGhee, & Schwartz, 1998) and the sequential priming paradigm (SPP; e.g., Bargh, Chaiken, Govender, & Pratto, 1992; Fazio, Sanbonmatsu, Powell, & Kardes, 1986). Another possibility is that the situation characteristics to which a person is sensitive may be related to that person's schematicity with regard to the characteristics. For example, sincerity of others may be a salient feature of social situations for those people who are themselves schematic for sincerity. If so, reaction time–based measures of schematicity (e.g., Fazio et al., 1986) may allow one to predict the situation features salient for a given individual. Finally, the paradigm can also be used in conjunction with psychophysiological responses, such as heart rate, skin conductance, and more advanced physiological measures, such as cardiac pre-ejection period, to situations as a function of the configuration of psychologically meaningful situation features. For example, a person might show a strong autonomic response to certain situation features of stressful situations, although his or her behavioral profile based on self-reports reveals little if any behavioral response to the same situation.

CONCLUSION

Intraindividual variations in behavior over time and across situations have long been considered antithetical to the construct of personality, imperfections in an otherwise neat and orderly world, and a "noise" that needs to be removed in order to obtain a clear signal about the true nature of persons. The central thesis of this chapter is to question this implicit assumption and to suggest changing or at least broadening how we approach personality science. From the beginning of modern psychology, when William James likened the ever-changing contents of consciousness to a stream and when Sigmund Freud focused on the mysterious vicissitudes of mental life, theorists of personality have acknowledged, at least tacitly, that understanding a person requires understanding the dynamics of that person's mental, behavioral, and emotional life, as great novels and plays attest. Doing so systematically and quantitatively, however, was difficult before the development of modern methodologies and information technology. Thus it is understandable that much of personality psychology has captured persons as a single point on a continuum. However, we believe that given the methodological sophistication the field has witnessed lately, it is time to revisit the study of people as they live their lives. Perhaps the dynamics of intraindividual variation in thoughts, feelings, and actions now can, and should, be a central subject matter of our field (e.g., Nowak, Vallacher, & Zochowski, Chapter 12, this volume).

Of course, the field's core mission is identifying the enduring and distinctive characteristics of each person that reflect a coherent intraindividual organization (Cervone & Shoda, 1999). But we suggest that constancy may be sought not only at the surface level in the form of stability and central tendencies but also in the regularities that are present in the pattern of intraindividual variation. Larsen (1990) used the term "second order consistency" to refer to the characteristic frequency with which an individual's experience varies over time. Inspired by this idea but broadening the concept to include not just distinctive frequencies of change but also other types of regularities, such as the behavioral signature in relation to active situation features just discussed, we propose the term *higher order consistency* to include the consistent way each person varies his or her behavior across situations.

The focus on intraindividual variability and the search for stable and distinctive patterns within it will in turn lead to a question about the cognitive–affective dynamics that produce them. What creates a pattern of higher order consistency in the changing stream of thoughts, feelings, and behaviors? We believe that such an understanding requires conceptualizing personality as a complex information processing system. The system of psychological processes that can account for such higher order regularity needs to take situations into account to explain why a particular person responds differently to different situations (Mischel & Shoda, 1995; Shoda & Mischel, 1998, 2000). The system needs to be dynamic in order to account for the way its states change. It also needs to be responsive to *internal* situations, such as what one is thinking, feeling, and doing at any given moment, as well as to external situations, so that the system is responsive to both internal and external situations in determining what the person will think, feel, and do next. Our hope is that identification of the regularity in the seemingly paradoxical variations of thoughts, emotions, and behaviors within each individual will facilitate explorations of personality as a dynamic social–cognitive–affective processing system.

Most research in personality and social psychology involves examining the relationship between one variable and another, which essentially amounts to making a scatterplot, as shown in Figure 10.5, in which each individual is represented by a single point. But if we unpack the point, there is, within it, intraindividual variability of experience and behavior. Two people who may be similar in terms of their average or overall characteristics may have quite different patterns of intraindividual variation, representing their characteristic social–cognitive–affective dynamics. By examining and understanding such dynamics, we may be one step closer to understanding the uniqueness in how each individual functions, not as a static object, but as a dynamic, thinking, feeling, behaving, and *living* system.

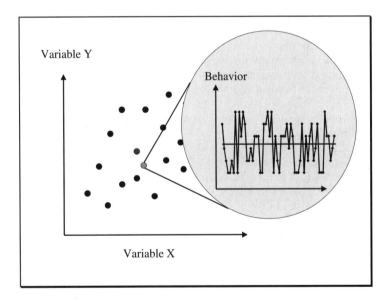

FIGURE 10.5. In a typical scatterplot, each person is represented by a point. When the point is "unpacked," there is, within it, intraindividual variability of experience and behavior, or "behavioral signature," potentially reflecting the individual's characteristic social–cognitive–affective dynamics.

ACKNOWLEDGMENTS

The study was supported in part by the University of Washington Royalty Research Fund, Grant H39349and NRSA Predoctoral Fellowship from the National Institute of Mental Health, as well as a Microsoft Fellowship in computer science and related fields. We are grateful to Ozlem Ayduk, Kathleen Cook, Rodolfo Mendoza-Denton, Walter Mischel, Jason Plaks, Naomi Zavislak, Vivian Zayas, and in particular Daniel Cervone and his colleagues at the University of Illinois at Chicago for their extensive and extremely constructive comments on earlier drafts, and Katja Brack and Kathleen Cook for making the data from their study of stressful situations available. Parts of this research were presented at the annual meeting of the Society of Personality and Social Psychology, 1999 and 2000.

REFERENCES

Bargh, J. A., Chaiken, S., Govender, R., & Pratto, F. (1992). The generality of the automatic attitude activation effect. *Journal of Personality and Social Psychology, 62*, 893–912.

Bolger, N., & Zuckerman, A. (1995). A framework for studying personality in the stress process. *Journal of Personality and Social Psychology, 69*, 890–902.

Brown, K. W., & Moskowitz, D. S. (1998). Dynamic stability of behavior: The rhythms of our interpersonal lives. *Journal of Personality, 66*, 105–134.

Carstensen, L. L., & Pasupathi, M., Mayr, U., & Nesselroade, J. R. (2000). Emotional experience in everyday life across the adult life span. *Journal of Personality and Social Psychology, 79*, 644–655.

Cervone, D., & Shoda, Y. (Eds.). (1999). *The coherence of personality: Social-cognitive bases of consistency, variability, and organization.* New York: Guilford Press.

Cote, S., & Moskowitz, D. S. (1998). On the dynamic covariation between interpersonal behavior and affect: Prediction from neuroticism, extraversion, and agreeableness. *Journal of Personality and Social Psychology, 75*, 1032–1046.

Eizenman, D. R., Nesselroade, J. R., Featherman, D. L., & Rowe, J. W. (1997). Intraindividual variability in perceived control in an older sample: The MacArthur successful aging studies. *Psychology and Aging, 12*, 489–502.

Fazio, R. H., Sanbonmatsu, D. M., Powell, M. C., & Kardes, F. R. (1986). On the automatic activation of attitudes. *Journal of Personality and Social Psychology, 50*, 229–238.

Feldman, L. A. (1995). Valence focus and arousal focus: Individual differences in the structure of affective experience. *Journal of Personality and Social Psychology, 69*, 153–166.

Fleeson, W. (2001). Toward a structure- and process-integrated view of personality: Traits as density distributions of states. *Journal of Personality and Social Psychology, 80*, 1011–1027.

Folkman, S., & Lazarus, R. S. (1985). If it changes it must be process: Study of emotion and coping in three stages of a college examination. *Journal of Personality and Social Psychology, 48*(1), 150–170.

Greenwald, A. G., McGhee, D. E., & Schwartz, J. L. K. (1998). Measuring individual differences in implicit cognition: The implicit association test. *Journal of Personality and Social Psychology, 74*(6), 1464–1480.

Kelly, G. (1955). *The psychology of personal constructs.* New York: Basic Books.

Kelley, H. H. (2000). The proper study of social psychology. *Social Psychology Quarterly, 63*(1), 3–15.

Kelley, H. H., & Thibaut, J. W. (1978). *Interpersonal relations: A theory of interdependence.* New York: Wiley.

Larsen, R. J. (1987). The stability of mood variability: A spectral analytic approach to daily mood assessments. *Journal of Personality and Social Psychology, 52,* 1195–1204.

Larsen, R. J. (1990). Spectral analysis of psychological data. In A. Von Eye (Ed.), *New statistical methods in longitudinal research, Vol. 2: Time series and categorical longitudinal data* (pp. 319–349). San Diego, CA: Academic Press.

Larsen, R. J., & Cutler, S. E. (1996). The complexity of individual emotional lives: A within-subject analysis of affect structure. *Journal of Social and Clinical Psychology, 15,* 206–230.

Larsen, R. J., & Kasimatis, M. (1990). Individual differences in entrainment of mood to the weekly calendar. *Journal of Personality and Social Psychology, 58,* 164–171.

Mendoza-Denton, R. (1999). *Lay contextualism in stereotyping: Situational qualifiers of stereotypes in intuitive theories of dispositions.* Unpublished doctoral dissertation, Columbia University.

Mischel, W., & Shoda, Y. (1995). A cognitive-affective system theory of personality: Reconceptualizing situations, dispositions, dynamics, and invariance in personality structure. *Psychological Review, 102,* 246–268.

Pelachaud, C., Badler, N. I., & Steedman, M. (1996). Generating facial expressions for speech. *Cognitive Science, 20*(1), 1–46.

Read, S. J., & Miller, L. C. (Eds.). (1998). *Connectionist models of social reasoning and social behavior.* Mahwah, NJ: Erlbaum.

Rhodewalt, F., & Morf, C. C. (1998). On self-aggrandizement and anger: A temporal analysis of narcissism and affective reactions to success and failure. *Journal of Personality and Social Psychology, 74,* 672–685.

Rusting, C. L., & Larsen, R. J. (1998). Diurnal patterns of unpleasant mood: Associations with neuroticism, depression, and anxiety. *Journal of Personality, 66,* 85–103.

Shoda, Y., & Mischel, W. (1998). Personality as a stable cognitive-affective activation network: Characteristic patterns of behavior variation emerge from a stable personality structure. In S. J. Read & L. C. Miller (Eds.), *Connectionist models of social reasoning and social behavior* (pp. 175–208). Mahwah, NJ: Erlbaum.

Shoda, Y., & Mischel, W. (2000). Reconciling contextualism with the core assumptions of personality psychology. *European Journal of Personality, 14,* 407–428.

Shoda, Y., Mischel, W., & Wright, J. C. (1994). Intra-individual stability in the organization and patterning of behavior: Incorporating psychological situations into the idiographic analysis of personality. *Journal of Personality and Social Psychology, 67,* 674–687.

Smith, E.R. (1996). What do connectionism and social psychology have to offer each other? *Journal of Personality and Social Psychology, 70(5),* 893–912.

Thibaut, J. W., & Kelley, H. H. (1959). *The social psychology of groups.* New York: Wiley.

Vansteelandt, K., & Van Mechelen, I. (1998). Individual differences in situation-behavior profiles: A triple typology model. *Journal of Personality and Social Psychology, 75,* 751–765.

Zelenski, J. M., & Larsen, R. J. (2000). The distribution of basic emotions in everyday life: A state and trait perspective from Experience Sampling data. *Journal of Research in Personality, 34,* 178–197.

CHAPTER 11

Integration and Compartmentalization
A Model of Self-Structure and Self-Change

CAROLIN J. SHOWERS

Traditional approaches to personality have focused on the higher order consistency in human behavior, rather than on intraindividual variability across situations (Cervone & Shoda, 1999a; 1999b). In this chapter, self-structure is viewed as a feature of personality that may speak to both the consistency and variability in behavior, broadly defined. On one hand, individuals may display relatively stable differences in the way they structure beliefs about the self. On the other hand, an understanding of self-structure may shed light on the *process* of how individuals change to fit the situation (Cantor & Kihlstrom, 1987; Showers & Ziegler-Hill, in press). When a person's behavior changes with the situation, what is changing is (at least in part) the *self*. Such change can be described in two ways: Either a particular domain or subset of the entire self-structure is activated, facilitating behaviors that may be specific to that context, or the self is actually restructured to fit that situation. In either case, the self-structure is an important element of people's discriminative facility in responding to specific contexts (cf. Mischel, 1973).

A fundamental feature of self-structure is evaluative organization. Whether we turn to psychodynamic theory or a trait approach for inspiration, the evaluative dimension is recognized as a basic way of categorizing beliefs about the self and others. From the psychodynamic perspective, the compartmentalization of positive and negative self-beliefs into the "good me" and the "bad me" is a primitive, but adaptive, defense designed to handle negative self-beliefs (Kernberg, 1984). From the trait perspective, evaluation is a key dimension of the semantic differential, which characterizes the major dimensions of meaning (Osgood, 1969). Ultimately, evaluative categorizations of self-beliefs have implications for self-evaluation at both global and specific levels. Global self-evaluations are believed to have important implications for a person's mood and motivation (Baumeister, 1998; Dutton & Brown, 1997; Tesser & Martin, 1996). However, many cognitive theorists emphasize the links between domain-specific self-evaluations and subsequent behavior (e.g., Harter, 1999; Marsh, Byrne, & Shavelson, 1992; Pelham, 1991).

Although most people's thoughts about the self are predominantly positive (e.g., Kendall, Howard, & Hays, 1989; Schwartz & Garamoni, 1986), it is features of *negative* self-beliefs (such as perceived importance and certainty) that are most strongly correlated with mood and self-esteem (e.g., Pelham & Swann, 1989; Showers, Abramson, & Hogan, 1998). Interest in the evaluative structure of the self (i.e., the organization of positive and negative self-beliefs) emerges when we recognize that most people have at least some important negative beliefs about the self. These negative beliefs potentially affect global self-evaluations and reactions to specific circumstances. If some negative beliefs about the self are virtually inevitable, the way they are organized within the overall cognitive structure of the self may be what moderates their impact. This perspective does not deny that the sheer number of negative beliefs in the self-concept has important consequences. Nonetheless, organizational factors may enhance or minimize the impact of that negative content.

EVALUATIVE COMPARTMENTALIZATION
AND INTEGRATION

This chapter focuses on a feature of evaluative organization of self-knowledge known as compartmentalization and integration (Showers, 1992a, 1995, 2000a). This perspective on the self has some underlying assumptions, starting with the belief that the self is multifaceted and consists of multiple selves or personae (Cantor & Kihlstrom, 1987; Markus & Wurf, 1987). This is an information processing perspective that views the self-concept as an enormous repertoire of self-relevant information, including both episodic and semantic knowledge. The repertoire of knowledge is organized into categories (or some kind of network structure). A person's multiple selves, then, are organizational structures that help to activate subsets of self-knowledge that might be relevant in specific contexts. The working self-concept, a person's possible selves, and the core self are examples of organizational structures (Cantor, Markus, Niedenthal, & Nurius, 1986; James, 1890; Markus & Nurius, 1987). Some of these structures are relatively stable; others may be constructed on-line.

Compartmentalization and integration refer to the evaluative organization of a person's multiple selves. These two types of self-organization can be illustrated by example. Table 11.1 presents examples of two individuals, Harry and Sally, who are describing the selves they experience in the academic domain. Each of them describes two distinct selves or personae. On a typical day at college, Harry experiences the self he calls "Renaissance scholar." This self is characterized by mostly positive attributes, such as *curious, disciplined, creative,* and *motivated.* However, during final exams, Harry experiences a very different self, the one he calls "taking tests and getting graded." This self is mostly negative and is characterized by attributes such as *worrying, distracted,* and *tense.* Harry's type of self-organization is called *compartmentalized,* because positive and negative attributes are segregrated into distinct self-aspect categories. In contrast, Sally's selves are an example of *evaluative integration.* Notice that Sally's selves contain all the same specific attributes as do Harry's; however, these attributes are organized quite differently. Sally defines her selves according to the type of college class she is in—either humanities classes or science classes. In each type of class, she experiences a mixture of positive and negative attributes—the defining characteristic of evaluative integration. In humanities classes, Sally feels creative and insecure; in science classes, she feels disciplined but tense.

TABLE 11.1. Examples of Compartmentalized Organization ("Harry") and Integrative Organization ("Sally") for Identical Items of Information about Self as Student

"Harry": Compartmentalized organization		"Sally": Integrative organization	
Renaissance scholar (+)	Taking tests, grades (−)	Humanities classes (+/−)	Science classes (+/−)
+ Curious	− Worrying	+ Creative	+ Disciplined
+ Disciplined	− Tense	− Insecure	+ Analytical
+ Motivated	− Distracted	+ Motivated	− Competitive
+ Creative	− Insecure	− Distracted	− Worrying
+ Analytical	− Competitive	+ Expressive	+ Curious
+ Expressive	− Moody	− Moody	− Tense

Note. A positive or negative valence is indicated for each category and each item. The symbol (+/−) denotes a mixed-valence category. Adapted from Showers (1992a). Copyright 1992 by the American Psychological Association. Adapted by permission.

Basic Model of Compartmentalization

Studies of compartmentalization and integration have examined the correlates and consequences of these two types of organization (Showers,
1992a; Showers & Kling, 1996b; Showers & Kevlyn, 1999). Returning
to the example of Harry and Sally, it seems that on a typical day at college when Harry experiences his positive "Renaissance scholar" self, he
would feel very good. The self-attributes that come to mind are purely
positive. In contrast, on a typical day at college, Sally will experience a
mixture of positive and negative self-beliefs, regardless of which type of
class she finds herself in, and so her feelings should be more neutral.
During final exams, however, when Harry experiences his negative self
("taking tests and getting graded"), he should feel extremely bad. At this
time, Harry may even feel worse than Sally who, on the way to her chemistry final, is still feeling disciplined and tense. Thus the association between a person's type of self-organization and overall feelings (i.e., mood
and self-esteem) may depend on the relative importance of different self-
aspect categories. If the self-concept is mostly positive and positive self-
aspect categories are highly important, then compartmentalized organization should be advantageous for mood and self-esteem, because it
relegates negative self-beliefs to categories that are not likely to be activated. The compartmentalized structure helps to minimize access to any
negative self-beliefs, essentially sweeping them under the rug.

However, when a person has many important negative self-beliefs,
it is likely that any negative compartments will be activated frequently,
flooding the individual with many specific negative self-beliefs. In this case,
the individual is likely to be better off (i.e., experience less negative mood
and higher self-esteem) if self-knowledge is organized in an integrative
fashion, so that negative attributes are closely linked to some positive
beliefs about the self. The advantage of integrative organization is that it
minimizes the impact of unavoidable negative self-beliefs.

The basic model of compartmentalization (Showers, 2000a) summarizes these predictions: When positive self-aspect categories are relatively
important or salient, compartmentalization should be associated with
more positive mood and higher self-esteem than should integrative organization; when negative self-aspects and attributes are relatively important or salient, integrative organization should be associated with more
positive mood and higher self-esteem. In other words, the basic model
holds that type of organization (integrative or compartmentalized) will
interact with the relative importance (or salience) of positive and negative aspects of self in predicting mood or self-esteem. For compartmentalized self-structures, the terms *positive compartmentalization* and *negative compartmentalization* are used to indicate whether positive or negative

self-aspects are more important and, therefore, whether that self-structure is likely to be advantageous. Similarly, integrative structures can be identified as positive integrative or negative integrative to indicate whether positive or negative aspects and attributes are most salient and, therefore, whether the integrative structure is likely to be effective.

As can be seen from the example, this is basically an information processing model in which activation of a particular self-aspect category brings to mind a set of attributes associated with that category. This information processing model could be applied to any knowledge structure, not just beliefs about the self. For example, a person's tendency to compartmentalize or integrate positive and negative beliefs about ice cream should be associated with his or her overall attitude toward (or emotional reaction to) ice cream, as predicted by the basic model. In fact, results confirming the hypotheses of the basic model have been obtained not only for the organization of self-knowledge (e.g., Showers, 1992a; Showers & Kling, 1996a; Showers, Abramson, & Hogan, 1998) but also for the organization of positive and negative beliefs about someone else, namely one's partner in a romantic relationship (Showers & Kevlyn, 1999). In the latter study, the organization of beliefs about one's romantic partner was associated with feelings of liking and loving for that partner.

Measurement of Evaluative Organization

The most commonly used measure of compartmentalization or integration is a self-descriptive card sorting task (Showers, 1992a; Showers & Kevlyn, 1999). Participants are provided with a stack of 40 cards, each containing the name of a specific attribute. Twenty attributes are positive and twenty are negative. Participants are told, "Think of the different aspects of yourself or your life, and sort the cards into groups so that each group represents an aspect of yourself or your life." They are told that they can use individual cards more than once and that they do not have to use all of the cards. Thus this task allows participants to generate their own self-aspect categories and to select as many or as few attributes as may fit each self-aspect. After completing the card sort, participants rate the importance, positivity, and negativity of each self-aspect category using 7-point Likert scales. A sample card sort appears in Table 11.2.

The task provides three important parameters of the self-concept. First, it provides the measure of compartmentalization, assessed by a phi coefficient (Cramer, 1945/1974; Everitt, 1977), which is based on a chi-square statistic. Given the proportion of negative attributes in the sort, the phi coefficient indicates the tendency for those attributes to be distributed equally across all self-aspects (phi = 0, the value that one would

TABLE 11.2. Actual Card Sort Illustrating Perfect Compartmentalization (Phi = 1.0)

Helpful	Not always "perfect"	Funny	Responsible	Lovable	Looking at the good in everyone
Giving	– Indecisive	Intelligent	Mature	Lovable	Optimistic
Friendly	– Lazy	Happy	Independent	Needed	Giving
Capable	– Isolated	Energetic	Organized	Friendly	Interested
Hardworking	– Weary	Outgoing	Interested		
	– Sad and blue	Fun and entertaining	Hardworking		
	– Insecure	Communicative			

Good work ethic	Making decisions	Taking disappointment hard	Good student	Talented
Hardworking	– Indecisive	– Sad and blue	Intelligent	Successful
Capable	– Uncomfortable	– Insecure	Interested	Capable
Intelligent	– Tense	– Like a failure	Organized	Confident
Interested	– Insecure	– Hopeless	Hardworking	Fun and entertaining
Successful		– Inferior		
Confident		– Isolated		
Mature		– Incompetent		
Independent				
Organized				
Energetic				

Note. Minus sign (–) indicates negative attributes. From Showers, Abramson, and Hogan (1998). Copyright 1998 by the American Psychological Association. Reprinted by permission.

expect if the cards were sorted by chance) or to be perfectly compartmentalized (phi = 1, all self-aspect categories are uniformly positive or uniformly negative). Phi is a continuous variable that ranges from 0 to 1, and the mean is typically around .7.

Other important parameters derived from the card sort are (1) the proportion of attributes that are negative, an index of self-concept content (i.e., the positivity or negativity of the self); and (2) the relative importance of positive and negative self-aspect categories, assessed by an index of differential importance (DI; Pelham & Swann, 1989).

Typically, the association between type of self-organization and a person's mood or self-esteem is examined by regressing a measure of mood or self-esteem onto phi, DI, and their interaction, with proportion of negatives held constant, to test whether evaluative organization explains variance in mood or self-esteem that cannot be accounted for by self-concept content (i.e., the overall positivity or negativity of self-beliefs). Figure 11.1 presents the results of such an analysis, showing results that

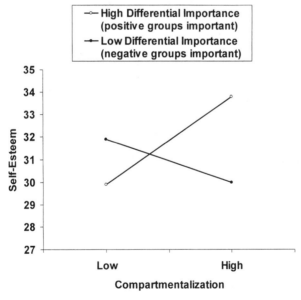

FIGURE 11.1. Adjusted predicted values for self-esteem (Rosenberg, 1965), supporting the basic model of compartmentalization. Predicted values are calculated at 1 *SD* above and below the means. For compartmentalization, *M* = .71, *SD* = .21; for differential importance, *M* = .46, *SD* = .42. Data from Showers (1992a); from Showers (2000a). Copyright 2000 by Cambridge University Press. Reprinted by permission.

are consistent with the basic model (Showers, 1992a). The open line represents individuals whose positive self-aspects are most important and indicates that greater compartmentalization is correlated with higher self-esteem. The closed line represents individuals whose negative self-aspects are more important and indicates that greater integration is correlated with higher self-esteem. Additional support for this basic model using the card sorting task to assess evaluative organization is reported by Showers, Abramson, and Hogan (1998), Showers and Kling (1996a), and Showers, McMahon, Sutton, and Davidson (1998).

ALTERNATIVE MEASURES OF COMPARTMENTALIZATION AND INTEGRATION

There are at least three alternative approaches to assessing compartmentalization and integration that have obtained results consistent with the basic model. One approach is to have participants list characteristics, behaviors, or attributes that describe them in a particular domain defined by the researcher (e.g., academic situations, social situations; Showers, 1992b, Studies 1 and 2). Analyzing the order of positive or negative items on the list should reveal the compartmentalization or integration of beliefs within that domain.

A second approach is to have participants write a paragraph about a specific negative attribute and then have judges code the content of those paragraphs for the presence or absence of integrative thoughts (Showers, 1992b, Study 2). This approach assesses the integrative thought process, that is, the stream of thought associated with a particular attribute. It may be thought of as a measure of a person's potential for integrative thinking. Some individuals with many salient positive attributes may be better off if their overall structure of the self is positive compartmentalized, but they have the ability to engage in integrative thinking when their attention is drawn to a specific negative attribute (McMahon, Showers, Rieder, Abramson, & Hogan, 1999). Although the card sort assesses abstract category structures, one might assume that these structures correspond to streams of interconnected thoughts (Showers, 1995). In individuals with compartmentalized self-structures, the stream of thoughts is uniformly valenced and may spiral upward or downward. In integrative self-structures, the stream of thought is mixed in valence and suggests a balanced, neutral, or possibly ambivalent reaction.

A third approach to assessing compartmentalization is simply to look at the extremity of a person's self-evaluations across a specific set of domains. This measure assumes that the greater the range of self-evaluations, the more likely it is that the person perceives different selves as extremely good or extremely bad. Such extreme ratings suggest compartmentalization of selves, and they have been associated with successful adjustment to relocation in elderly women (Showers & Ryff, 1996).

THE POSSIBILITY OF CHANGE IN SELF-ORGANIZATION

A careful reading of the predictions of the basic model suggests the possibility that self-organization may change. Whereas a compartmentalized self-structure should be advantageous in some circumstances (namely, when positive self-aspects are most central to the self), integrative organization may be beneficial in other circumstances (namely, when negative self-aspects are salient). Hence, if changing circumstances alter the perceived importance or salience of positive and negative aspects of self, then the most adaptive type of organization may be one that can change. If people have sufficient flexibility to shift their type of self-organization to fit the circumstances, then changes in self-organization may allow a higher level of functioning and maintain the most positive view of self overall.

To examine the possibility of self-change, self-organization was assessed in a sample of individuals at two points in time. These individuals were participating in a longitudinal, prospective study of depression (Showers, Abramson, & Hogan, 1998).[1] The sample had been selected for high (top quartile) or low (lowest quartile) cognitive vulnerability to depression. Participants were interviewed every 6 weeks for a period of 2 years. At each 6-week interval, they completed measures of negative life events that had occurred during that interval and made retrospective reports of mood for each 2-week period. The first assessment of self-structure came at the outset of the study, which happened to be a high-stress interval for most participants. This assessment coincided with participants' final exams for the first semester of college. The second assessment came, on average, 2 years later, at a time when the number of stressful life events was typically quite low.

Figure 11.2 presents the results of this self-change study, showing mean levels of compartmentalization at time 1 and time 2 for individuals who were either high or low in cognitive vulnerability to depression as a function of whether they reported high levels of major negative life events or only minor negative events at time 1 (first-year final exams). Among individuals who were low in vulnerability to depression but were reporting major negative events at time 1, there was a significant change in type

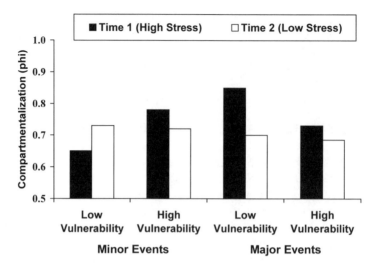

FIGURE 11.2. Self-change study. Mean values of compartmentalization (phi), illustrating change in compartmentalization from time 1 to time 2 for individuals low in cognitive vulnerability to depression who experienced major events at time 1. Data from Showers, Abramson, and Hogan (1998).

of organization from time 1 to time 2, $F(1,75) = 5.86$, $p < .02$. Specifically, these individuals were more compartmentalized when stress was high than when stress was low $(t(13) = 2.71, p < .02)$. With the exception of the low vulnerability, minor events group, there was a tendency for all groups to be more compartmentalized when stress was high than when stress was low.

To understand this result, it is important to recognize that the low vulnerability, major events group may be viewed as unusually good copers. They were experiencing high levels of stress yet had low vulnerability to depression. Although they indeed reported more negative mood at time 1 than at time 2, their mood was not nearly so negative at time 1 as that of the high vulnerability group, who reported similar life events. Moreover, a regression analysis of mood scores for the entire sample at time 1 indicated that, among those who were experiencing high levels of stress, greater compartmentalization was associated with less negative mood.

Although these data are correlational and must be interpreted cautiously, they are consistent with the notion that increases in compartmentalization may be an effective response to stressful life events. Individuals who have the flexibility to change their type of self-organization may experience less negative mood when stressful events occur.

ADDITIONAL EVIDENCE FOR INCREASED
COMPARTMENTALIZATION UNDER STRESS

Findings from a second longitudinal study also suggest that compartmentalization of negative beliefs may help individuals cope when stressful events occur. This study did not examine self-organization but rather the organization of positive and negative beliefs about someone else, namely one's partner in a romantic relationship (Showers, 2000b; Showers & Kevlyn, 1999). Participants in this study had been in an exclusive dating relationship for 3 months or more. They performed the card sorting task to generate a description of their romantic partner at the outset of the study and again 1 year later.[2] The average length of the relationships was 21 months at the outset of the study, and 64% of these relationships were intact at the 1-year follow-up. There were no main effects for change in type of organization over the 1-year period, either for participants who were still together or for those who had ended their relationships. However, at the 1-year follow-up, participants completed measures of the stressors (relationship problems and conflicts) experienced over the past year (until the point of breakup, if that had occurred). Regression analyses indicated that individuals in newer relationships (here, less than 2 years) experiencing high relationship stress showed substantial change in the structure of beliefs about their partner, $\beta = -.53$, $p < .03$. Figure 11.3 illustrates this result. Individuals who described their partners in relatively negative terms showed an increase in compartmentalization from time 1 to time 2 under conditions of high relationship stress.

Follow-up analyses suggested that increases in compartmentalization under these conditions were associated with a greater likelihood of remaining in the relationship and a more positive attitude toward one's partner (greater liking) at time 2, $\beta s > .25$, $p s < .05$. Hence, similar to the self-change study, the findings of the relationship study are consistent with the view that increased compartmentalization may be an effective response to the dual challenges of high relationship stress and a negative perception of one's partner.

Figure 11.3 also shows that two groups shifted to a more integrative type of organization over time. These individuals were in newer relationships and experienced either many negative attributes in their partner or high levels of stress (but not both). Under these moderately negative circumstances, perhaps salient negative beliefs received the extra attention needed for integrative thinking. Follow-up analyses indicated that these changes in partner structure were associated with greater likelihood of staying together (for the high negativity, low stress group) and greater liking (for the low negativity, high stress group). These shifts toward integrative organization are reminiscent of a similar trend ($t(21) = 1.56$,

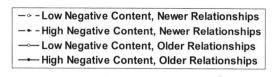

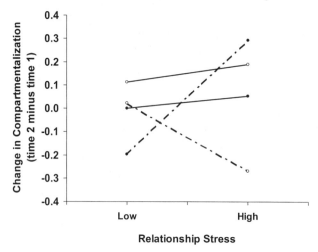

FIGURE 11.3. Relationship study. Change in structure of knowledge about a romantic partner over 1 year as a function of relationship stress, length of relationship, and the negativity of perceptions of the partner. Positive change indicates increased compartmentalization, and negative change indicates increased integration. These are predicted values calculated at 1 *SD* above and below the means. Negative content refers to the proportion of negative attributes in the card sort.

$p < .14$) in the self-change study for individuals with low vulnerability to depression and only minor stressors. These exceptions to the general pattern of increased compartmentalization under stress are discussed below.

WHY INCREASED COMPARTMENTALIZATION MAY BE AN EFFECTIVE RESPONSE TO STRESS

In both the self-change and the relationship studies, change in type of organization under conditions of extreme negativity (and high stress) was in the direction of greater compartmentalization. At first glance, this finding does not seem consistent with the basic model, which suggests that integrative organization should be more effective when negative self-aspects are salient, a condition that is likely to be met under stress. Yet both studies also provided evidence that people who were increasingly compartmentalized under high stress were coping well; that is, they were less depressed in the self-change study and were more likely to stay together in the relationship study. Hence, it seems that compartmentalization may be an effective style of organization in a wider range of contexts than the predictions of the basic model imply. After all, both compartmentalization and integration can be effective strategies for handling negative beliefs. The exact conditions under which one type of organization should be preferred to the other remain to be defined.

With hindsight, two important factors may contribute to the preference for compartmentalization as a response to stress in these studies. First, it is important to consider the relative effort that compartmentalized versus integrative organization entails. Evaluation is a natural basis for categorization (Osgood, 1969), and so compartmentalization may generally require less effort, because attributes of similar valence should be closely linked in an associative network (Bower, 1981; Fiske, 1982; Halberstadt & Niedenthal, 1997). In contrast, integrative organization may require more effort. When a negative belief is activated, spreading activation may prime other similarly valenced beliefs. An individual may have to override the emotional reaction to an initial negative belief in order to activate knowledge that is relevant but positive. Therefore, if integration requires greater cognitive resources, people may act like cognitive misers (Fiske & Taylor, 1984). They may use compartmentalization to the greatest extent possible, exerting the extra effort to create integrative associations only when compartmentalization is no longer successful.[3]

A second reason that compartmentalization may be so pronounced in these studies may have to do with the nature of the stressors (and the negative beliefs that come to mind) for these college student samples. Specifically, the stressors and negative self-beliefs experienced by many college students may be especially easy to compartmentalize. The life events reported by students in the self-change study included problems with course work, professors, friends, and so on. In a college student's very complex life, failing a single course or ending a romantic relationship may be readily compartmentalized while performance in other classes or other social relationships remain intact. Similarly, in the relationship study, college students may find it easier to compartmentalize a romantic partner's negative attributes than would older couples who share a range of long-term adult responsibilities. Thus compartmentalization may be especially effective for the stressors and life contexts of the college-student populations examined in these studies.

EVIDENCE THAT PEOPLE SOMETIMES SHIFT
TOWARD INTEGRATIVE ORGANIZATION

Despite the major findings of the longitudinal studies, there is some evidence that people who are well adjusted can shift from a compartmentalized self-structure to an integrative style of thinking when negative attributes are salient. This evidence seems more consistent with the predictions of the basic model. In one study, participants completed a card sorting task to describe the self as a whole, then performed the paragraph task to describe one of their most negative attributes. The paragraphs were coded for the presence of integrative thoughts. Participants who were positive compartmentalized on the card sort but displayed integrative thinking in their paragraphs were those who reported the least negative mood (McMahon et al., 1999).[4]

It is not surprising that results of the paragraph task are not always consistent with the card sort. The paragraph task necessarily focuses the participant's attention on a negative attribute. Compartmentalization of the attribute (which would minimize the likelihood of activation) is not possible, because the attribute has already been activated. Hence people who handle negative attributes well should display integrative thinking on this task. However, if they have many important positive attributes, they may benefit from a compartmentalized structure for the self as a whole (as measured by the card sort).

Moreover, as indicated previously, evidence that some individuals become more integrative under stress also emerged in both longitudinal studies. In both cases, the groups that displayed this type of change in organization were experiencing circumstances that were only moderately negative. In the self-change study, the individuals who were most integrative under stress were those low in vulnerability to depression and who were experiencing only minor stressors (Showers, Abramson, & Hogan, 1998). In the relationship study, the groups that became integrative under stress were experiencing either a negative perception of their partner or high stress, but not both (Showers, 2000b). One explanation for these trends toward integration is that, at the outset of their respective studies, these groups' perceptions of self or partner were unrealistic. Over time, they added negative attributes or took the time to process those they already knew. Newly discovered negative beliefs may attract a great deal of attention and interest, and individuals may make the effort to incorporate them into a previously unmarred view of self or partner via integrative thinking when circumstances afford that opportunity. Under these conditions, negative beliefs may receive the attention and effort that facilitates integrative processing.

A DYNAMIC MODEL OF SELF-STRUCTURE

A dynamic model of self-structure brings together the results of the longitudinal studies, allowing for both the prevalence of compartmentalization under stress and the exceptional groups that showed shifts toward integration. It also incorporates the idea that integration may require unusual effort and attention and is consistent with the apparent ability of well-adjusted, positive compartmentalized individuals to shift to integrative thinking when they focus on a negative attribute. One theme of this model is that shifts toward integration tend to be short-lived and may emerge primarily when individuals are focusing a great deal of attention on negative attributes. Because maintaining integrative structures may be difficult, many people eventually revert to a compartmentalized style of organization. This dynamic view of self-structure is diagrammed in Figure 11.4.

At the top of Figure 11.4, positive compartmentalization is depicted as the baseline style of organization for most individuals. The assumption is that most people construct self-concepts that are basically positive and construct their lives to maintain relatively low levels of stress. Under these conditions, they take advantage of the effectiveness and efficiency of compartmentalization. From the top, moving down either side of the diagram, Figure 11.4 depicts how self-structures may change when negative attributes become salient (e.g., when stressful events occur).

The left side of the diagram shows the hypothesized shift in self-structure for individuals who are not handling their stress or salient negative attributes especially well. These individuals may shift to a negative compartmentalized style of organization. This shift simply entails a change

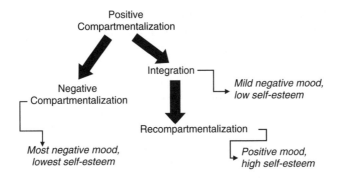

FIGURE 11.4. A dynamic model of self-organization, illustrating how self-structure may change in response to stressful life events.

in the perceived importance of positive and negative self-aspect categories. Along this path, the evaluative structure remains the same, and there is merely a shift from positive compartments being most salient to activation of negative compartments. The leftmost line indicates that such a shift should be associated with extremely low self-esteem and the most negative mood.

The right side of the diagram shows the pattern of change hypothesized for individuals who are coping relatively well with stress or salient negative beliefs. When negative attributes become salient, these individuals may focus attention on them and engage in integrative thinking in an attempt to minimize their impact. However, this effort will use cognitive resources. Individuals who shift to integrative thinking may eventually become worn out both by the difficulty of maintaining integrative thoughts and the continued focus on their negative attributes and beliefs. Thus many individuals may revert to a compartmentalized style of organization. This process may involve recompartmentalizing the stresses or negative attributes that they have experienced; in other words, it may correspond to a restructuring of one's life. As shown by the lower right line, people who succeed in recompartmentalization should be the happiest and experience the highest self-esteem and the greatest psychological well-being.

As an example, consider positive-compartmentalized Harry (Table 11.1). He may cope best if, during final exams, he shifts to an integrative structure that helps to remind him of his scholarly attributes despite his current stress ("I may feel tense about these tests, but I know my intellectual curiosity will return"). However, maintaining that integrative structure throughout the semester would require considerable effort and would promote continued awareness of his negative attributes. If Harry can adopt a positive compartmentalized structure during the semester and shift to an integrative structure during final exams, he may be able to maximize his experience of his positive attributes with minimal cognitive effort.

As the upper right line suggests, however, there may be some individuals who remain committed to integrative styles of thinking. These individuals (1) may actually prefer integrative thinking (i.e., are more practiced and find it less effortful than do others); or (2) may have negative attributes (or negative experiences) that are especially difficult to compartmentalize. For example, the loss of a child or parent or a difficult divorce may make it difficult to segregate attributes of self associated with these events from more positive self-domains. In these cases, integration may be a "best-one-can-do" strategy. The upper right line indicates that individuals who remain integrative will experience some degree of residual negative mood or lower self-esteem as a result of the focus on negative attributes that this style of organization implies. Integration may be preferable to negative compartmentalization with its strong focus on negative attributes, but over the long term it may never compare to positive compartmentalization in terms of feeling good.

DYNAMICS OF SELF-ORGANIZATION: A DIFFERENT VIEW

Recently, Nowak, Vallacher, Tesser, and Borkowski (2000) performed computer simulations of the dynamic process of self-organization. In their view, self-integration is a process motivated by a press toward greater self-organization. Integration resolves evaluative inconsistencies between related items of self-knowledge, leading to a self-structure that has local areas of evaluative coherence (much like the compartmentalized structures described here). This dynamic systems view of self is consistent with Showers's dynamic model in that it implies a general preference for compartmentalized structures (i.e., the press toward greater self-organization). Nowak et al. also characterize the self-system as a dynamic equilibrium, which fits the process described here of temporarily shifting from a baseline compartmentalized structure to a more integrative one, followed by a return to the baseline structure when possible. Moreover, according to their model, some individuals who have a weak press for self-organization could maintain a structure with low evaluative coherence, like those individuals identified here as integrative.[5]

LONG-TERM SELF-CHANGE

The emphasis here on the transience of integrative structures does not mean that long-term change in self-organization does not occur. One possibility is that the nature of stressful experiences over the life span tends to facilitate the development of integrative thinking either as a cumulative response to life stress or in response to rare traumatic events. Psychological treatment may increase flexibility by encouraging clients to develop an alternative structure or style of thinking (i.e., compartmentalization or integration, whichever one they do not use). So far, the stability of evaluative organization in college students appears to be moderate. In the 2-year self-change study, Showers, Abramson, and Hogan (1998) found that the test–retest reliability for compartmentalization over 22 months was $r = .56$ ($n= 79$; individuals selected for high and low cognitive vulnerability to depression). In contrast, for these individuals' DI scores, $r = .07$; for the proportion of negative attributes in the card sort, $r = .71$.[6] Future work should examine non–college-student samples that represent the entire lifespan, testing both the stability of self-structure and the possibility that integrative organization is a more common response to stresses experienced after college than is indicated by the college-student data reported here.

SUMMARY

To date, the literature on self-structure has demonstrated both good stability in self-organization (consistent with a higher order view of personality) and the possibility of self-change. Because self-structure is so fundamental to cognition, emotion, and motivation, it may be appropriate to expand the notion of situation-behavior profiles (Mischel & Shoda, 1995) to situation-structure-behavior profiles. The dynamic model proposed here describes a characteristic pattern of structural change that corresponds to the changing salience of negative attributes, such as might occur under stress. However, on closer inspection, the changes observed should be idiographic, with some individuals increasing their compartmentalization under stress and others shifting toward integrative styles. It is important to be mindful that both compartmentalization and integration are effective strategies for handling negative beliefs. Ultimately, the researcher's task is to understand how individuals choose the type of organization that best fits their current circumstances and their organizational strategies.

NOTES

1. This sample came from the Cognitive Vulnerability to Depression Study, funded by National Institute of Mental Health Grant 1R01MH43866, awarded to Lyn Y. Abramson, and National Institute of Mental Health Grant 1R01MH48216, awarded to Lauren B. Alloy. Collection of the self-organization data described here was supported by National Institute of Mental Health Fellowship F32MH10058 and funds from the University of Wisconsin Graduate School, awarded to Carolin J. Showers.
2. Analyses of the card sorting data at time 1 are reported by Showers and Kevlyn (1999).
3. The findings of Showers and Kling (1996a) are consistent with the notion that integrative thinking requires greater cognitive resources than compartmentalization. In Study 2, participants exposed to a sad mood induction either completed the Twenty Statements Test (focusing attention on the self) or performed complex arithmetic problems (distraction) while recovering from the sad mood. Evaluative organization of the self had been assessed at a prior session. Those individuals with an integrative self-structure recovered more quickly from the sad mood, but only in the self-focused condition.

4. The participants in this study (McMahon et al., 1999) were females who had been screened on measures of disordered eating and body dissatisfaction. There were three groups: Positive Beliefs (low body dissatisfaction, no disordered eating); Dissatisfied (high body dissatisfaction, no disordered eating); and Disordered (high body dissatisfaction, disordered eating). Most of the participants who displayed the combination of positive compartmentalization on the card sort and high integration on the paragraph task were from the Positive Beliefs group.

5. Note that in Nowak et al.'s model, the process of integration is said to resolve evaluative inconsistencies, leading to a coherent (compartmentalized) structure. In Showers's model, integrative thinking preserves the evaluative inconsistency of individual items of self-knowledge, leading to coherence only at the category level. Whereas in the former model, evaluative inconsistencies imply a disorganized self, in the latter model, integrative self-structures are considered to be highly organized.

6. Here, differential importance is calculated by correlating importance and positivity–negativity ratings across each individual's card sort groups. This measure may be less reliable than the DI scores generated by the Self-Attributes Questionnaire (Pelham & Swann, 1989), which asks about 10 nomothetic self-domains.

REFERENCES

Baumeister, R. F. (1998). The self. In D. T. Gilbert, S. T. Fiske, & G. Lindzey (Eds.), *The handbook of social psychology* (Vol. 1, 4th ed. pp. 680–740). New York: McGraw-Hill.

Bower, G. H. (1981). Mood and memory. *American Psychologist, 36,* 129–148.

Cantor, N., & Kihlstrom, J. F. (1987). *Personality and social intelligence.* Englewood Cliffs, NJ: Prentice-Hall.

Cantor, N., Markus, H., Niedenthal, P., & Nurius, P. (1986). On motivation and the self-concept. In R. M. Sorrentino & E. T. Higgins (Eds.), *Handbook of motivation and cognition: Foundations of social behavior* (pp. 96–121). New York: Guilford Press.

Cervone, D., & Shoda, Y. (1999a). Beyond traits in the study of personality coherence. *Current Directions in Psychological Science, 8,* 27–32.

Cervone, D., & Shoda, Y. (Eds.). (1999b). *The coherence of personality: Social-cognitive bases of consistency, variability, and organization.* New York: Guilford Press.

Cramer, H. (1974). *Mathematical methods of statistics.* Princeton, NJ: Princeton University Press. (Original work published 1945)

Dutton, K. A., & Brown, J. D. (1997). Global self-esteem and specific self-views as determinants of people's reactions to success and failure. *Journal of Personality and Social Psychology, 73,* 139–148.

Everitt, B. S. (1977). *The analysis of contingency tables.* London: Chapman & Hall.

Fiske, S. T. (1982). Schema-triggered affect: Applications to social perception. In M. S. Clark & S. T. Fiske (Eds.), *Affect and cognition* (pp. 55–78). Hillsdale, NJ: Erlbaum.

Fiske, S. T., & Taylor, S. E. (1984). *Social cognition.* New York: Random House.

Halberstadt, J. B., & Niedenthal, P. M. (1997). Emotional state and the use of stimulus dimensions in judgment. *Journal of Personality and Social Psychology, 72,* 1017–1033.

Harter, S. (1999). *The construction of the self: A developmental perspective.* New York: Guilford Press.

James, W. (1890). *The principles of psychology.* New York: Henry Holt.

Kendall, P. C., Howard, B. L., & Hays, R. C. (1989). Self-referent speech and psychopathology: The balance of positive and negative thinking. *Cognitive Therapy and Research, 13,* 583–598.

Kernberg, O. F. (1984). *Object relations theory and clinical psychoanalysis.* New York: Aronson.

Markus, H., & Nurius, P. (1987). Possible selves. *American Psychologist, 41,* 954–969.

Markus, H., & Wurf, E. (1987). The dynamic self-concept: A social psychological perspective. *Annual Review of Psychology, 38,* 299–337.

Marsh, H. W., Byrne, B. M., & Shavelson, R. J. (1992). A multidimensional, hierarchical self-concept. In T. M. Brinthaupt & R. P. Lipka (Eds.), *The self: Definitional and methodological issues* (pp. 44–95). Albany, NY: State University of New York Press.

McMahon, P. D., Showers, C. J., Rieder, S. L., Abramson, L. Y., & Hogan, M. E. (1999). *Integrative thinking and flexibility in the organization of self-knowledge.* Unpublished manuscript.

Mischel, W. (1973). Toward a cognitive social learning reconceptualization of personality. *Psychological Review, 80,* 252–283.

Mischel, W., & Shoda, Y. (1995). A cognitive-affective system theory of personality: Reconceptualizing situations, dispositions, dynamics, and invariance in personality structure. *Psychological Review, 102,* 246–268.

Nowak, A., Vallacher, R. R., Tesser, A., & Borkowski, W. (2000). Society of self: The emergence of collective properties in self-structure. *Psychological Review, 107,* 39–61.

Osgood, C. E. (1969). On the whys and wherefores of E, P, and A. *Journal of Personality and Social Psychology, 12,* 194–199.

Pelham, B. W. (1991). On confidence and consequence: The certainty and importance of self-knowledge. *Journal of Personality and Social Psychology, 60,* 518–530.

Pelham, B. W., & Swann, W. B., Jr. (1989). From self-conceptions to self-worth: On the sources and structure of global self-esteem. *Journal of Personality and Social Psychology, 57,* 672–680.

Rosenberg, M. (1965). *Society and the adolescent self-image.* Princeton, NJ: Princeton University Press.

Schwartz, R. M., & Garamoni, G. L. (1986). A structural model of positive and negative states of mind: Asymmetry in the internal dialogue. *Advances in Cognitive Behavioral Research and Therapy, 5,* 1–62.

Showers, C. (1992a). Compartmentalization of positive and negative self-knowledge: Keeping bad apples out of the bunch. *Journal of Personality and Social Psychology, 62,* 1036–1049.

Showers, C. (1992b). Evaluatively integrative thinking about characteristics of the self. *Personality and Social Psychology Bulletin, 18,* 719–729.

Showers, C. J. (1995). The evaluative organization of self-knowledge. In M. Kernis (Ed.), *Efficacy, agency, and self-esteem* (pp. 101–120). New York: Plenum Press.

Showers, C. J. (2000a). Self-organization in emotional contexts. In J. P. Forgas (Ed.), *Feeling and thinking: The role of affect in cognition and judgments* (pp. 283–307). Paris: Cambridge University Press.

Showers, C. J. (2000b, July). *Social-cognitive perspectives on the dynamic self: The organization of self-knowledge.* Paper presented at the 10th European Conference on Personality, ECP10, Cracow, Poland.

Showers, C. J., Abramson, L. Y., & Hogan, M. E. (1998). The dynamic self: How the content and structure of the self-concept change with mood. *Journal of Personality and Social Psychology, 75,* 478–493.

Showers, C. J., & Kevlyn, S. B. (1999). Organization of knowledge about a relationship partner: Implications for liking and loving. *Journal of Personality and Social Psychology, 76,* 958–971.

Showers, C. J, & Kling, K. C. (1996a). Organization of self-knowledge: Implications for recovery from sad mood. *Journal of Personality and Social Psychology, 70,* 578–590.

Showers, C. J., & Kling, K. C. (1996b). The organization of self-knowledge: Implications for mood regulation. In L. L. Martin & A. Tesser (Eds.), *Striving and feeling: Interactions among goals, affect, and self-regulation* (pp. 151–174). Mahwah, NJ: Erlbaum.

Showers, C. J., McMahon, P. D., Sutton, S. K., & Davidson, R. J. (1998). *Cognitive compensations for negative mood: The interplay of self-structure and brain activation.* Unpublished manuscript.

Showers, C. J., & Ryff, C. D. (1996). Self-differentiation and well-being in a life transition. *Personality and Social Psychology Bulletin, 22,* 448–460.

Showers, C. J., & Zeigler-Hill, V. (in press). Organization of self-knowledge: Features, functions, and flexibility. In M. R. Leary & J. P. Tangney (Eds.), *Handbook of self and identity.* New York: Guilford Press.

Tesser, A., & Martin, L. (1996). The psychology of evaluation. In E. T. Higgins & A. W. Kruglanski (Eds.), *Social psychology: Handbook of basic principles* (pp. 400–432). New York: Guilford Press.

CHAPTER 12

The Emergence of Personality
Personal Stability through Interpersonal Synchronization

ANDRZEJ NOWAK
ROBIN R. VALLACHER
MICHAL ZOCHOWSKI

Humans revel in their uniqueness. They profess disdain for conformity and dependence on others, preferring to think of themselves instead in terms of personal abilities, talents, interests, and traits that distinguish them from their social surround. Yet humans are undeniably among the most social of animals, spending the majority of their time in the presence of other people, thinking about and interacting with them in one way or another, with interludes of true solitude being few and far between. Considerable theory and research have documented the overarching importance of interdependence, social support, and intimacy to virtually every indicator of subjective well-being (e.g., Baumeister & Leary, 1995; Myers & Diener, 1995; Rogers, 1961; Zimbardo, 1977). It is doubtful, in fact, that humans could have survived as a species in our ancestral environment, let alone risen to preeminent status in the animal kingdom, were it not for their propensity for social coordination (e.g., Caporael & Brewer, 1995). The idealization of individuality may seem out of touch with the reality of social embeddedness, but in a fundamental sense these two pillars of psychology are mutually reinforcing. The propensity for coordinating with others plays a key role in creating individuality, and the distinct personalities that are shaped in this fashion constrain the nature of social interactions and hone relationship preferences. Our aim in this chapter is to delineate the nature of this reciprocal linkage between social coordination and individual variation.

We begin by reframing social interaction in terms of synchronization, a phenomenon central to the study of nonlinear dynamical systems. The core idea is that individuals are not static or passive entities but rather can be viewed as separate systems capable of displaying complex patterns of thought and behavior over time. In social interaction, mutual influence between the individual systems promotes synchronization of their respective dynamics, resulting in a higher order system (e.g., a dyad) with its own dynamic properties. In essence, the individuals establish a common rhythm or temporal pattern of thought and behavior. To achieve synchronization, each individual adjusts the internal states responsible for his or her own dynamics. With repeated episodes of the synchronization process, each individual's setting of internal parameters becomes increasingly engraved in his or her system, thereby creating a particular propensity for social interaction. In effect, these settings constitute a latent structure of personality that fosters both uniqueness and stability in the surface structure of interpersonal behavior.

To test the assumptions and implications of this scenario, we introduce a formal model of synchronization based on the interaction or "coupling" of separate dynamical systems. Each system, representing an individual, has its own dynamic tendency, which is regulated by the setting of a control factor for the system. When coupled, the separate systems adjust their respective control factors—which represent individuals' internal states—in an attempt to achieve a synchronized temporal pattern in their behavior. Computer simulations of this scenario are employed to investigate the development of stable internal states through social relations, the role of personality in shaping social interaction, and the conditions fostering expression of individual differences in interpersonal contexts. In a concluding section, we summarize the implications and benefits of framing personality and social interaction in terms of synchronization dynamics. We suggest that conceptualizing social interaction as the progressive coordination of separate dynamical systems provides insight into several perennial issues in personality theory and serves as a useful heuristic for charting new lines of research concerning the interplay between the individual and his or her social context.

SYNCHRONIZATION IN SOCIAL RELATIONSHIPS

If there is anything worse than being physically isolated from other people, it is being socially isolated while surrounded by others. The mere presence of others is clearly not sufficient to satisfy basic social needs. Rather, people strive to have meaningful interactions, engage in common action, and exchange thoughts and feelings. Interpersonal experiences do not have to be verbal in nature, nor do they have to be pleasant or otherwise positive—although that it is no doubt preferable—for people to feel connected to others. Even an asymmetric power relationship, in which one is consistently in the weaker or more dependent position, may be preferable to having no relationship at all. The defining feature of any relationship—whether a momentary interaction or a long-term relationship—is some degree of temporal coordination among the words, gestures, and actions of the people involved. A simple conversation, for example, is defined in terms of turn-taking in speaking and the coordination of various nonverbal cues, such as gestures, bodily movements, and eye contact. Two individuals talking on their respective cell phones to different people, for example, can hardly be described as having a meaningful interaction, even if they are standing shoulder to shoulder. Although both are engaged in the same activity and occupy the same physical space, their respective words and gestures are completely decoupled and devoid of meaningful coordination.

The Nature of Synchronization

The significance of social interaction has hardly been lost on psychologists. To a large extent, however, interactions and relationships have been conceptualized in terms of global properties that characterize the interaction or relationship as a whole. Thus dyadic and group interactions are commonly investigated with respect to such dimensions as cooperation versus competition, compatibility of goals and motives, the suspension of self-interest, and the structure of roles and norms (e.g., Biddle & Thomas, 1966; Dawes, 1980; Levine & Moreland, 1998; Berkowitz & Walster, 1976; Wish, Deutsch, & Kaplan, 1976). In approaches that emphasize the temporal evolution of social interactions, the focus is usually restricted to the development of strategies for achieving personal or social goals (e.g., Axelrod, 1984; Messick & Liebrand, 1995; Thibaut & Kelley, 1959). Interpersonal behavior, however, involves the temporal coordination of behavior at divergent levels of analysis, from basic movements and utterances to broad action categories reflecting momentary goals and long-range plans. Even something as elemental as leaving a room, after all, requires that the room's occupants coordinate their physical movements so as not to stumble over each other. As group action becomes more complex, the ability of group members to coordinate their activities in time becomes correspondingly more important.

To distinguish the dynamic aspects of coordination from its conventional interpretation, we employ the term *synchronization*. Synchronization refers to the fact that the actions, thoughts, and feelings of one person are temporally related to the actions, thoughts, and feelings of one or more other people. Synchronization may arise as a result of mutual influence in social interaction but also may be the result of each individual reacting in a similar fashion to a salient external factor, such as an outside person (e.g., a speaker), music, threats, and so forth. Synchronization can take different forms. Perhaps the most basic form is positive correlation, such that the overt behaviors, attitudes, or emotions of one person induce similar behaviors or states in the other person. Imitation and empathy epitomize this form of synchronization. Synchronization can also be manifested as negative correlation. In an antagonistic relationship, for instance, the sadness of one person might induce satisfaction in the other and vice versa. Synchronization can also take on more complex forms that reflect nonlinear relationships and higher order interactions between the partners' respective behaviors and internal states (see Nowak & Vallacher, 1998; Nowak, Vallacher, & Borkowski, 2000). Sometimes the synchronization that characterizes a relationship may be sufficiently subtle and complex to confuse observers or perhaps the partners themselves.

In its most basic form, synchronization refers to the coupling of behavior patterns, with particular emphasis on movement coordination (e.g., Beek & Hopkins, 1992; Newtson, 1994; Rosenblum & Turvey, 1988; Schmidt, Beek, Treffner, & Turvey, 1991; Turvey, 1990). Pairs of individuals, for example, might simply be asked to swing their legs. One person swings his or her legs in time to a metronome and the other person tries to match those movements. This simple paradigm reveals several phenomena concerning synchronization of individuals' movements. First, synchronization may be in phase, with people swinging their legs in unison, or in antiphase, with people swinging their legs with the same frequency but in the opposite direction. Second, hysteresis is commonly observed. When participants are instructed to synchronize out of phase and the frequency of movement increases, at some tempo they are no longer able to synchronize antiphase and they switch their synchronization mode to in phase. When the tempo decreases again, at some value they are able to coordinate out of phase again, but this tempo is significantly lower than the point at which they originally started to synchronize in phase. The appearance of hysteresis shows that coordination in movement can be analyzed as a nonlinear dynamical system (cf. Kelso, 1995). The crucial variable in this case is the tempo of movement. Yet more complex modes of coordination have been captured in this line of research (cf. Baron, Amazeen, & Beek, 1994; Kelso, 1995; Turvey, 1990).

These seemingly simple findings may be reflected in more complex social situations. When the tempo of behavior is increased, such as in a high stress or panic situation, it may prove impossible for people to co-ordinate their respective behaviors in any other than an in-phase manner. In a crowded disco that suddenly bursts into flames, for example, it may be impossible for people to take turns leaving the room, although that is the only mode of coordination that would make evacuation possible. Instead, everyone tries to match the behavior of everyone else, thus pre-venting more complex modes of coordination from developing. In simi-lar fashion, it may be difficult for members of a dyad to take turns in speaking in a stressful or otherwise emotion-inducing situation. Argu-ments have this quality, of course, but so do contexts defined in terms of excitement, anticipation, and other positive forms of affect.

Synchronization in Relationships

Any two people picked at random can usually manage to synchronize with respect to rudimentary movements, such as leg swinging, clapping, and exiting rooms (e.g., Dittman & Llewellyn, 1969). Synchronization for these individuals, however, is likely to become more difficult as the ac-tion in question becomes more complex. It may be impossible, for ex-ample, for two unacquainted people to synchronize their efforts suffi-ciently to assemble a mechanical device or create a piece of art. The ability to synchronize in more complex modes requires at least some semblance of concordance in the requisite internal states of each person. Thus, in assembling the mechanical device, each person should have similar or complementary knowledge and a common plan, and in creating a piece of art each person should have similar esthetic preferences. Even synchro-nization with respect to simple spontaneous acts in social interaction is facilitated by similarity in internal states (e.g., Tickle-Degnen & Rosenthal, 1987). Whether two people can joke around effectively, for example, will depend on their respective moods and humor preferences. Such synchro-nization might be next to impossible if one person has just viewed "Spinal Tap" while the other person has been busy reviewing the Sierra Club's latest list of ozone-destroying agents.

The importance of similarity in facilitating synchronization is ap-parent with respect to stable characteristics such as attitudes, values, talents, temperament, and personality traits. Indeed, similarity with re-spect to such characteristics has been shown consistently to be among the strongest preconditions for interpersonal attraction (cf. Byrne, Clore, & Smeaton, 1986; Newcomb, 1961). By the same token, individuals avoid forming relationships with people who appear to be different from them in their personal characteristics (e.g., Rosenbaum, 1986). The significance of similarity to synchronization potential, and hence to interpersonal attraction, applies as well to transient internal states such as moods, momentary motives, and current concerns. When in a good mood, a person may be disinclined to seek out someone who is ruminating over his or her most recent setbacks in life. A despondent person, in turn, may keep his or her distance from other people who are busy savoring their successes.

There are occasions in which a person is motivated to interact with another person despite perceived dissimilarity in their respective internal states. For that matter, circumstances sometimes mandate interactions with dissimilar others, whether or not the person desires such contact. Under these conditions, people are often capable of adjusting their internal state to maximize the likelihood of achieving synchronization with their interaction partners. This ability underlies people's potential for empathy and perspective taking in social relations. Research has demonstrated that people sometimes prepare themselves for social interaction by changing their internal state to match the anticipated state of the interaction partner, even if this means toning down a positive mood in favor of a more subdued one (e.g., Erber, Wegner, & Thierrault, 1996).

Not all internal states, however, are equally amenable to this process. Some internal states of interaction partners are difficult, if not impossible, to observe directly (cf. Jones & Davis, 1965). Moods and emotions are easy to detect, for example, but mood volatility is difficult to discern from a single observation. Attempts to match someone's mood based on faulty assumptions can clearly hinder the development of long-term synchronization with the person. Even if someone's internal state is readily detectable, it may prove difficult to modify one's own state to match it. It is hard to change one's cognitive style or temperament, for example, regardless of how pragmatic it would be do so in preparing for an interaction with someone whose way of thinking and tempo of expression is markedly different from one's own. There is evidence, for example, that differences in temperament can hinder effective emotional and behavioral coordination (e.g., Dunn & Plomin, 1990). In this sense, personality sets constraints on social interaction. People's stable characteristics—traits, values, and the like—bias the choice of interaction partners and dictate the likely success of establishing relationships with those who are chosen.

But one can look at the process in reverse to ask how social interactions shape personality. Personality, after all, comes from somewhere. To be sure, a wide variety of individual differences can be traced to genetics, but even in these cases considerable variance remains to be explained—presumably in terms of social forces. We propose that individual differences are shaped by the history of social interactions. In such interactions, individuals set their internal states to synchronize with others. To the extent that these interactions are sustained over time, the associated internal settings become engraved in the person's cognitive–affective system. These engraved settings operate as ready parameters for subsequent interactions, thus promoting efficiency in one's social relations.

We suggest that a person's stable internal settings function as equilibrium values in the person's cognitive–affective system. This means that these settings represent stable states to which the system returns if perturbed by external factors. A highly optimistic person, for example, may experience deep sadness in reaction to a bad life event, but over time such a person will engage in a variety of mechanisms—both adaptive (e.g., seeking social support, reframing the event in terms of its potential for personal growth) and defensive (e.g., denial, rationalization)—that function to reinstate his or her optimistic style. A person with depressive tendencies, on the other hand, will more readily embrace the bad news, avoiding opportunities to become comforted and even seeking further news that would support the negative view triggered by the initial event. So although both the optimistic and depressed individuals can experience both happy and sad states, these states are psychologically reversed in terms of their transient, as opposed to attracting, equilibrium qualities.

This proposed reciprocal relationship between personality and social interactions has intuitive appeal, but the mechanisms responsible for it are unclear. To provide the missing precision, we propose a computational model of interpersonal synchronization that incorporates basic principles forthcoming from the work on nonlinear dynamical systems. We present the results of computer simulations that test the viability of key assumptions in the model and hypotheses regarding the relationship between personality and the history of interpersonal synchronization.

A FORMAL MODEL OF SYNCHRONIZATION

Synchronization is critical for the function of biological and physical systems (cf. Glass & Mackey, 1988; Haken, 1982; Turvey, 1990). Synchronization underlies such physical phenomena, for example, as laser pulsation (e.g., Haken, 1982) and autocatalysis in chemical reactions (e.g., Prigogine & Stengers, 1984). With respect to biological systems, there is evidence that the generation of coherent mental states from neural activity is critically dependent on the synchronization of neural assemblies in the brain (e.g., Tononi & Edelman, 1998). Even the functioning of a single neuron depends on the synchronization in the opening and closing of ion channels (e.g., Lowen, Liebovitch, & White, 1999). The remarkable feature of synchronization in these cases is that the elements in question (e.g., physical particles, neurons, ion channels) tend to synchronize by virtue of their mutual influences without the control of a higher order agent. This propensity for self-organization has been extensively modeled in physics and mathematics as the "coupling" of separate dynamical systems.

These features of synchronization provide the foundation for a formal model of personality and social interaction. In essence, the model envisions social interaction as a vehicle for coupling the dynamics of individuals. Each individual brings his or her personal dynamic tendencies to social interaction and attempts to synchronize these tendencies with his or her interaction partner. As a result of these attempts, social interaction revises the settings for each individual, or engraves entirely new settings, which then provide the foundation for subsequent social interactions. In principle, this reciprocal relation between settings of internal parameters and social interaction iterates continuously throughout social life. In reality, the engravings of some tendencies are likely to become particularly stable and thus resistant to modification in the ordinary course of social encounters. To set the stage for the formal model, we describe next the essence of nonlinear dynamical systems and the potential for synchronization of such systems that results from their coupling.

Humans as Nonlinear Dynamical Systems

The approach of dynamical systems was developed in mathematics and the physical sciences to provide formalisms regarding the nature of change over time of phenomena. Hence, to explain any process of change is tantamount to identifying the equations characterizing the change. In this sense, the notion of dynamical systems refers to a set of equations describing a system's dynamics. In a less formal sense, a dynamical system is a set of interconnected elements that undergo change by virtue of their mutual influences. In the absence of external influences, a dynamical system may display a pattern of sustained change in some system-level property that reflects the mutual adjustment of elements at each moment in time. Although dynamical systems have been the primary tool for describing processes in the physical and natural sciences for centuries, only recently have scholars discovered that very simple rules of interaction among system elements can produce highly complex dynamics on the system level, provided the interactions are nonlinear in nature. In a nonlinear system, the effects of changes in one variable are not reflected in a proportional manner in other variables. The relations among variables, moreover, usually depend on the values of other variables in the system, and thus are interactive in nature (cf. Nowak & Lewenstein, 1994; Schuster, 1984).

Perhaps the most remarkable discovery emanating from the investigation of nonlinear dynamical systems was that the behavior of such systems does not depend on the nature of the specific system in question but rather reflects invariant principles that transcend traditional scientific boundaries (cf. Schuster, 1984). Thus laser pulsation, chemical reactions, weather patterns, and heart rate dynamics all share common properties despite the enormous differences in the elements and variables associated with each phenomenon. Because of this potential for capturing general features of change, the nonlinear dynamical systems approach has become increasingly popular in the neural, behavioral, and social sciences. This approach, in fact, has demonstrated considerable utility in capturing the dynamism and complexity inherent in a wide variety of psychological and social processes, including political behavior (e.g., Hegselman, Troitzch, & Muller, 1996), organizational behavior (Axelrod & Cohen, 1999), cognitive processes (cf. Port & van Gelder, 1995), human development (e.g., Fischer & Bidell, 1997; Thelen & Smith, 1994; van Geert, 1991), and social psychological phenomena (cf. Arrow, McGrath, & Berdahl, 2000; Guastello, 1995; Nowak & Vallacher, 1998; Read & Miller, 1998; Smith, 1996; Vallacher & Nowak, 1994, 1997).

Humans are clearly dynamical systems in the sense that they display change over time. The abundance of interactions among variables underlying psychological phenomena, meanwhile, clearly indicates that humans are nonlinear systems. Yet the enormous complexity of human thought and behavior would seem to render the modeling of human systems in their entirety an impossible task. As it happens, however, the qualitative behavior of a nonlinear system does not depend on the nature of the elements that compose the system or on precise specification of all the factors that influence the system. Rather, the system's qualitative behavior usually depends on the nature of the interactions among a small set of variables that are critical for describing the system's behavior. In this sense, the nonlinear dynamical systems approach typically concentrates on building models that describe the most important relations among elements. Such models of qualitative understanding are ideally suited to capture the fundamental dynamic properties of even quite complex systems.

All dynamical systems are composed of a set of *dynamical variables* (x) that change in time, and one or more *control parameters* (r) that play a decisive role in influencing the dynamical variables. The simplest dynamical system capable of complex (e.g., chaotic) behavior is the logistic map (Feigenbaum, 1978; Schuster, 1984). The logistic map involves repeated iteration, which is basic to all discrete dynamical systems. This simply means that the output value of the dynamical variable (x) at one step (n) is used as the input value at the next step $(n + 1)$. In other words, the current value of the dynamical variable (which varies between 0 and 1) depends on the variable's previous value—that is, $x_{n+1} = f(x_n)$. The logistic map represents this dependency in two opposing ways. First, the higher the previous value, the higher the current value—specifically, x_{n+1} equals x_n multiplied by the value of r. Second, the higher the previous value, the lower the current value—specifically, x_{n+1} equals $(1- x_n)$ multiplied by the value of r. The combined effect of these two forces is represented in the logistic map and is expressed as $x_{n+1} = rx_n(1- x_n)$, where x_{n+1} is the value of a dynamical variable at one time, x_n is the value of the same variable at the preceding time, and r is the control parameter (the crucial variable influencing changes of x over time). Depending on the value of r, the logistic equation may display qualitatively different patterns of behavior (i.e., patterns of changes in x), such as convergence on a single value, oscillatory (periodic) changes between two or more values, and very complex patterns of evolution resembling randomness (i.e., deterministic chaos). These patterns are invariant in a host of systems that transcend traditional topical boundaries in science (cf. Gleick, 1987).

With respect to modeling human dynamics, the dynamical variable (x) can be interpreted as behavior. Changes in x thus reflect variation in the intensity of behavior. The control parameter, r, corresponds to internal states (e.g., personality traits, moods, values, etc.) that shape the person's pattern of behavior (i.e., changes in x over time). The representation of opposing forces in the equation epitomizes the idea of conflict, a key concept in many theoretical treatments of psychological process. In the approach–avoid situation (Miller, 1944), for example, movement toward a goal increases both approach and avoidance tendencies. In analogous fashion, the work on achievement motivation (e.g., Atkinson, 1964) has identified two concerns, the desire for success and the fear of failure, that combine in different ways to produce resultant motivation. Theory and research on the dynamics of suppression, meanwhile, suggest that attempts at action suppression activate an ironic process that works at cross-purposes with the attempted suppression (cf. Wegner, 1994). It is fair to say, in fact, that most theories and issues in psychology are defined in terms of conflicting tendencies or forces (e.g., impulse vs. self-control, autonomy vs. social identity, short-term vs. long-term self-interest, egoism vs. altruism). The logistic equation captures this basic feature of human systems and provides insight into the internally generated dynamics that result from the operation of conflicting forces and processes.

It is important to note that the logistic equation is generic in form, is intended to reflect basic processes involving the conjunction of conflicting forces, and does not depend on specific identities of x and r. Thus x can refer to behavior at various levels of identification, from simple movements to broad action categories, each of which may be associated with a correspondingly different time scale (e.g., seconds vs. days). The identity of r is similarly flexible and can refer to a wide variety of internal states, from momentary concerns and moods to basic dimensions of temperament and personality. The key point is that a person described by this simple equation can display a pattern of changes in behavior without any influence from outside. In this view, external factors do not induce activity in an otherwise passive person but rather exert their influence by modifying the person's *intrinsic dynamics*—his or her internally generated patterns of behavior (cf. Nowak & Vallacher, 1998).

Social Interaction as the Coupling of Nonlinear Dynamical Systems

If two dynamical systems signal their respective states to each other, their activity tends to become synchronized such that they display the same pattern of changes in their system-level properties (Kaneko, 1989, 1993; Shinbrot, 1994). Two pendulums suspended from a common cable, for example, tend to become synchronized in their respective rhythms if their respective strings are the same length. This happens because the movement of each pendulum gets transmitted to the other by virtue of the common cable. The potential for self-organized synchronization is not limited to oscillatory behavior but also characterizes nonlinear dynamical systems capable of producing very complex temporal patterns of behavior (e.g., deterministic chaos). This property provides a useful prototype for understanding the synchronization underlying various collective processes in physics, chemistry, and biology (cf. Shinbrot, 1994).

Against this backdrop, coupled logistic maps can be used to model the synchronization of people in social interaction (Nowak & Vallacher, 1998; Nowak, Vallacher, & Borkowski, 2000). The dynamics of each interaction partner are represented by a logistic equation. To capture interpersonal synchronization, the behavior of each person not only depends on his or her preceding state but also on the preceding state of the other person. Formally, such influence is introduced by the assumption that the behavior of each partner at a given moment depends to a certain degree on the behavior of the other partner at the preceding moment. The coupling is done in a simple way, according to the following equation:

$$x_1(t+1) = \frac{r_1 x_1(t)(1-x_1(t)) + \alpha r_2 x_2(t)(1-x_2(t))}{1+\alpha}$$

$$x_2(t+1) = \frac{r_2 x_2(t)(1-x_2(t)) + \alpha r_1 x_1(t)(1-x_1(t))}{1+\alpha}$$

To the value of the dynamical variable representing one person's behavior (x_1), one adds a fraction, denoted by α, of the value of the dynamical variable representing the behavior of the other person (x_2). The size of this fraction (α) corresponds to the strength of coupling and reflects the mutual interdependency of the relationship. When the fraction is 0, there is no coupling on the behavior level. When the fraction is 1, each person's behavior is determined equally by his or her preceding behavior and the preceding behavior of the other person. Intermediate values of this fraction correspond to intermediate values of coupling.

Modeling the Synchronization of Behavior

When the control parameters in a coupled system have the same value, the dependence between the respective dynamical variables causes the maps to fully synchronize, so that the values of x_1 and x_2 become identical (Kaneko, 1993). Obviously, the respective control parameters of two individuals are rarely, if ever, identical, nor do all relationships have the same degree of interdependence. In computer simulations (Nowak & Vallacher, 1998), we systematically varied the similarity of partners' control parameters (r), representing their internal states, and their degree of coupling (α), representing partners' mutual influence (e.g., intensity of communication). For each simulation, we started from a random value of x for each person, drawn from a uniform distribution that varied from 0 to 1. We let the two coupled systems run for 300 steps, so that each system had a chance to come close to its pattern of intrinsic dynamics and both systems had a chance to synchronize. For the next 500 simulation steps, we recorded the values of x for each system and measured the degree of synchronization.

   The main results were straightforward. In general, the degree of synchronization between partners' behaviors increased both with α and similarity in r. This implies that similarity in internal states and interdependence can compensate for one another in achieving or maintaining a given level of synchronization. For two people to achieve a high degree of synchronization, then, relatively little coupling is necessary if their respective control parameters are similar. Conversely, if the partners are different in their respective internal states, high mutual influence (constant monitoring, communication, mutual reinforcement, etc.) is necessary to maintain the same level of synchronization. Results also revealed that for very low values of coupling, the two systems evolved independently, but that for relatively weak coupling, complex forms of synchronization were achieved. Interestingly, for moderate values of coupling, the systems tended to stabilize one another's behavior, such that each system behaved in a considerably more regular manner than it would have without the coupling (cf. Ott, Grebogi, & York, 1990).[1]

Modeling the Synchronization of Internal States

Modeling the direct synchronization of control parameters is relatively straightforward. One need only assume that on each simulation step, the value of each person's control parameter drifts somewhat in the direction of the value of the partner's control parameter. The rate of this drift and the size of the initial discrepancy between the values of the respective control parameters determine how quickly the control parameters begin to match. This mechanism assumes that both interaction partners can directly estimate the settings of one another's control parameters. In many types of relationships, considerable effort may be focused on communicating or inferring these settings (cf. Jones & Davis, 1965; Kunda, 1999; Nisbett & Ross, 1980; Wegner & Vallacher, 1977). Even with such effort, however, the exact values of the relevant control parameters may be difficult or impossible to determine.

Control parameters can also become synchronized through behavioral coordination. Research concerning the facial feedback hypothesis, for instance, has established that when people are induced to mechanically adopt a specific facial configuration linked to a particular mood (e.g., disgust), they tend also to adopt the corresponding affective state (e.g., Strack, Martin, & Stepper, 1988). This matching of internal states to overt behavior is enhanced when the behavior is interpersonal in nature. Even role playing, in which a person simply follows a behavioral script in social interaction, often produces pronounced changes in attitudes and values on the part of the role player (e.g., Zimbardo, 1970).[2]

In terms of our model, behavioral coordination occurs when each person modifies the value of his or her own control parameter in order to match the other person's pattern of behavior. The exact value of the partner's control parameter is invisible to the person, but he or she remembers the partner's most recent set of behaviors (i.e., the most recent values of x), as well as his or her own most recent behaviors. By comparing his or her own behavior with that of the partner, the person adjusts his or her own control parameter until there is a match in their respective behavior patterns (cf. Zochowski & Liebovitch, 1997, 1999). If the pattern of the partner's observed behavior is more complex than his or her own pattern of behavior, the person slightly increases the value of his or her own control parameter. If the partner's behavior is less complex than one's own behavior, on the other hand, the person slightly decreases the value of his or her own control parameter. In effect, each person can discover one another's internal state by monitoring the evolution of one another's behavior.

Figure 12.1 shows the time course of synchronization as two maps progressively match each other's control parameters in the manner de-

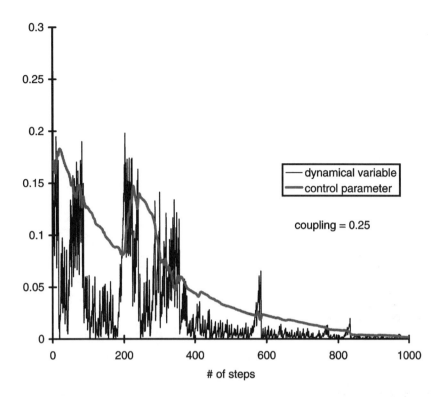

FIGURE 12.1. Development of synchronization under weak coupling.

scribed previously (Nowak & Vallacher, 1998). This simulation was run for relatively weak coupling ($\alpha = 0.25$). The x-axis corresponds to time in simulation steps, and the y-axis portrays the value of the difference between the two maps. The thin line corresponds to the difference in the dynamic variables, whereas the thicker line corresponds to the difference in r. Over time, the difference in the respective control parameters of the two maps decreases and the maps become perfectly synchronized in their behavior. This suggests that attempting behavioral synchronization with weak levels of influence and control over one another's behavior will facilitate matching of one another's internal states.

Figure 12.2 shows the results when the simulation was run with a stronger value of coupling ($\alpha = 0.7$). Note that although coordination in behavior develops almost immediately, the control parameters fail to converge, even after 1,000 simulation steps. This is because strong coupling causes full synchronization of behavior, even for maps with quite

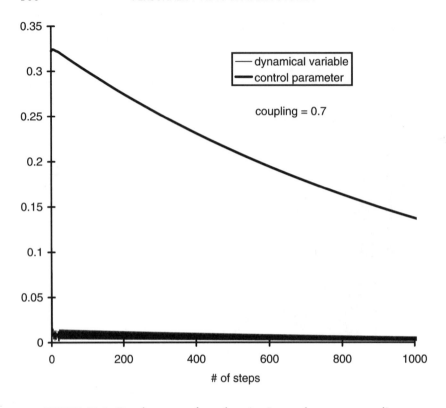

FIGURE 12.2. Development of synchronization under strong coupling.

different control parameters. Once the behavior is in full synchrony, the two maps do not have a clue that their control parameters are different. Hence, if the coupling were removed, the dynamics of the two respective maps would immediately diverge. This result suggests that using very strong influence to obtain coordination of behavior may effectively hinder synchronization at a deeper level. More generally, there is optimal level of influence and control over behavior in relationships. If influence is too weak, synchronization may fail to develop. Very strong influence, on the other hand, can prevent the development of a relationship based on mutual understanding and empathy. Although highly controlled partners may fully synchronize their behavior, they are unlikely to internalize the values of control parameters necessary to maintain such behavior in the absence of interpersonal influence. For such internalization to occur, intermediate levels of mutual influence would seem to be most effective. On balance, then, the most advantageous degree of coupling is the minimal amount necessary to achieve synchronization.

These findings may shed light on a puzzling conclusion concerning the relative impact of parents and peers on children's personality development (e.g., Harris, 1995; Scarr, 1992). Despite the disproportionate amount of time that children spend with their parents as opposed to any single peer—particularly when they are very young and thus most impressionable—there is reason to think that children develop personality traits that are more similar to those of their peers than to those of their parents. This conclusion is controversial, to say the least, but it is not particularly surprising in light of the simulation results. Because of the strong coupling that characterizes parent–child relationships, children have little need to internalize the values of their parents' control parameters in order to develop and maintain behavioral coordination with them. In monitoring a child's behavior, praising it when it is deemed appropriate and attempting to redirect it when it is less so, parents exert fairly constant and strong influence over what the child does. Because parents' behavior control is obvious to the child, he or she learns to act in accordance with the underlying reinforcement contingencies, rules, expectations, and the like.

To be sure, children internalize certain lessons from these experiences and thus may develop various control parameters that resemble their parents'. The need for adopting parents' internal states, however, pales in comparison to the strategic value of matching the internal states of their peers. Peers, unlike parents, are not in a position to monitor a child's behavior, let alone control it on a daily basis. Peers are also far less faithful interaction partners than are parents, and the surface structure of their behavior is more erratic as well. These features of peer relations—the relatively weak coupling, the uncertain stability of the relationship, and the potential for unpredictable action—all suggest the practical value of learning the bases for peers' behavior. Beyond that, it is easier to synchronize with the interests, moods, and thoughts of someone who is similar to oneself in age, life experiences, competencies, and power. Children no doubt love, and may even appreciate, their parents, but they probably don't empathize and identify with them as readily as they do with their peers. Synchronization with peers, in short, has all the ingredients for convergence on common control parameters and thus may be especially influential in engraving the values of such parameters in children's cognitive–affective systems.[3]

SYNCHRONIZATION AND INDIVIDUAL DIFFERENCES

Each social interaction provides the opportunity to learn how best to set one's control parameters in service of synchronization, but this process takes considerable time and effort. Efficient functioning in social relations requires a more rapid means of achieving synchronization. We propose that this efficiency is provided by the stabilization of certain settings of control parameters in the person's cognitive–affective system at the expense of other settings. The idea is that prolonged synchronization with respect to specific settings of control parameters produces a preference for these settings. The internal states established over time to facilitate synchronization in a particular relationship, in other words, will carry over to other interactions or to situations in which the person is alone. In effect, these settings become engraved in the person's mental and behavioral repertoire. This does not mean that the person becomes fixated at these settings but rather that, in the absence of other factors, these settings are readily adopted in preference to other settings.

The ready activation of these settings enables rapid resynchronization on successive interactions with the people responsible for their initial generation and creates the potential for efficient synchronization with other people who share similar settings. By the same token, though, the engraving of particular settings can make it difficult for the person to achieve synchronization with other people whose own settings are different from his or her own. This proposed scenario provides a basis for the generation of stable individual variation with respect to internal states, as well as preferences for other people and interaction contexts.

Personality Variables as Synchronization Equilibria

Social interaction with any one person is never exactly the same from one time to the next. This means that the settings of control parameters that result from prolonged interaction are not fixed values but rather may be portrayed as system equilibria, in the vicinity of which the system resides most of the time and to which the system returns if perturbed by an external force (cf. Nowak, Vallacher, & Burnstein, 1998; Nowak, Vallacher, Tesser, & Borkowski, 2000). It is possible for a person to have multiple equilibria for a given control parameter, each corresponding to a mode of synchronization achieved in interaction with a specific person or group or with the same person or group in different settings. These equilibria—corresponding to fixed-point attractors in nonlinear dynamical systems (cf. Nowak & Vallacher, 1998)—may vary in strength, such that certain equilibria are more likely to capture and maintain the dynamics of the person's behavior than are other equilibria.

The strength of a given equilibrium is dictated by three properties—its *basin of attraction*, its *depth*, and its *shape*. The basin of attraction represents the range of values surrounding an equilibrium that eventually converge on the equilibrium. An equilibrium with a wide basin will "attract" a relatively large range of nearby values. A highly optimistic person, for example, might react to neutral or even moderately bad news with strong evidence of his or her tendency to view the world positively. If the width of the basin covers the whole range of values that can be adopted, the system will be pulled toward the equilibrium regardless of its starting value. For the highly optimistic person, even seemingly devastating news (e.g., the loss of his or her job) may be reframed in positive terms (e.g., an opportunity to travel, learn new skills, and get to know his or her children). An equilibrium with a narrower basin, in contrast, will attract a smaller range of nearby values. A person with an equally strong tendency to stabilize on high optimism, for example, may display this tendency only in reaction to very positive events. When the person is in a pessimistic or even a neutral mood, then, his or her optimism may not be evident. However, if truly good news puts the person in the vicinity of his or her narrowly defined equilibrium, he or she will be highly effective in stabilizing on optimism.

Depth corresponds to the force required to move the system out of the equilibrium. A deep equilibrium is one that can resist relatively strong forces in the direction of some other value outside the basin of attraction. If a person's equilibrium for optimism is very deep, for example, once the person is within the basin of attraction, very strong inducements from outside this range are required to change his or her mental state. A shallow equilibrium, meanwhile, is one that is more readily destabilized by forces associated with a contradictory setting of the control parameter. Thus, if a person's optimism is not especially well entrenched, even a brief encounter with a skeptical person might be sufficient to dampen or eliminate the person's rosy view of the world.

Finally, shape describes how the system reacts to various deviations from its equilibrium and how strongly each deviating state will be pulled back to the equilibrium. Some equilibria may react very weakly to small deviations but may react in a disproportionately stronger fashion for larger deviations. With respect to optimism, for example, such an equilibrium would allow the person to move almost freely through a range of positive moods but strongly restrict him or her from moving into a range of negative moods. A contrasting example is an equilibrium in which the forces that return the system to its equilibrium are very strong in the immediate vicinity of the equilibrium but become progressively weaker with increasing distance from the equilibrium. An optimistic person may very strongly stabilize on a very positive view of the world, for example, but once the person is induced to adopt a moderately optimistic view, he or she may be less inclined to resist an outright negative worldview.

Energy Landscapes for Personality

An equilibrium and its associated basin of attraction can be depicted with an energy landscape metaphor. Imagine a landscape in which hills correspond to high energy and valleys correspond to low energy. Figure 12.3 portrays different versions of such a landscape. The x-axis in each figure corresponds to values of the control parameter, and the y-axis corresponds to the energy associated with these values. Each valley corresponds to a local minimum of the energy function (i.e., an equilibrium state), with the depth of each valley depicting the strength of the attracting equilibrium. Equilibrium-driven behavior can be described as a search for local minima in the landscape. Dynamics of the control parameter consist of the descent of the system from any state to the closest equilibrium. Metaphorically, one can envision a ball rolling on a hilly landscape. The ball rolls down a hill until it reaches a valley, at which point it comes to rest. Different factors—such as an attempt to synchronize with a new person— can move the value of the control parameter away from its current equilibrium, but if the force is not too strong, the system will eventually return to this equilibrium (i.e., the ball will roll back down the slope). The strength of the force necessary to move the control parameter out of its equilibrium must equal (or exceed) the energy differential between the top and bottom of the valley.

The four equilibria depicted in Figure 12.3a differ with respect to depth, basin of attraction, and shape. *A* portrays a weak equilibrium that is shallow and has a narrow basin of attraction, *B* portrays an equally narrow but deeper equilibrium, *C* portrays a relatively shallow equilibrium with a wide basin of attraction, and *D* portrays an equilibrium that

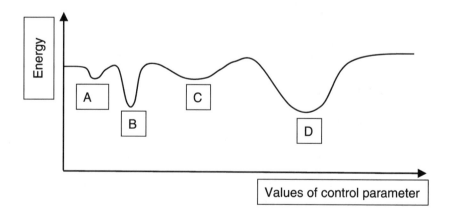

FIGURE 12.3a. Energy landscapes for personality.

is both deep and has a wide basin of attraction. The shape of the basin of attraction for each equilibrium is represented by the slope of its hills and valleys.

Slope can show local variation, with steeper slopes corresponding to stronger forces associated with equilibrium. E, F, and G in Figure 12.3b illustrate this feature. E shows an equilibrium with a weak stabilizing tendency near the equilibrium, which gets progressively stronger with distance from the equilibrium. F shows an equilibrium with the opposite tendencies—that is, a strong stabilizing tendency near the equilibrium, which becomes progressively weaker with distance from the equilibrium. The configuration in G depicts a small local equilibrium existing within the general basis of attraction of a wider and stronger equilibrium. Yet other configurations representing depth, basin of attraction, and shape can be envisioned, each capturing a potential type of equilibrium dynamics.

The exact value of a control parameter is always influenced by a host of biological, cognitive, environmental, and social factors. The joint effect of all these forces may be represented as a random influence or "noise." In the energy landscape metaphor, noise can be envisioned as "shaking up" the landscape and thus qualitatively changing the dynamics of the system. In the presence of small noise, the value of the control parameter will hover around its equilibrium rather than remain at its precise value. For stronger values of noise, weaker equilibria in the energy landscape may become unstable and lose their ability to capture the dynamics of the system. This scenario provides insight into the well-documented tendency for people to engage in dominant responses under conditions of stress and other forms of arousal (e.g., Zajonc, 1965). Because weak equilibria, representing nondominant responses, are destabilized under such conditions, the person is left with only his or her strongest equilibrium. For very high values of noise, however, even strong equilibria may

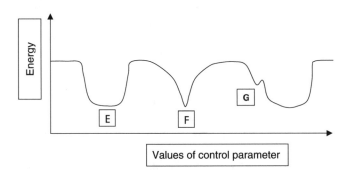

FIGURE 12.3b. Shapes of basins of attraction for equilibria.

become unstable, and the system may be unable to achieve any coherent mode of synchronization. Internal preferences, in other words, no longer provide cues to synchronization under high values of noise. This scenario corresponds to the heightened attention to situational cues and loss of individuality under high stress or other "noisy" circumstances that can destabilize internalized bases for action (e.g., Diener, 1980; Turner & Killian, 1957; Zimbardo, 1970). In a panic situation, for example, everyone may engage in a similar fashion (e.g., running), despite considerable variation among them in their personal behavioral styles and values.

The energy landscape metaphor makes interesting predictions about the conditions under which personality is likely to be apparent in behavior. In particular, it suggests a curvilinear relationship between noise and the manifestation of individual differences. Under low levels of noise (e.g., few outside influences, low levels of stress), most people can adopt a wide variety of internal states, even those that reflect a relatively weak equilibrium. Hence, the manifestation of clear individual differences is thus unlikely to be observed, and most people can modify their internal states to match the norms and expectations they experience from one context to the next. People are also unlikely to display a great deal of individual variation under conditions of high noise, as even strong personal equilibria are destabilized. Instead, people are likely to behave in a reactive fashion to the forces acting on them. Personality under such conditions thus represents a fairly weak force in generating behavior. Personality is likely to be a strong causal factor, however, under moderate levels of noise, because of the tendency for such conditions to destabilize all but the strongest equilibria in people's energy landscape. In this case, behavior is likely to reflect a person's most deeply engraved control parameters, with weaker settings being psychologically unavailable.

Modeling Individual Differences in Social Interaction

To model equilibrium dynamics, we modified the original model so that two logistic equations can change each other's control parameters by trying to synchronize at the behavioral level. All the simulations testing the revised model were run under moderate values of coupling ($\alpha = 0.25$). The first set of simulations examined the effect of equilibria on synchronization. The first system (A) always had a control parameter with a fixed value ($p_A = 3.65$), whereas the second system (B) changed its own control parameter in an attempt to synchronize with A. The starting value for B's control parameter was $p_B = 3.55$, which is in the lower range of the chaotic regime. We examined the time course of the convergence of B's control parameter to A's, as well as the time course of synchronization of the two systems. As an index of synchronization, we measured the momentary difference between the control parameters of A and B. Synchronization was considered to be established when the absolute value of the difference between iterates of the two systems, $(|x_A - x_B|)$, was less then 0.01 for at least 500 iterations. It is important to note that B does not directly observe A's control parameter. Rather, B changes the value of its own control parameter so that the dynamics of its behavior (i.e., the values of its dynamical variable) match the dynamics of A's behavior. If an attracting equilibrium exists for B, it exerts a pulling force on B when B is in its basin of attraction.

In the first set of simulations, we measured how long it took the two systems to synchronize, depending on the presence and location of B's attractor. Figure 12.4 compares the time it took two systems to synchronize when there was no attractor for B, when B's attractor was located at the value of A's control parameter, and when there was a weak attractor for B in a different location. The bars represent an average of $n = 7$ simulation runs. Synchronization was achieved most quickly when the position of B's attractor overlapped with the value of A's control parameter and most slowly when the attractor was in a different location. This result is very intuitive—in the first case, the attractor facilitated faster alignment of A's and B's control parameters, whereas in the second case it hampered the process.

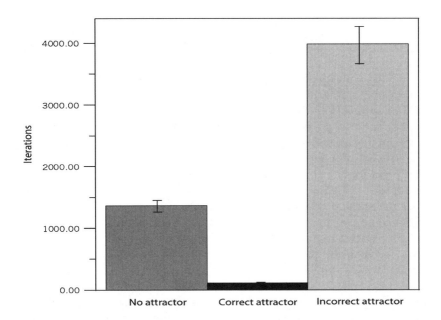

FIGURE 12.4. Time to achieve synchronization.

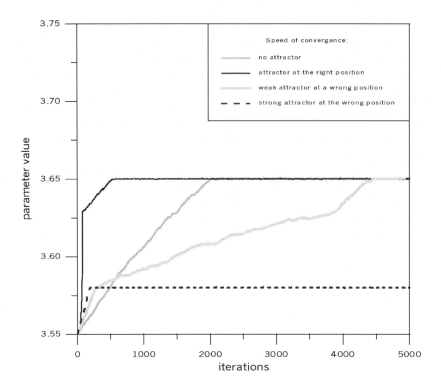

FIGURE 12.5. Evolution of synchronization.

This result can be easily seen in Figure 12.5, which depicts the evolution of *B*'s control parameter in the three cases described previously, and additionally in the case in which *B*'s attractor is strong enough to keep *B*'s control parameter from aligning to *A*'s. The *x*-axis in Figure 12.5 corresponds to time (in simulation steps) and the *y*-axis corresponds to the value of *B*'s control parameter. As in the simulations described previously, the initial value of *A*'s control parameter was set to $p_A = 3.65$, and the value of *B*'s control parameter was set to $p_B = 3.55$. In the first three cases (black and gray lines), the systems achieved synchronization. Synchronization was achieved most quickly (after 600 steps) in the case in which *B*'s attracting equilibrium matched that of *A* (black line). The force exerted within *B*'s basin of attraction added to the changes of parameter caused by *B*'s synchronization attempts, which in turn resulted in the fastest changes in *B*'s control parameters. Synchronization took the longest (4,500 steps) in the third case (light gray line), in which *B*'s equilibrium was different from *A*'s, because the force within *B*'s basin of attraction counteracted the (bigger) parameter changes due to synchronization attempts. In the fourth case (dashed line), in which B's equilibrium was not only different from A's but also relatively strong, the systems failed to achieve convergence in control parameters and thus failed to synchronize. In this case, the forces within B's basin of attraction were stronger than the force associated with synchronization attempts, so that the system was unable to leave its equilibrium in order to synchronize.

Taken together, these simulations show the facilitative effect of compatible equilibria and the hindering effect of incompatible equilibria on synchronization. As long as the synchronization force is stronger than that of the force within the basin of attraction, the control parameters will eventually converge, and the systems will synchronize. When forces associated with a basin of attraction exceed synchronization forces, however, the respective control parameters of two systems are unlikely to converge, and the systems will fail to synchronize in their behavior.

In these simulations, we always started with a preset value of B's control parameter, which was far away from its equilibrium. This state of affairs may be rare in real life, because people's control parameters are likely to remain in the vicinity of their respective attracting equilibria much of the time (even in the absence of synchronization attempts). In the second set of simulations, then, we investigated the consequences of stabilizing B's control parameter on its equilibrium value. This value corresponded closely to the equilibrium value for A's control parameter. This scenario corresponds to a situation in which previous interactions with the same partner had established a stable attracting equilibrium corresponding to the partner's value. Even in the absence of interaction with the partner, then, B's control parameter usually resides within the basin of attraction of this equilibrium. To stabilize B's control parameter in this way, we let B's system run for 2,000 iterations without being coupled to the other system. Only then did we engage coupling between A and B (dashed line). As Figure 12.6 reveals, there is rapid onset of synchronization, because B's control parameter is already very similar to that of A at the onset of interaction.

Taken together, these simulations demonstrate the advantages of establishing control parameters with attracting equilibria that enable one to synchronize with other people. Such values allow one to achieve faster synchronization, even if the initial values of people's control parameters are quite different. A recent interaction may have changed the value of a person's control parameter, for example, but the person will still quickly converge on his or her equilibrium value when interacting with someone who shares this particular setting.

The third set of simulations portrays the development of equilibria as a result of prolonged social interaction. Figure 12.7 illustrates the progressive development of an attracting equilibrium as B attempts to syn-

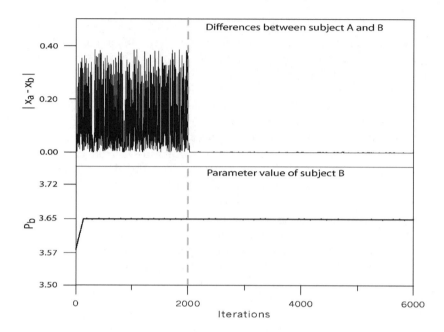

FIGURE 12.6. Onset of synchronization through coupling.

chronize with *A*. Over time, *B* digs a progressively deeper attractor in whatever region it resides. Not only are the successive equilibria progressively deeper, but they may also slightly change their values (see also Figure 12.8) as *B* progressively approaches the value of *A*'s equilibrium with greater precision.

In the fourth set of simulations, we examined synchronization with similar versus dissimilar others. In these simulations, we followed changes of the attractor landscape when the position of *A*'s attractor is close to the position of *B*'s attractor, and when the position of *A*'s attractor is far away from *B*'s attractor. In other words, Figure 12.8 depicts the effects observed for similarity versus dissimilarity. In interaction with a similar other, the value of an existing attracting equilibrium moves gradually to match the value of the interaction partner (see Figure 12.8, left panel). This can be interpreted as slight adjustment of individual difference variables to enable more effective interaction with those who are already fairly similar to oneself. The right panel in Figure 12.8 demonstrates a completely different scenario when interacting with someone whose equilibrium is dissimilar to one's own. In order to interact with a dissimilar other, the person leaves his or her equilibrium and changes his or her equilibrium to match that of the other person. After establishing synchroniza-

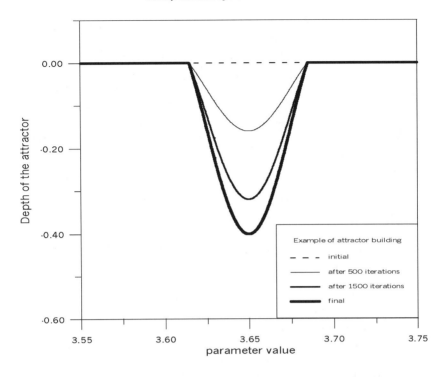

FIGURE 12.7. Development of attractor in social interaction.

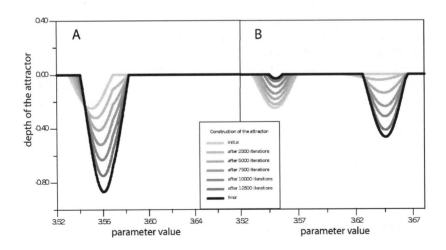

FIGURE 12.8. The development of equilibria in interaction with similar and dissimilar others.

tion, a new equilibrium is engraved in the person's energy landscape. Instead of trying to adjust a current equilibrium, in other words, the person establishes an alternative equilibrium to match that of the interaction partner. In this way, multiple equilibria can be established, with each equilibrium stabilizing the values of a control parameter for a specific type of interaction partner or a specific type of interaction setting.

This perspective reveals how behavior may be situation specific yet still governed by individual differences. Individual differences with respect to specific values of a control parameter are thus revealed not by its average value but rather by the nature of the attractor landscape for control parameters. The person's preferred and avoided values in this landscape specify a unique configuration that defines the person's pattern of behavior across different interaction partners and contexts. This scenario is consistent with the perspective that emphasizes personal patterns of behavior across situations developed by Mischel and Shoda (1995; Shoda, Mischel, & Wright, 1994).

Because prolonged social interaction engraves values of equilibria for control parameters, these parameters are likely to govern the person's behavior toward others in subsequent social interactions. These people, in turn, may engrave these parameters in their own system and employ them in their subsequent interactions with others, and so on. In effect, the engraving of values for control parameters gives rise to the social transmission of individual difference variables. Having a long-term relationship with a friend during adolescence, for example, may have the effect of generating several stable internal states by means of the synchronization dynamics we have described. Those characteristics, in turn, may cause engravings of similar characteristics in subsequent friends later in life. To illustrate this possibility, we ran a final set of simulations in which a strong equilibrium was engraved in one person (A) and no equilibrium was engraved in the other person (B). The simulations ran until the systems synchronized. We then removed A and coupled B with a new system, C, that did not have a preset equilibrium. As Figure 12.9 reveals, the equilibrium of A was transmitted through B to C without much change in its value. The slight change that did occur during social transmission reflected refinement of the equilibrium over time. Thus A's equilibrium changed slightly to foster synchronization with B, and B's equilibrium changed slightly to foster his or her synchronization with C.

CONCLUSIONS, IMPLICATIONS, AND FUTURE ITERATIONS

People are highly social animals, and as such they are deeply invested in establishing stable and meaningful relationships with one another. Far

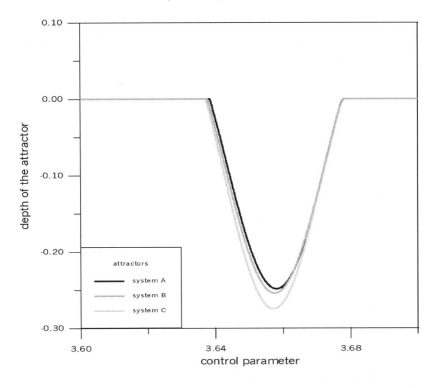

FIGURE 12.9. Social transmission of equilibria through synchronization.

from fostering herd-like homogeneity, the concern with interpersonal relations provides an important mechanism for the generation of individual differences with respect to a variety of internal states. Individual differences, in turn, are manifested in the choice of relationship partners and shape the course of social interactions with them. This feedback loop between social interaction and personality carries with it a number of implications for personality science—and for social psychology, as well—that we develop below. We also call for empirical research to validate these implications and to test the assumptions underlying this model.

Personality and Social Interaction

A defining feature of social interaction is the temporal coordination of expressed thoughts, feelings, and actions between the parties to the interaction. To a certain extent, the synchronization of interpersonal experience can be achieved through mechanisms of direct influence, such as communication, monitoring, and reinforcement. In the context of ongoing social relations, however, successful synchronization is more efficiently attained by the matching of relevant internal states that dictate the tempo and content of social interaction. By achieving concordance in internal states, interaction partners do not need to expend as much energy monitoring and influencing each other's actions directly but rather can spontaneously synchronize their verbal and motoric output over time by virtue of having a common wellspring for action.

To the extent that a person's internal states promote prolonged synchronization, they become engraved as equilibria in his or her cognitive–affective system, thereby providing for regularity and consistency in behavior. Once specific internal states are established as equilibria, moreover, they guide the choice of subsequent interaction partners. Because these choices are based on the potential for effective synchronization, people seek out others with similar equilibria for internal states. Interaction with these partners, in turn, tunes and reinforces the person's equilibria. This positive feedback loop between social interaction and personality may serve as an important mechanism providing for stability in personality, despite the fairly continual turnover in relationships that characterizes social life.

If this feedback loop is broken, however, the decoupling of the individual from similar others has the potential for producing a drift in the individual's equilibrium values. The reason is the internal forces within the person's cognitive–affective system that operate independently of incoming information or social influences. The intrinsic dynamics of thought produced by these forces can take the form of attitude polarization (cf. Tesser, 1978), sustained oscillations between evaluatively conflicting judgments (cf. Vallacher, Nowak, & Kaufman, 1994), and repeated episodes of thought deconstruction and emergent understanding (cf. Vallacher & Nowak, 1997). To be sure, the intrinsic dynamics of thought are critically important for establishing and maintaining coherence in the cognitive–affective system as a whole (Vallacher & Nowak, 1999). If unchecked by social reality, however, such processes may cause the control parameters that enable synchronization to drift to new values that hinder future interactions, which in turn can reinforce the person's social isolation (Vallacher, Nowak, Markus, & Strauss, 1998). It's interesting in this regard that perpetrators of random acts of violence (e.g., shooting rampages) are commonly described in seemingly benign terms as loners who don't bother other people. The existence of social relations, then, is critical not only for the development of personality structure but also for its maintenance.

Personality and Consistency

People may desire to interact with similar others, but often their choice in these matters is limited. One can choose with whom to strike up a conversation at a party or establish an intimate relationship, for example, but one has little control over the identities of one's parents, teachers, and coworkers. To the extent that these partners have different equilibria for control parameters, the person's interaction with them may cause the formation of new equilibria in his or her system. Thus, for every control parameter there is a potential for the coexistence of different equilibria, corresponding to the history of synchronization in social interactions. If the person has synchronized with a relatively homogenous collection of individuals and groups, of course, then a single equilibrium is to be expected. But to the extent that relationships of various kinds are formed with widely different and incompatible individuals and groups, the person is likely to have formed multiple equilibria for various internal states.

In different situations and with different interaction partners, then, different equilibria may exert their influence on the person. The reason is that each equilibrium attracts states within its basin of attraction. Thus the same person may actively pursue very volatile interactions in one setting but very relaxed interactions in another setting, depending on which basin of attraction captures the person's internal state in each setting. By this reasoning, cross-situational consistency in behavior would be indicative of a single equilibrium for the dimension in question. Even here, though, the degree of consistency would depend on the strength of the equilibrium. If the equilibrium is relatively weak and thus easily destabilized, the person may appear to be governed by forces in the situation. A person might be inclined to pursue relaxed social interactions, for example, but if the basin of attraction for this equilibrium is narrow or the equilibrium value is easily destabilized, he or she might display little evidence of relaxation when the situation is tense or otherwise calls for more volatile behavior.

By the same token, the meaning of temporal and situational variability on a dimension of interest is not always clear. Although high consistency of a given behavior over time and across contexts indicates that the system is stabilized within a strong and narrow equilibrium, the lack of such consistency is open to three alternative interpretations. First, a high degree of variability could simply mean that the person does not have an equilibrium for this parameter but rather is responsive to external forces and noise in his or her behavior. A second, equally plausible interpretation, however, is that high variability reflects the presence of a single, relatively flat equilibrium with a wide basin of attraction. In this case, variability would signal flexibility in the person's control parameter for behavior rather than the absence of the corresponding internal state. The third possibility is that high variability indicates the presence of two or more equilibria, with noise or a consistent external influence moving the system between their respective basins. A person characterized by such a landscape may have two or more quite distinct—even conflicting—settings with respect to a particular control parameter, each of which provides a stable platform for action. The availability of multiple equilibria means that the person may display noteworthy variability in his or her social behavior, depending on the interaction partner and social context, yet act in accordance with his or her personality in each instance.

More generally, the notion of equilibrium implies that a person's standing on a dimension of individual difference does not simply represent some aggregate value or central tendency of the person's behavior (cf. Caprara & Cervone, 2000; Mischel & Shoda, 1995). Not everyone, first of all, can be characterized in terms of preferences on every possible dimension (cf. Bem & Allen, 1974; Markus, 1980). For some people, the ability to synchronize may require settings of some parameters (e.g., independence) but not of others (e.g., conscientiousness). Only with respect to those parameters that develop energy landscapes can one detect internal forces attributable to personality. For those parameters without pronounced energy landscapes, the person's behavior is likely to reflect the impact of forces in the immediate situation. Even when a person has developed stable equilibria on a given dimension, the existence of multiple equilibria would render the description of average tendencies misleading, as such values may represent a setting the control parameter never adopts. A person who has tendencies toward both aggressive and conciliatory behavior may never demonstrate the average of these two tendencies, for example, although an approach emphasizing aggregation would make this prediction.

The Self and Synchronization

Achieving and maintaining interpersonal synchronization can prove to be difficult and time-consuming. This is true when interacting with someone for the first time, of course, but even in a close relationship sustained synchrony can prove to be a fragile phenomenon, open to a host of disrupting influences (stresses, distractions, mood swings, etc.). To a certain extent, people can automatically adjust their internal states to achieve or reinstate effective synchronization. Frequent and spontaneous fine-tuning of control parameters, in fact, is probably inherent in the ebb and flow of most social encounters. Sometimes, however, synchronization can prove especially difficult to achieve in the first place or is not easily reinstated after being seriously derailed. We propose that under these conditions, control processes are engaged whose function it is to consciously adjust one's internal settings in an attempt to establish or reestablish effective synchronization (cf. Vallacher & Nowak, 1999; Vallacher et al., 1998).

Specifically, synchronization gone awry promotes a special form of negative arousal in the cognitive–affective system that is subjectively experienced as self-consciousness (e.g., Vallacher, Wegner, & Somoza, 1989). Embarrassment, for example, is a negative self-conscious emotion that signals disruption in ongoing social interaction (cf. Tangney & Fischer, 1995). Beyond its signaling function, self-scrutiny focuses conscious attention on one's internal states in an effort to find different settings that can restore interpersonal synchrony. In effect, self-consciousness plays the role of an outside agent that adjusts control parameters on-line, thereby exercising direct control over the system's dynamics. The self, from this perspective, does not simply mirror one's experiences but also performs an "executive function" in ongoing thought and behavior (cf. Baumeister, 1998; Carver & Scheier, 1998). By the same token, self-consciousness dissipates when interpersonal synchronization is reestablished (Vallacher et al., 1998). With this in mind, the experience of spontaneous synchrony in social interaction may represent a special manifestation of "flow" (Csikszentmihalyi, 1990), a state commonly depicted, in part, as the loss of self-awareness while engaged in activities that match one's personal capacities and reflect one's preferences.

Caveats and Future Iterations

Our aim in this chapter was not to propose a new set of individual difference variables. The approach we have outlined simply provides a formal framework for describing how individual differences both arise from and shape social interactions. We propose that individual differences may be described as equilibria for control parameters that allow for synchronization of thought, feeling, and behavior in social interaction. Because this is a formal model, it does not make claims as to the specific nature of the control parameters, nor of the classes of behavior they control. By the same token, though, the model provides a heuristic for rethinking the nature of individual differences and the relation between internal states and overt behavior.

One possibility we feel merits investigation is that the identity of internal states is directly related to the identity of the dynamical variables they control. Specifically, the motoric and verbal output that defines the stream of action in social encounters can be viewed as relatively low-level identities of action that provide the basis for the emergence of progressively higher level action identities, which are engraved as stable settings for subsequent action maintenance (cf. Vallacher & Wegner, 1987). In the emergence process, higher level identities crystallize as lower level identities are repeatedly enacted under conditions that reliably point to one set of implications and consequences rather than to others. A person might synchronize with a particular interaction partner with respect to speaking rapidly, for example, and begin to develop a higher level representation for this relatively basic act that reflects the consequences of these interaction episodes. Thus the person may come to represent speaking rapidly as "expressing one's opinions," "engaging in persuasion," or "dominance attempts," depending on the tenor of his or her repeated interactions with the partner. High-level identities established in this fashion are relatively resistant to change and function as internal states that provide a stable platform for action in the future (cf. Vallacher, 1993). Through the emergence process, then, people's cognitive–affective systems may become populated with a wide variety of goals, traits, and values, each providing a platform for specific acts in the course of social interaction.

Despite the press for emergent understanding, there is no guarantee that basic actions will give rise to stable (maintainable) higher level identities for what one does or intends to do (cf. Vallacher, 1993; Vallacher & Kaufman, 1996). This perspective raises the specter that some people may fail to achieve highly stable equilibria with respect to any internal state relevant to social interaction. In research relevant to this possibility, Vallacher and Wegner (1989) found that people differ in the extent to which they characteristically identify their behavior in relatively low-level, mechanistic terms as opposed to higher level, comprehensive terms reflecting consequences and self-evaluative implications. Compared to "high-level agents," the "low-level agents" in this research were less certain of their standing on common trait dimensions and demonstrated greater openness to social feedback regarding their self-perception with respect to certain personality traits. Interestingly, the low-level agents were more likely than the high-level agents to have experienced environmental and interpersonal instability during childhood. This association is consistent with the synchronization perspective, as prolonged interaction with specific others fosters the engraving of equilibrium values for internal states. In effect, then, people may vary in the extent to which they develop stable higher level identities for their actions that function as equilibrium values in their social interactions.

Equating the emergence of high-level identities with the engraving of internal settings in the person's cognitive–affective system has certain advantages. First, because this perspective defines control parameters and dynamical variables in terms of shared properties, the dynamics of mind and action can be discussed within a common realm of discourse. The categorical distinction between action systems and cognitive–affective systems, in other words, may be more illusory than real (cf. Vallacher, 1993). Second, this perspective allows for considerable flexibility in the identity status of personality variables. The reason is that high-level identities for action are not defined in terms of any single category but rather

reflect the entire panoply of mental states—traits, values, goals, anticipated consequences (negative as well as positive)—that populate the
myriad taxonomies proposed in personality theory and research. Thus
a person might have a control parameter that reflects a common self-
perceived trait (e.g., sincerity) for some social interactions, but also one
that reflects an idiosyncratic goal (e.g., get others to laugh at themselves)
in other social interactions. Finally, this perspective has the distinct virtue
of specifying a plausible mechanism by which stable internal states become engraved in people's personalities.

At this point, though, we do not wish to claim that the process of
action emergence is the only mechanism—or even the primary mechanism—by which specific settings of internal states become engraved as
equilibria in people's personalities. Contemporary personality research
is replete with well-documented models and taxonomies (e.g., Atkinson,
1964; Buss & Plomin, 1984; Costa & McCrae, 1995; Wiggins, 1980),
each with its own assumptions regarding the genesis of individual differences. Several personality traits and temperament variables have a genetic
basis (cf. Plomin, Owen, & McGuffin, 1994), for example, and thus may
represent prewired equilibria for personal and interpersonal behavior that
are relatively impervious to experiences in social interaction. If this is the
case, people may experience difficulty achieving synchronization on these
dimensions with dissimilar others, regardless of the stability of the interaction context (e.g., Dunn & Plomin, 1990; Harris, 1998). Synchronization experiences, whether successful or unsuccessful, may well promote
the emergence of higher level identities for one's social behavior (e.g.,
impressing vs. disappointing someone), but if the operative control
parameter is under biological (i.e., hormonal or genetic) control, it may
continue to direct one's actions despite the availability of these new mental
representations.

A final caveat is in order. We do not claim that interpersonal synchronization is the only means by which social experiences engrave specific settings of control parameters in people's cognitive–affective systems.
Theory and research in personality science have identified a host of other
plausible mechanisms of personality development and maintenance, including direct reinforcement, social learning and modeling, labeling and
self-fulfilling prophecies, identification, and guilt induction. It may be
possible, of course, to reframe such processes as specific synchronization
mechanisms, each associated with a particular balance of coupling and
progressive matching of internal states. But this is hardly a foregone conclusion. Hopefully, research in the years to come will establish the fundamental social mechanisms responsible for individual variation and identify
the interactions among these mechanisms that give rise to each person's
uniqueness. Only through repeated iterations of the scientific method can

we hope to achieve a stable equilibrium in our theoretical understanding of the interplay between personality and social interaction.

NOTES

1. For a complete description of these simulations and the results they produced, see Nowak and Vallacher (1998, pp. 194–199).
2. The tendency for overt behavior to resynchronize one's internal states provides an explanation for the effectiveness of various indoctrination techniques and social rituals in forging interpersonal bonds among people who barely know one another. Many techniques and rituals are designed to establish group cohesiveness by inducing the coordination of motor activities. Dancing, for example, has been employed in virtually all societies throughout history as a means of establishing relationships—whether an intimate relationship between two people or group solidarity in a preliterate culture preparing for war. In similar fashion, group singing is not only popular among friends but also plays an important role in cultural institutions as seemingly diverse as religious groups and military organizations. Particularly when accompanied by simple patterns of motor movements—clapping and moving in unison in church, marching in the military—the effectiveness of this strategy in inducing a sense of group identity and shared values is often truly impressive.
3. It is interesting to consider these findings in light of the sustained interest in social psychology in the effects of incentives on personal motivation (cf. Lepper & Greene, 1978). There is abundant evidence from several independent research traditions suggesting that the use of material rewards and the threat of punishment are effective in securing compliance but that they tend to do so at the expense of creating personal desires that match one's action (cf. Vallacher, Nowak, & Miller, in press). Within the present framework, this is tantamount to enhancement of behavioral synchronization through strong coupling (e.g., high levels of monitoring and influence, the use of rewards and punishments, etc.), without the creation of an internal state that can produce the behavior in the absence of coupling.

REFERENCES

Arrow, H., McGrath, J. E., & Berdahl, J. L. (2000). *Small groups as complex systems*. Thousand Oaks, CA: Sage.

Atkinson, J. W. (1964). *An introduction to motivation*. Princeton, NJ: Van Nostrand.

Axelrod, R. (1984). *The evolution of cooperation*. New York: Basic Books.

Axelrod, R., & Cohen, M. D. (1999). *Harnessing complexity: Organizational implications of a scientific frontier*. New York: Free Press.

Baron, R. M., Amazeen, P. M., & Beek, P. J. (1994). Local and global dynamics of social relations. In R. R. Vallacher & A. Nowak (Eds.), *Dynamical systems in social psychology* (pp. 111–138). San Diego: Academic Press.

Baumeister, R. F. (1998). The self. In D. T. Gilbert, S. T. Fiske, & G. Lindzey (Eds.), *The handbook of social psychology* (Vol. 1, pp. 680–740). Boston: McGraw-Hill.

Baumeister, R. F., & Leary, M. R. (1995). The need to belong: Desire for interpersonal attachments as a fundamental human motivation. *Psychological Bulletin, 117,* 497–529.

Beek, P. J., & Hopkins, B. (1992). Four requirements for a dynamical systems approach to the development of social coordination. *Human Movement Science, 11,* 425–442.

Bem, D. J., & Allen, A. (1974). On predicting some of the people some of the time: The search for cross-situational consistencies in behavior. *Psychological Review, 81,* 506–520.

Berkowitz, L., & Walster, E. (Eds.). (1976). *Advances in experimental social psychology* (Vol. 9). New York: Academic Press.

Biddle, B. S., & Thomas, E. J. (Eds.). (1966). *Role theory: Concepts and research.* New York: Wiley.

Buss, A. H., & Plomin, R. (1984). *Temperament: Early developing personality traits.* Hillsdale, NJ: Erlbaum.

Byrne, D., Clore, G. L., & Smeaton, G. (1986). The attraction hypothesis: Do similar attitudes affect anything? *Journal of Personality and Social Psychology, 51,* 1167–1170.

Caporael, L. R., & Brewer, M. B. (1995). Hierarchical evolutionary theory: There *is* an alternative, and it's not creationism. *Psychological Inquiry, 6,* 31–34.

Caprara, G. V., & Cervone, D. (2000). *Personality: Determinants, dynamics, and potentials.* Cambridge, UK: Cambridge University Press.

Carver, C. S., & Scheier, M. F. (1998). *On the self-regulation of behavior.* Cambridge, UK: Cambridge University Press.

Costa, P. T., Jr., & McCrae, R. R. (1995). Primary traits of Eysenck's P-E-N system: Three- and five-factor solutions. *Journal of Personality and Social Psychology, 69,* 308–317.

Czikzentmihalyi, M. (1990). *Flow: The psychology of optimal experience.* New York: Harper & Row.

Dawes, R. M. (1980). Social dilemmas. *Annual Review of Psychology, 31,* 169–193.

Diener, E. (1980). Deindividuation: The absence of self-awareness and self-regulation in group members. In P. Paulus (Ed.), *The psychology of group influence* (pp. 209–242). Hillsdale, NJ: Erlbaum.

Dittman, A. T., & Llewellyn, L. G. (1969). Body movement and speech rhythm in social conversation. *Journal of Personality and Social Psychology, 11,* 98–106.

Dunn, J., & Plomin, R. (1990). *Separate lives: Why siblings are so different.* New York: Basic Books.

Erber, R., Wegner, D. M., & Thierrault, N. (1996). On being cool and collected: Mood regulation in anticipation of social interaction. *Journal of Personality and Social Psychology, 70,* 757–766.

Feigenbaum, M. J. (1978). Quantitative universality for a class of nonlinear transformations. *Journal of Statistical Physics, 19,* 25–52.

Fischer, K. W., & Bidell, T. R. (1997). Dynamic development of psychological structures in action and thought. In W. Damon (Series Ed.) & R. Lerner (Vol. Ed.), *Handbook of child psychology: Vol. 1. Theoretical models of human development* (pp. 467–561). New York: Wiley.

Glass, L., & Mackey, M. C. (1988). *From clocks to chaos: The rhythms of life.* Princeton, NJ: Princeton University Press.

Gleick, J. (1987). *Chaos: The making of a new science.* New York: Viking-Penguin.

Guastello, S. J. (1995). *Chaos, catastrophe, and human affairs: Applications of nonlinear dynamics to work, organizations, and social evolution.* Mahwah, NJ: Erlbaum.

Haken, H. (Ed.) (1982). *Order and chaos in physics, chemistry, and biology.* Berlin: Springer.

Harris, J. R. (1995). Where is the child's environment? A group socialization theory of development. *Psychological Review, 102,* 458–489.

Harris, J. R. (1998). *The nurture assumption: Why children turn out the way they do.* New York: Free Press.

Hegselman, R., Troitzch, K., & Muller, U. (Eds.). (1996). *Modeling and simulation in the social sciences from the philosophy of science point of view.* Dordrecht, The Netherlands: Kluwer Academic.

Kaneko, K. (1989). Chaotic but regular Posi-Nega Switch among coded attractors by clustersize variation. *Physical Review Letters, 63,* 219–223.

Kaneko, K. (Ed.). (1993). *Theory and applications of coupled map lattices.* Singapore: World Scientific.

Kelso, J. A. S. (1995). *Dynamic patterns: The self-organization of brain and behavior.* Cambridge, MA: MIT Press.

Kunda, Z. (1999). *Social cognition: Making sense of people.* Cambridge, MA: MIT Press.

Jones, E. E., & Davis, K. E. (1965). From acts to dispositions: The attribution process in person perception. In L. Berkowitz (Ed.), *Advances in experimental social psychology* (Vol. 2, pp. 220–266). New York: Academic Press.

Lepper, M. R., & Greene, D. (Eds.). (1978). *The hidden costs of reward.* Hillsdale, NJ: Erlbaum.

Levine, J. M., & Moreland, R. L. (1998). Small groups. In D. T. Gilbert, S. T. Fiske, & G. Lindzey (Eds.), *The handbook of social psychology* (4th ed., Vol. 2, pp. 415–469). New York: McGraw-Hill.

Lowen, S. B., Liebovitch, L. S., & White, J. A. (1999). Fractal ion-channel behavior generates fractal firing patterns in neuronal models. *Physical Review E, 59,* 5970–5980.

Markus, H. (1980). The self in thought and memory. In D. M. Wegner & R. R. Vallacher (Eds.), *The self in social psychology* (pp. 102–130). New York: Oxford University Press.

Messick, D. M., & Liebrand, V. B. G. (1995). Individual heuristics and the dynamics of cooperation in large groups. *Psychological Review, 102,* 131–145.

Miller, N. E. (1944). Experimental studies of conflict. In J. M. Hunt (Ed.), *Personality and the behavior disorders* (pp. 431–465). New York: Ronald.

Mischel, W., & Shoda, Y. (1995). A cognitive–affective system theory of personality: Reconceptualizing situations, dispositions, dynamics, and invariance in personality structure. *Psychological Review, 102,* 246–268.

Myers, D. G., & Diener, E. (1995). Who is happy? *Psychological Science, 6,* 10–19.

Newcomb, T. M. (1961). *The acquaintance process.* New York: Holt, Rinehart, & Winston.

Newtson, D. (1994). The perception and coupling of behavior waves. In R. R. Vallacher & A. Nowak (Eds.), *Dynamical systems in social psychology* (pp. 139–167). San Diego: Academic Press.

Nisbett, R., & Ross, L. (1980). *Human inference: Stategies and shortcomings of social judgment.* Englewood Cliffs, NJ: Prentice-Hall.

Nowak, A., & Lewenstein, M. (1994). Dynamical systems: A tool for social psychology? In R. R. Vallacher & A. Nowak (Eds.), *Dynamical systems in social psychology* (pp. 17–53). San Diego, CA: Academic Press.

Nowak, A., & Vallacher, R. R. (1998). *Dynamical social psychology.* New York: Guilford Press.

Nowak, A., Vallacher, R. R., & Borkowski, W. (2000). Modeling the temporal coordination of behavior and internal states. In G. Ballot & G. Weisbuch (Eds.), *Applications of simulation to the social sciences* (pp. 67–86). Oxford, UK: Hermes Science.

Nowak, A., Vallacher, R. R., & Burnstein, E. (1998). Computational social psychology: A neural network approach to interpersonal dynamics. In W. Liebrand, A. Nowak, & R. Hegselman (Eds.), *Computer modeling and the study of dynamic social processes* (pp. 97–125). New York: Sage.

Nowak, A., Vallacher, R. R., Tesser, A., & Borkowski, W. (2000). Society of self: The emergence of collective properties in self-structure. *Psychological Review, 107,* 39–61.

Ott, E., Grebogi, C., & York, J. A. (1990). Controlling chaos. *Physics Review Letters, 64,* 1196–1199.

Plomin, R., Owen, M. J., & McGuffin, P. (1994). The genetic basis of complex behaviors. *Science, 264,* 1733–1739.

Port, R. F., & van Gelder, T. (Eds.). (1995). *Mind as motion: Explorations in the dynamics of cognition.* Cambridge, MA: MIT Press.

Prigogine, I., & Stengers, I. (1984). *Order out of chaos.* New York: Bantam.

Read, S. J., & Miller, L. C. (Eds.). (1998). *Connectionist models of social reasoning and social behavior.* Mahwah, NJ: Erlbaum.

Rogers, C. R. (1961). *On becoming a person.* Boston: Houghton Mifflin.

Rosenblum, L. D., & Turvey, M. T. (1988). Maintenance tendency in coordinated rhythmic movements: Relative fluctuations and phase. *Neuroscience, 27,* 289–300.

Rosenblum, M. E. (1986). The repulsion hypothesis: On the nondevelopment of relationships. *Journal of Personality and Social Psychology, 61,* 1156–1166.

Scarr, S. (1992). Developmental theories for the 1990s: Development and individual differences. *Child Development, 63,* 1–19.

Schmidt, R. C., Beek, P. J., Treffner, P. J., & Turvey, M. T. (1991). Dynamical substructure of coordinated rhythmic movements. *Journal of Experimental Psychology: Human Perception and Performance, 17,* 635–651.

Schuster, H. G. (1984). *Deterministic chaos.* Vienna: Physik Verlag.

Shinbrot, T. (1994). Synchronization of coupled maps and stable windows. *Physics Review E, 50,* 3230–3233.

Shoda, Y., Mischel, W., & Wright, J. C. (1994). Intraindividual stability in the organization and patterning of behavior: Incorporating psychological situations into the idiographic analysis of personality. *Journal of Personality and Social Psychology, 67,* 674–687.

Smith, E. R. (1996). What do connectionism and social psychology offer each other? *Journal of Personality and Social Psychology, 70,* 893–912.

Strack, F., Martin, L. L., & Stepper, S. (1988). Inhibiting and facilitating conditions of the human smile: A nonobtrusive test of the facial feedback hypothesis. *Journal of Personality and Social Psychology, 54,* 768–777.

Tangney, J. P., & Fischer, K. W. (Eds.). (1995). *Self-conscious emotions: The psychology of shame, guilt, embarrassment, and pride.* New York: Guilford Press.

Tesser, A. (1978). Self-generated attitude change. In L. Berkowitz (Ed.), *Advances in experimental social psychology* (Vol. 11, pp. 85–117). New York: Academic Press.

Thelen, E., & Smith, L. B. (Eds.) (1994). *A dynamic systems approach to the development of cognition and action.* Cambridge, MA: MIT Press/Bradford Books.

Thibaut, J. W., & Kelley, H. H. (1959). *The social psychology of groups.* New York: Wiley.

Tickle-Degnen, L., & Rosenthal, R. (1987). Group rapport and nonverbal behavior. *Review of Personality and Social Psychology, 9,* 113–136.

Tononi, G., & Edelman, G. M. (1998). Consciousness and complexity. *Science, 282,* 1846–1851.

Turner, R. H., & Killian, L. M. (1957). *Collective behavior.* Englewood Cliffs, NJ: Prentice-Hall.

Turvey, M. T. (1990). Coordination. *American Psychologist, 4,* 938–953.

Vallacher, R. R. (1993). Mental calibration: Forging a working relationship between mind and action. In D. M. Wegner & J. W. Pennebaker (Eds.), *The handbook of mental control* (pp. 443–472). New York: Prentice-Hall.

Vallacher, R. R., & Kaufman, J. (1996). Dynamics of action identification: Volatility and structure in the mental representation of behavior. In P. M. Gollwitzer & J. A. Bargh (Eds.), *The psychology of action* (pp. 260–282). New York: Guilford Press.

Vallacher, R. R., & Nowak, A. (Eds.). (1994). *Dynamical systems in social psychology.* San Diego, CA: Academic Press.

Vallacher, R. R., & Nowak, A. (1997). The emergence of dynamical social psychology. *Psychological Inquiry, 8,* 73–99.

Vallacher, R. R., & Nowak, A. (1999). The dynamics of self-regulation. In R. S. Wyer, Jr. (Ed.), *Advances in self-regulation* (Vol. 12, pp. 241–259). Mahwah, NJ: Erlbaum.

Vallacher, R. R., Nowak, A., & Kaufman, J. (1994). Intrinsic dynamics of social judgment. *Journal of Personality and Social Psychology, 66,* 20–34.

Vallacher, R. R., Nowak, A., Markus, J., & Strauss, J. (1998). Dynamics in the coordination of mind and action. In M. Kofta, G. Weary, & G. Sedek (Eds.), *Personal control in action: Cognitive and motivational mechanisms* (pp. 27–59). New York: Plenum Press.

Vallacher, R. R., Nowak, A., & Miller, M. E. (in press). Social influence. In I. Weiner (Series Ed.) & M. J. Lerner & T. Millon (Vol. Eds.), *Comprehensive handbook of psychology: Vol. 5. Personality and social psychology.* New York: Wiley.

Vallacher, R. R., & Wegner, D. M. (1987). What do people think they're doing? Action identification and human behavior. *Psychological Review, 94,* 1–15.

Vallacher, R. R., & Wegner, D. M. (1989). Levels of personal agency: Individual variation in action identification. *Journal of Personality and Social Psychology, 57,* 660–671.

Vallacher, R. R., Wegner, D. M., & Somoza, M. P. (1989). That's easy for you to say: Action identification and speech fluency. *Journal of Personality and Social Psychology, 56,* 199–208.

van Geert, P. (1991). A dynamic systems model of cognitive and language growth. *Psychological Review, 98,* 3–53.

Wegner, D. M. (1994). Ironic processes of mental control. *Psychological Review, 101,* 34–52.

Wegner, D. M., & Vallacher, R. R. (1977). *Implicit psychology: An introduction to social cognition.* New York: Oxford University Press.

Wiggins, J. S. (1980). Circumplex models of interpersonal behavior. In L. Wheeler (Ed.), *Review of Personality and Social Psychology* (Vol. 1, pp. 265–292). Beverly Hills, CA: Sage.

Wish, M., Deutsch, M., & Kaplan, S. J. (1976). Perceived dimensions of interpersonal relations. *Journal of Personality and Social Psychology, 33,* 409–420.

Zajonc, R. B. (1965). Social facilitation. *Science, 149,* 269–274.

Zimbardo, P. G. (1970). The human choice: Individuation, reason, and order versus deindividuation, impulse, and chaos. In W. J. Arnold & D. Levine (Eds.), *Nebraska Symposium on Motivation* (Vol. 17, pp. 237–307). Lincoln: University of Nebraska Press.

Zimbardo, P. G. (1977). *Shyness: What it is and what you can do about it.* Reading, MA: Addison-Wesley.

Zochowski, M., & Liebovitch, L. S. (1997). Synchronization of the trajectory as a way to control the dynamics of the coupled system. *Physical Review E, 56,* 3701.

Zochowski, M., & Liebovitch, L. S. (1999). Self-organizing dynamics of couple map systems. *Physical Review E, 59,* 2830.

Index

Personality coherence, 241
  intraindividual variability as
    indicator of, 241–242, 265–
    267
Personality development, 13–14,
  83–84
  agency, development of,
    188–189
  cross-sectional versus
    longitudinal research, 198–
    199, 226
  dynamical systems model of,
    312–318
  environmental model (and
    contextual influences), 158–
    161, 169–172, 197–198,
    211
  goodness-of-fit model, 162–163
  interactional model, 161–162
  organismic metatheory, 177–178,
    187
  stability of individual differences,
    165–167, 170–171
  trait model, 155–158, 167–168
  traits, mean levels of, 219–220,
    222–225
  transformation (versus stability),
    55
  transformational model, 164–
    165
  vulnerability model, 163–164
Personality psychology
  boundaries of academic
    discipline, 2–3
  history, 12–13
  social contexts for, 17–18
Personality science, 4–6
  defined, 4
  interdisciplinary advances and,
    6–12
Piaget, Jean, 154, 188
Positron emission tomography
  (PET), 133

Prosocial behavior, 181–182
  prosocial strategies of resource
    control, 184–186
Psychodynamic theory, 271–272

S

Self-concept, structure of
  assessment, 275–279
  and intraindividual variability in
    behavior, 271
  dynamic model of, 285–287
  evaluative organization
    (compartmentalization and
    integration), 272–275
  information-processing
    perspective, 272–273, 275
  in psychodynamic theory, 271–272
  stress and, 281–283
  and synchronization in social
    interaction, 322–323
  in trait theory, 272
Self-consciousness, 323
Self-esteem, 206
Serotonin. *See* Neurotransmitter
  systems and personality
Shyness, 84–85
  behavioral and physiological
    correlates, 89–91
  definition, 84–85
  environmental experience and
    change, 93–94
  genetic bases, 98
  neural substrates of, 85–86
  startle eyeblink response and, 88–89
  temperamental antecedents, 86–89
  types of, 94–96
Simulated situations paradigm.
  See Situations
Situations
  psychological features, 245–248,
    256–259